NATURAL THERAPEUTICS

Volume 2

PRACTICE

HENRY LINDLAHR, M.D.

EDITED AND REVISED BY

JOCELYN C. P. PROBY,
M.A., M.Litt. (Oxon), D.O. (Kirksville, U.S.A.)

SAFFRON WALDEN

THE C. W. DANIEL COMPANY LIMITED

First published in this edition by
The C. W. Daniel Company Limited,
1 Church Path, Saffron Walden, Essex, CB10 1JP, England

© Henry Lindlahr 1919
Revisions and Additions © Jocelyn C. P. Proby 1981

ISBN 0 85207 320 8

Printed in Great Britain by
Hillman Printers, Frome, Somerset

CONTENTS

EDITOR'S INTRODUCTION

As its name implies, this second volume of Lindlahr's work is mainly concerned with the practical application of the ideas and methods of treatment set forth in the first volume. It does, however, do more than this in that it considerably develops and adds to what is said in the first volume, and is a mine of information on a number of points which are scarcely touched on there. The work is divided into five parts and some comments should perhaps be made on each of these.

Part I is concerned with the regimen which, in Lindlahr's view, should be followed for the creation and maintenance of health and for the prevention of disease. It is, of course, the basis of his philosophy that health is produced and maintained by the individual himself living or learning to live in accordance with natural laws. Unless he happens to be lucky enough to be born into an environment and a community in which the living habits are thoroughly healthy, this means that thought and effort on his part are necessary. He has to make up his mind that he cannot be healthy merely by conforming to what is considered the norm in living and eating habits or by following his tastes and inclinations at all times. The way we live is very much a question of habit and habits can be good or bad. Tastes, too, are very much a question of habit and it is very easy to acquire tastes which are vitiated and harmful. It is for this reason that Lindlahr lays so much emphasis on the bringing up of children on natural lines, so that their tastes and habits should be good and conducive to health.

The regimen here drawn up and recommended by Lindlahr does undoubtedly appear extremely formidable and rigorous and it would seem doubtful whether it would be possible, or even desirable, for everyone to carry it out rigidly and in its entirety. It is, however, clear that modern civilized man cannot hope to have good health himself or to hand it on to his children unless he does something to care for his body and to subject it to some kind of routine or discipline. Bad health being something which we mostly bring on ourselves, the pursuit of health can be regarded as a kind of virtue which we should seek to practise. This does not mean that we should worry and fuss about our health all the time and become hypochondriacal; nor, I think, should it mean that we should cease altogether to take a full part in the work and social activities of our communities even though this may sometimes involve us in things which are inimical to health or which make it harder to maintain. Rather we should seek so to look after ourselves that we can be fit in mind and body to lead a full and useful life in our own chosen sphere of activity.

In addition to acquiring good habits of eating and drinking in accordance with the principles of natural dietetics, Lindlahr lays emphasis on the importance of a number of other matters which are essential to be considered in relation to the maintenance of health. (1) We must train ourselves to have a right mental attitude, to be able to relax and to be able to sleep in a satisfactory manner. (2) We must pay attention to the care of the skin not only for the purpose of keeping it clean, but also to maintain its efficiency as an eliminative and temperature response mechanism. It is important to give special care also to the eyes and the nasal passages. (3) Exercise, preferably in the fresh air, is of great importance and the best form of exercise apart from running and walking is the playing of games and sports of various kinds. However, even those who have healthy outdoor occupations and recreations do require to some extent to do special exercises in order to maintain harmonious and balanced conditions in the body with good posture and flexibility of the whole musculature. This is because civilized life and work almost invariably involve a use of the body in ways which are inharmonious, unbalanced and incomplete. This must be countered by some sort of exercise routine such as that which Lindlahr describes and advocates and of which breathing exercises are an important part. The sections of the book in which he discusses Breathing and Exercises, how they should be performed and their physiological and psychological effects, are worthy of careful study and are very stimulating to thought. I am not, however, entirely convinced that the exercises which he advocates are the best which could be devised or that they are suitable for all people in all situations. Lindlahr displays a certain suspicion of yoga which would appear to be somewhat exaggerated, though there are some yogic practices which are capable of arousing or liberating forces which are dangerous if not under proper control; but the simpler routines of hatha yoga and the deep breathing which goes with them would seem to be about the best kind of exercising which one could hope to find. The great advantage of them is that there is, or should be, no straining or jerking involved and their aim is to produce flexibility and harmonious working of the joints and musculature rather than overdevelopment or overstimulation of any particular muscle groups or parts of the body. It should be noted that most of the best exercises which are recommended and used by "keep fit" enthusiasts and teachers, including to some degree Lindlahr himself, would appear to be derived from yoga in a more or less modified form. The truth may be that those who seek good health should develop some sort of exercise routine suited to themselves and their way of life based on the principles which Lindlahr lays down. To do this they can seek the help of books, classes or experts and would be wise to do so if they are old, weak or infirm in any special way.

Parts II and III are concerned with the practical application of the principles of Natural Therapeutics to the treatment of acute and chronic diseases respectively. There is not much to be said about this except that there are certain points to be noted. Lindlahr lays very great emphasis on the importance of hydrotherapy in the treatment of both classes of disease. In the case of acute disease it is mainly used for the purpose of keeping fever within safe limits without suppressing it, as well as helping and promoting the eliminative efforts of the body. In the case of chronic disease it is used for the purpose of restoring the health and functioning of the skin as an eliminative organ. Indeed the principal aim of Natural Therapeutics is to ensure the efficient working of the four great emunctories of the body, skin, kidneys, bowels and lungs, and by regulation of the food intake to reduce the burdens which those organs have to undertake. As Lindlahr points out, the principles of treatment in all forms of disease are essentially the same, and it is possible, within limits, by applying those principles, to treat successfully any kind of disease without having necessarily been able to give it a name or fully to diagnose it in terms of orthodox medicine. However, in some of the sections Lindlahr has some excellent information on how to deal with certain common symptoms and with certain organs and parts of the body in a natural manner.

The sections on insanity and on mental, emotional and psychical disorders require and deserve careful and thoughtful study. The main thing which would seem to emerge in this connection is that the treatment of such conditions should begin with the treatment of the physical body, which will, in many cases, bring about a cure and will in any case provide a sound basis on which psychological and mental forms of treatment can operate. It is interesting to note that there does now seem to be a movement in orthodox psychiatric circles towards physical and chemical methods of treating mental disorders rather than relying solely on psychological techniques. Unfortunately, the physical and chemical methods generally used, such as shock treatment, leucotomy and powerful and prolonged drugging, are very far removed from the kind of treatment of the physical body which Lindlahr advocates.

It should also be noted that Lindlahr did apparently intend to publish another volume (Vol. V of his series) in which he planned to deal more in detail with the treatment of certain grave conditions.

Part IV is concerned with the procreation, birth and care of babies. There is no doubt that this part of the work is in a sense incomplete. Lindlahr states in various places in his writings that he intended to bring out a volume entitled "Nature Cure Eugenics", but it did not in fact appear. This volume would undoubtedly have had much more to say on many of the subjects touched on here, and its non-appearance is the more unfortunate because some of the ideas put forward are controversial and others require further development and elucidation in the light of modern practice and research. I have thought it proper, therefore, to try to deal further with some of these matters in notes and appendices.

Part V is mainly concerned with first aid and contains useful information in this field, some of which is unusual. The section on the care of teeth and how to prevent the almost universal bad condition of them is very worthy of study. The section on growing old is also full of interest.

Since the publication of Vol. 1, an interesting autobiographical article published by Henry Lindlahr in a Nature Cure magazine, shortly before his death, has come into my hands. I have felt that this should be included in this volume as giving readers a better understanding of Lindlahr as a person and as showing how he arrived at his conclusions:

He writes:

In our halcyon days of youthful vigour we are apt to look upon health culture, mind culture and higher philosophy with contempt and derision, but suffering is the great awakener, revealer and teacher. So long as we are prosperous and suffering does not overtake us, we are content to jog along in the old ruts and to live in "the good old ways" to the very limit of Nature's endurance.

In my youth I had learned the ten commandments, but neither in church, school nor college had I been taught that there is a decalogue and a morality of the physical as well as of the spiritual. Left in total ignorance of the laws of natural living and following the example of friends and boon companions, I imagined that the highest philosophy of life is "to have a good time while it lasts" and to "let tomorrow take care of itself".

I accepted the popular belief that life and death, health and disease are largely matters of chance or dependent upon draughts, wet feet, germs and bacteria or upon the will of a capricious Providence.

My friends of the medical profession assured me that eating and drinking and the use of liquor and tobacco had little to do with physical condition. Their advice was "Eat and drink what agrees with you (that is, what tastes good and makes you feel good), satisfy your physical appetites and cravings to the fullest extent; it is only natural to do so.

If you get into trouble, come to us and we will fix you up all right." Again the comfortable doctrine of "do as you please" and of vicarious salvation. Such advice is administered constantly and indiscriminately to the youth of our country, in private consultations and in open clinics by physicians of good repute.

As a result of all these teachings and examples of personal irresponsibility and ethical and moral nihilism, chaos filled my mind and soul. I did not know what to believe or what to disbelieve and, as a natural result, ceased to care how I lived. My only concern was the gratification of my physical appetites and my desires for diversion and amusement.

My early life was a sort of experiment to see how far I could go in violating the rules of wholesome living without suffering immediately and intensely Nature's penalties.

Finally, however, I reached the limits of Nature's endurance and began to suffer greatly from the results of my ignorance and foolishness.

Following the advice of my friends, the doctors, I sought relief and cure in drugging. But though I consulted one after another of the "best" physicians, their pills and potions gave only slight temporary relief. At the age of thirty-five I found myself a physical and mental wreck without faith in God, in Nature or in myself. Many times the desire to end my miserable existence threatened to overwhelm me. The terror of it all was my utter ignorance and helplessness. I failed to see the causes of my troubles, much less the way out of them. However, the darkest hours are just before the dawn.

The Beginning

One day I confided my deplorable condition to a sympathetic friend. He handed me a book and expressed the wish that its perusal might do me some good. It proved to be one of the first publications dealing with the laws of natural living and healing and was written by Louis Kuhne, a humble weaver, the great pioneer of Nature Cure.

In simple but convincing language it taught that all disease, barring accidents and surroundings hostile to human life, is due to violations of nature's laws in habits of living; and that, therefore, the fundamental principle of true healing must consist in a return to natural habits of living.

His simple means of cure consisted in pure food diet, free from morbid matter of the animal carcass; water, air and sun baths; massage and systematic exercise.

As I read the book, it was as though a great light were arising before me and illuminating my darkened consciousness. For the first time I realized that the process of life and death, health, disease and cure are subject to the workings of natural laws, as definite and exact as the laws of gravitation and chemical affinity; that there is a decalogue and a morality of the physical as well as of the spiritual, and that if I would faithfully comply with the laws of my physical nature, there was still hope of regeneration and the recovery of health — physical, mental and spiritual.

I read on eagerly through the night and into the morning hours, until I had absorbed the contents of the book. The next morning at my bath and at breakfast I began to practise the natural regimen and have carried it out to the best of my ability from that time to this.

The results were most gratifying. There were ups and downs and healing crises, but all along, to my great joy, I experienced a steady improvement. The satisfaction and happiness this gave me were indescribable. I was conscious that I was working out my own salvation through my own knowledge and personal effort. I realized that I had arisen out of utter ignorance and helplessness and become independent of the quacks of philosophy, religion and medicine — that I was indeed the master of my fate.

While the home regimen of natural living wrought a decided improvement in my health, it was not sufficient to entirely overcome the deepseated chronic ailments from which I was suffering. The same was true in the case of my wife. She had been an invalid for years before our marriage and several years later she had been rejected by the New York Insurance Company as a victim of Bright's disease. The examining physician for the Company assured me it was no use to try again and pronounced her case incurable.

At that time I had already become acquainted with Nature Cure and we were living strictly in harmony with its teachings; therefore I could not accept the verdict of the doctor, and I said to him: "You will take her within two years." "Never," he insisted. "Once albumin, always albumin." He had to retract his prognosis, however. After another year of natural living, not a trace of albumin was to be found and the New York Life Insurance Company accepted the risk without hesitation. I may add that she has ever since enjoyed perfect health.

My Experiences in European Sanitoria and Schools for Nature Cure

About six months after I became acquainted with Nature Cure philosophy, I disposed of all my possessions, severed my business connections, and with my family departed for Europe, principally to seek treatment for both my wife and myself in the Nature Cure sanitoria. I had intended to remain in Europe about three months, but became so enthusiastic over the improvement we both experienced and the wonderful things I learned about Nature Cure that I lost interest in everything else. I realized that commercial pursuits, no matter how remunerative, could never again satisfy me. Moneymaking had lost its charm. Higher and finer ideals had taken its place. I had grasped the law of service which ordains that we achieve content and happiness only as we make others happy. "Freely ye have received, freely give." In compliance with this injunction of the Master, I decided to make Nature Cure my life work.

Instead of three months, I spent a year in Nature Cure schools and sanitoria, studying as well as benefiting by treatment. At the end of the first really happy year of my life, I returned to this country and began the study of osteopathy and medicine.

After I had obtained my diploma and become a licensed osteopathic physician, I continued the study of medicine, practising natural methods of treatment in my leisure hours. In that way I had the opportunity of comparing the results of my own work with those obtained by medical and surgical treatment in the clinics and hospitals of the medical schools I attended.

In the class rooms and the clinics I listened with two ears and saw with two eyes. That is to say, all I heard and saw had for me two meanings — the one intended by the books and professors on the lecture platforms; and the other my own interpretation of their theories and practices in the light of Nature Cure philosophy. I reserved the right to be the judge of all that transpired before me.

Though already advanced in years, I thoroughly enjoyed these belated school days. The study and research proved so intensely interesting that I would not have forgone the pleasure of a lecture or clinic for the best "show" in Chicago.

Compare my experience with that of the average student on the benches of our great medical schools, drinking in, as gospel truth, every word uttered by the teachers; not able to judge between truth and error; not allowed to entertain an independent opinion; helplessly swayed by the power of suggestion. In four or five years he is hopelessly hypnotized and obsessed by the one-sided theories of a particular school.

This explains why we find it easy to convince any person endowed with common intelligence and good sense, of the simple truths of Nature Cure, and why we find it almost impossible to change the dogmatic beliefs of the trained nurse, the medical student or the practising physician. Their brains are so stuffed and befuddled with the "theories of the schools" that they have lost the power of common sense reasoning. As an old proverb puts it, "For the many trees they cannot see the forest."

In due time I graduated in allopathy, homoeopathy and eclectic medicine, passed the examination of the State Board of Health of Illinois, and obtained my licence to practise as allopathic physician and surgeon.

Nature Cure Truly Eclectic

During my search for health and knowledge in European Nature Cure schools and sanitoria I found that all these institutions were teaching and practising only a part of the truth. They would emphasize one or more of the natural methods of living and of treatment and ignore others just as important. Some of the things they did were all right, others all wrong. Not one of them measured up to my ideal of an all-round Nature Cure institution.

The Return to America

These experiences inspired me with the idea of founding in this country an institution that should teach and practise all that is good in natural living and healing.

For the last sixteen years I and my good helpers have been trying out, sifting and selecting the true and practical from that which proved irrelevant, harmful and destructive. We are determined to continue this process of natural selection indefinitely. It is this which makes Nature Cure the only evolutionary and truly eclectic system of therapeutics ever formulated.

In our Nature Cure institutions representatives of the allopathic, homoeopathic, osteopathic, neuropathic, chiropractic and naprapathic schools of healing work side by side in the practice of Nature Cure, magnetic, mental and spiritual healing, year in and year out in perfect harmony, without a shadow of misunderstanding, jealousy or intolerance. There is not another institution on earth that exemplifies true eclecticism in a similar way.

INTRODUCTION

WHAT IS NATURAL THERAPEUTICS?

The Lindlahr System of Natural Therapeutics represents the first effort ever made to combine in one system all that is good in the various methods of treating human ailments. It is, therefore, the only true eclectic system of therapeutics in existence. It takes in all that is true in old school medical theories and practice, as well as all that is valuable in modern drugless healing methods. On the basis of a few fundamental natural laws, it brings order out of chaos, simplicity and unity out of complexity and confusion. It reduces the multiplicity of medical and drugless theories and healing methods to a few simple principles and applications. It represents one of the most far-reaching revolutionary movements in the history of mankind — fundamental to all other reforms, individual as well as social. It searches for causes and for rational treatment on the physical, mental, moral, spiritual, psychical and social planes of being. It reveals with irrefutable logic that the causes of disease and the effects of natural and unnatural treatment are identical in all domains of human life.

One of the pioneers in the Nature Cure movement summarized the philosophy of health, disease and treatment in the epigram, "Health is cleanliness". Orthodox medical science has learned that this is true as far as surroundings are concerned, but has not yet applied this principle to internal conditions, which is proved by the fact that instead of purifying human bodies of morbid waste, systemic poisons and disease taints, it saturates them with drug poisons and disease products, under the guise of medicines, vaccines, serums and antitoxins.

The following may serve to define more clearly the difference between the old and new philosophy of disease and treatment. The old school of medicine teaches that practically all diseases are caused by minute living beings specially created by nature for this malign purpose; and that human bodies are the helpless, chance victims of these destructive, invisible enemies. On this germ theory of disease is based the slogan of modern medical science, "Paralyse or kill the germ (with ice, poisons, serums, antitoxins, vaccines or surgical operations) and cure the disease."

1

Natural Therapeutics, or the science of natural healing, does not deny the existence of disease germs and parasites, but claims, and proves beyond the possibility of doubt, that these germs and their seed spores, or micro-zymes, grow and multiply only in bodies heavily encumbered with and weakened by food, drink and drug poisons, morbid taints and various disease products in the form of vaccines, serums and antitoxins. Further-more, this new interpretation of disease makes it clear that these much maligned bacteria and parasites feed on, digest and decompose the morbid encumbrances or pathogenic material in animal and human bodies.[1]

These are bold claims in view of the adverse opinion held almost unani-mously by the old schools of medicine. The first theory is equivalent to saying: "There is no need to clean your house in order to prevent moulds, fungi and vermin. All that is necessary is diligently to soak the premises with antiseptics and germ killers." Such practice may succeed for a while, but what condition will the house be in if dirt and poisonous chemicals are allowed to accumulate? The better practice endeavours to keep the house scrupulously clean by the use of water, soap, brush and broom, and by flooding it with fresh air and sunlight. If this is done, can there be any danger of moulds, fungi and vermin, or invasion from with-out? In like manner the drugless healer purifies the human body by natural methods of living and of treatment, by adjusting mechanical lesions and harmonizing mental and emotional discord.

The following revelations concerning the true character of germs and their functions in the economy of nature may enable the reader to decide for himself which one of these theories is most rational. Professor Béchamp, a contemporary of Pasteur and Metchnikoff, taught as long as sixty years ago that normal cells of living bodies as well as bacteria and other micro-organisms were not the smallest living bodies, but that they were made up of infinitely more minute beings which he called "micro-zymes" — minute ferment bodies. He proved that these microzymes are the primal units of life which, under normal conditions, develop into the normal cells of living bodies, but which, under abnormal conditions, as in dead bodies or in accumulations of morbid materials in living bodies, may develop into bacteria and parasites, whose natural function it is to con-sume and decompose putrefying materials into their component elements. In other words it can be said that every disease germ lives on its own particular kind of disease matter, and if it does not find this it has to leave for pastures new (or it is eaten up by its own microzymes). For when the morbid material is consumed, the microzymes feed on the protoplasm of

[1]
An appendix on the subject of Parasitism appears in Volume I of this series (Philosophy of Natural Therapeutics).

2

their own bacteria until there is nothing left but the microzymes themselves. These may again develop into bacteria in contact with other morbid material.

It will be seen that according to this rational theory of germ activity the much dreaded bacteria and parasites, instead of being the deadly enemies of living beings are nature's scavengers, on whose activity depends the removal of dead and putrefying matter, and therefore the very existence of living beings. In other words, they are nature's provision for keeping the earth clean and sweet. Furthermore, we know that, barring accident, all disease in human bodies is caused by the excessive accumulation of morbid waste (pathogenic matter), which clogs and obstructs the capillary circulation, thus interfering with cell nutrition and drainage; that the white blood corpuscles or leucocytes, which were mistaken by medical science for living cells and germ destroyers (phagocytes), are in reality particles of mucoid matter condensed in the tubular structures of the spleen and the lymph nodes into comparatively compact bodies for the purpose of keeping the blood serum fluid and facilitating its transfusion through the membranes of the blood vessels and cells (osmosis). If these white corpuscles remained in the circulation in diffused form they would thicken the blood serum to such an extent that it would prevent cell nutrition and drainage. It is, in fact, such obstruction by pathogenic materials in the tissues of the body which interferes with the nutrition of the cells. Thus the cells, on the one hand, are starved, and on the other are poisoned by their own excrements. No wonder they lose vitality, deteriorate and putrefy, thus calling into action bacteria and parasites, the minute scavengers and destroyers of morbid matter and white blood corpuscles. For these reasons the natural therapist does not fill human bodies with drug poisons and disease products to "kill the germs", but purifies the blood and tissues, adjusts mechanical lesions, and harmonizes mental and emotional activities so that there is no necessity for the development of normal microzymes into bacteria, and no food for disease germs invading the system from without. That it is indeed possible to develop such natural immunity to infectious diseases is being proved by ever increasing numbers of faithful adherents to natural ways of living and of treating human ailments.

The conclusion of the matter is that all acute diseases start with obstruction of the capillary circulation by accumulation of mucoid matter and white corpuscles. The white corpuscles instead of being valiant little germ hunters and germ eaters (phagocytes) are in reality eaten and decomposed into pus by the bacteria. Succeeding blood counts of our chronic patients who improve under natural treatment show invariably a very marked decrease in white corpuscles and an increase in red corpuscles. It

3

may be asked, if this is true, and if disease arises within the organism rather than through invasion from without, why it is that epidemics occur and many people become affected at the same time by similar kinds of disease germs. The answer to this is that the majority of people in a certain locality are addicted to the same unnatural habits of living and of treating their ailments, thus producing in many of them the same kind of morbid soil and the same kind of bacterial and inflammatory action. There is also no doubt that atmospheric and cosmic influences which are at present little understood have a bearing on the periodic appearance of epidemic and endemic diseases. It is, however, becoming clear that immunity to disease can be acquired by the careful observance of nature's laws. Through right living and following the natural regimen which is outlined in this volume the system may be brought into such a state of purity and health that bacteria will find no congenial soil for development.([1])

As evidence I give the story of an osteopathic physician who was a member of our staff. He enlisted in the marines, and described his experiences in the following letter: "... I never felt finer in my life than Friday a week ago. On that day I received my first shot of serum. It was the 'three-in-one', a mixture of typhoid, paratyphoid and meningitis sera. As usual when the filthy stuff is injected into a clean body, purified by years of natural living, the reaction was powerful. It made me deathly sick. I felt nauseated and had a terrible headache. After taking a few cold sprays on the quiet during the night I felt better in the morning. Then I was vaccinated. This was my finish. Within a few hours I developed temperature and became so weak that I had to go to bed. Next morning the lymphatic glands all over my body, especially in the neck, were swollen, my tongue was thickly coated, and I vomited several times. My temperature went up to 102. I was still in the barracks and treated myself as best I could with throat packs, cold compresses over the chest and abdomen, and cut out the eats. Monday brought no improvement. I tried to hide my condition to avoid being taken to hospital. Tuesday night my temperature went up and I became delirious. The boys told me I left my bed and shouted at the top of my voice that I was choking and needed help. Next morning I became conscious and found myself on a hospital cot. — At regular intervals one of the medical assistants made the rounds with a quart bottle full of a grayish, vile tasting, mixture. Everybody in the place, no matter what ailed him, had to take a dose. I kept mine in my mouth until I had an opportunity to spit it into my handkerchief and then

([1])
    An appendix on the subject of Epidemics appears in Volume I of this series (Philosophy of Natural Therapeutics).

cleansed my mouth with water as best I could. Later on one of the doctors told me that it was a mixture of aconite, gelsemin and phenacetin. In between times calcium iodide was passed round in a coffee cup. I realized that if I took the stuff, the fever caused by the blood poisoning might be suppressed, and the disease and drug poisons sent to the brain and spinal cord, with paralysis or death as the finish. After I had become quite friendly with the doctors they agreed to let me off from the dope and I was not offered any more of it. This was rather a lucky escape considering that only a few days before (one fellow was court martialled and given twenty-five days for insisting on having an enema instead of cathartics). The doctors were also kind enough to place a wash basin of cold water under my cot so that I could renew my throat packs and abdominal compresses from time to time. I succeeded, also, in fasting a short time longer, pleading that food would nauseate me and not stay down anyway. After a few days, however, they insisted that I must eat to keep up my strength or the 'disease' would get the best of me. To avoid trouble I took the food, but when unobserved passed it on to my neighbours, who, though sick as dogs, swallowed it greedily.

"After I became able to talk to the doctors more freely I mentioned that my fever was due to blood poisoning from the serums and vaccine. At this they expressed great surprise. It seems that such a possibility had never entered their heads. They evidently didn't know what was the matter with me nor with many others in the ward. The only thing they seemed to know was that we had fever, and for this everybody received at regular intervals the same dope. When a patient in the ward neared the end he was taken to a room upstairs for the finish.

"An osteopathic friend called on me several times and when the internes were not looking, gave me a good head and neck treatment, and the glands a good draining, which of course relieved me wonderfully. During the daytime the doctors would not let me go to the bathroom upstairs because there was a lot of 'draught' and I might 'take cold'; but I made good by slipping up there during the night and taking a few cold sprays, and then going back to bed without drying. These whole body packs gave me great relief. While lying in that ill ventilated room, surrounded by influenza, pneumonia and meningitis cases, it made me furious to think that after trying for years to keep my body in a clean and healthy condition, it had been saturated with these filthy poisons. If anything had been needed to convince me of the sanity and efficacy of Nature Cure, this experience surely would have done it. I have learned since that many of our company became sick after the injections; twenty-four were taken to the hospital and three of these died. But after all I am thankful for the great house-cleaning. I'm better off than many of the fellows who

5

did not work up an acute reaction, but still have the filth in their systems."

This experience of Dr. X throws an interesting light on the origin and spread of the epidemic of influenza and pneumonia in the fall of 1918. It started almost simultaneously in practically all the army and navy camps in the United States. From the camps it spread to the neighbouring country and cities. Why should this occur among young men who were the pick of the country for health and youthful vigour, living in the best hygienic surroundings that science could establish, leading wholesome outdoor lives with plenty of vigorous exercise? Without doubt, an over-abundance of nitrogenous starchy foods, coffee and tobacco, plus disease products in the form of serums, antitoxins and vaccines, had created the morbid soil for the propagation of the germs of influenza, pneumonia, meningitis and of other infectious diseases. While some of the serums, antitoxins and vaccines may not contain live bacteria, they do contain the microzymes which, under favourable conditions, will develop into bacteria and parasites. Bacteriologists admit that bacteria become more malignant as they pass through disease-encumbered bodies. The foregoing would explain not only the simultaneous outbreak in the home camps of the army, but also its extraordinary virulence, unequalled in any former outbreak.

The press for December 5, 1918, carried a report from the U.S. Health Department giving the estimates of deaths from influenza and pneumonia during the preceding epidemic. "Since September 15, between 300,000 and 350,000 deaths from influenza and pneumonia have occurred among the civilian population of the United States. About 20,000 deaths occurred in the camps of the United States." The number of soldiers in the home camps during the period covered by this report was approximately 1,500,000. The population of the United States is about 110,000,000. Using these figures we have the following percentages: mortality among civilians would be 302 in 100,000 living; among soldiers in camp, 1,333 per 100,000 living; or more than four times that of the civilian death rate. What an astonishing revelation this is when we consider that the civilian population includes the very old and the very young, those whose resistance has been weakened by chronic disease, lack of proper nourishment and unhygienic surroundings; while the camp population includes only the physically fit, living under the most favourable conditions. The medical profession claims that the serum and vaccine practice has prevented the spread of typhoid fever and smallpox in the late war. This we are not ready to admit, believing that these diseases, like yellow fever, cholera, bubonic plague, etc., have yielded to better hygiene, scientific drainage, and other common sense and practical methods. But suppose they are

6

right in their claim — it remains a fact that a larger percentage of soldiers have lost their lives through disease during this war than in any other modern war. The latest statistics tell us that in France 16,000 American soldiers died of disease, while only 40,000 were killed in the hard fought battles or died from wounds. The loss from disease in American camps has been just as great as in Europe. What difference did it make to these victims of disease whether they died of typhoid or smallpox, or of influenza, pneumonia, meningitis or other disease, bred and nourished in the morbid soil created by serums, antitoxins and vaccines?

Another bit of evidence comes from an entirely different source unbiased by nature cure doctrines. A friend from an eastern city writes: "An undertaker from here who volunteered for duty at Camp — —, and who has done most of the embalming there, says that in his opinion the deaths were not caused by pneumonia, as evidenced by the fact that no pus was present in the lungs as is always the case following this disease. He said big, strong, robust fellows would die in three days after being taken down, and in the greatest agony; that their lungs were filled with gas, they could not get their breath, and strangled to death. He also said that in his judgement the trouble was caused by the serums that were being injected into them — that these serums were impregnated with the germs or poisons that caused all the trouble."

PART I

SECTION I

A GENERAL REGIMEN FOR WHOLESOME LIVING AND FOR PREVENTION OF DISEASE

The following is an outline of a daily regimen for natural living and home treatment which will prove fully sufficient to maintain good health and ensure physical and mental efficiency, provided, however, the system is in good condition to begin with. In order to cure acute or deep-seated chronic conditions it is necessary to apply thorough systemic natural treatment as outlined under the respective headings. The regimen may have to be modified somewhat to suit various constitutions and changing conditions.

1. **Mental Adjustment.** When your mental alarm clock has awakened you in the morning from sleep, lie flat on your back in a perfectly relaxed position. For a few minutes let the feeling of rest, peace and goodwill permeate your whole being. Then in a prayerful attitude of mind make your affirmations and denials according to your daily need.[1]

2. **Water Sniffing.** Then arise without further delay and after washing your face and hands in cold water, sniff cold water from the hollow of your hand through your nose until the water passes freely through the nasal passages into the mouth. Repeat this in the beginning six times, and gradually increase to twelve times. The water sniffing should be repeated three or four times a day, every time one has occasion to wash, and before retiring in the evening. At first this practice may have an irritating effect, but this will soon be overcome. If in the beginning the water cannot be taken cold it should be tempered. Within a few days or weeks, however, it should be used as it comes from the tap. Water sniffing is an excellent means for cleansing the nasal passages of all ob-

[1]
The use of prayers and affirmations is dealt with in Volume I of this series (Philosophy of Natural Therapeutics), particularly Chapters XLI and XLIII.

9

struction. It is the best treatment for catarrh and a splendid natural stimulant to the membranes and nerve endings in the nasal passages. Through stimulation of these nerve endings it has a tonic effect upon the brain and nervous system.

3. **Eye Bath.** Follow the instructions under Sec. XXV. In case of weak eyes, follow the eye massage and exercises.

4. **Morning Drink.** After the water sniffing and eye bath, and after cleaning the teeth and mouth with dilute lemon juice (one fourth of a lemon to one half glass of water), sip slowly a glass or two of fresh, cold water. In the water, unless otherwise ordered, you may take the juice of half a lemon or lime. Do not use warm or hot water for drinking. Warm water is weakening and enervating inside as well as outside the body. The hot water drinking fad is all wrong, though it may be temporarily indicated under certain disease conditions.

5. **Morning Cold Rub and Air Bath** (Secs. XIII and XX). After the bath, exercise nude before an open window, if the outside temperature permits. Soon the circulation and skin action will improve to such an extent that you can do this with impunity in midwinter as well as in summer time. After the cold rub, go through the breathing exercises and curative gymnastics. If possible, exercise from fifteen to thirty minutes. Also pinch, slap and massage the fleshy parts of the body vigorously, from the feet up. Rub the back with a flesh brush or with a rough towel. The breathing exercises and internal massage are given in Sec. XXI, the physical exercises in Sec. XXIII and the psychological exercises in Sec. XXIV. Study these sections carefully, especially what is said about changing and alternating the exercises from week to week. Begin with the lighter exercises and from day to day take more difficult ones. The time to be spent in exercise must be determined by your occupation and other individual conditions. Do not exercise immediately before or after eating, nor when very tired.

6. **Morning Walk.** After dressing, if the weather permits, take a brisk walk or short run in the open air. Otherwise spend from ten to fifteen minutes in bag punching or other exercises adapted to your individual requirements.

7. **Exercise.** Exercise is one of the most important factors in the daily natural regimen and one that is too much neglected. Normal, healthy life means that there must be activity of each individual cell in order to promote the assimilation of food and the eliminations of waste products from the cells and tissues. Performing ordinary daily routine work, such as housework, even hard labour, does not accomplish the desired result. It exercises only certain sets of muscles and leaves others undeveloped. In order to be effective exercise should be undertaken with enthusiasm and

energy. Outdoor field sports and games are best, and should be continued until profuse perspiration comes. Where that is not possible some regular substitute should be used, and the will power should be directed to that set of muscles or that part of the body which is being exercised at any given time. Walking is a splendid form of exercise, provided it is made vigorous enough to set in motion all the muscles of the body and to produce perspiration. There is no better form of elimination than natural perspiration.

8. **Sun and Air Baths.** Sun and air baths are important for reviving the dead skin and for keeping it in normal condition. They should be taken every day. This can be done in combination with your regular exercise, but may be taken at a separate time and place (Sec. XX). Vitality or life force comes to us through the sun; and the direct action of sun, light and air on the skin is very beneficial. Do not expose your body to the direct rays of the sun for too long a time at the start, as the sun's rays have a powerful stimulating effect. You should begin with moderate exposure and gradually increase until you get the amount suited to your individual condition. If no special provision is made for outdoor air baths, take all exercise nude before an open window. The cold spray or sponge bath taken during exposure to the sun and air will increase skin action. Let the body dry in the air, rubbing it with the hands to increase its magnetism. Before going to sleep, take a short air bath in front of the open window. This may be combined with breathing exercises, internal massage or a few corrective movements; but care must be taken not to drive away sleep by over-strenuous exercise.

9. **The Evening Cold Sitz Bath.** This important application is described later in Sec. XIII. It should be taken regularly as long as there are no bad after-effects. A few people become stimulated by this bath instead of being soothed and quieted, and complain of disturbed sleep. In such cases the bath may have to be taken lukewarm or omitted entirely. Women must not take the cold sitz bath during the menstrual period and should cease cold water applications a few days before the arrival of the period and not resume until a day or two after. If you do not react well to the sitz bath, try the air bath with self-massage as described under "morning cold rub". The cold sitz bath is beneficial in the majority of cases. It draws the blood from the brain and spinal cord into the abdominal parts and organs where it is most needed, thus inducing quiet, dreamless sleep. If you suffer from cold feet due to defective circulation follow the directions for Foot Baths and Barefoot Walking, in Sec. XIII.

10. **Eating and Drinking.** Wrong eating and drinking is the most prolific of all the causes of disease, and therefore regulation of the diet in harmony with nature's laws and principles becomes of prime importance

11

in the treatment of acute and chronic disease. In case of chronic disease every drop of blood and every cell is affected and in order to produce a cure complete regeneration has to take place. The greater the change in food, provided you select foods that are pure and eliminating, the greater and faster will be the changes in the blood and tissues. A carefully selected balanced diet containing the neutralizing and eliminating elements provides one of the most important means for complete regeneration of the human organism. It requires steady, persistent use of will power and self-control to arrive at the proper daily quantity and kind of food and to maintain that schedule, but the results obtained are well worth the effort.

There are certain kinds of foods and drinks which have no place in the strict natural regimen. These are coffee, tea and all kinds of alcoholic and fermenting drinks. Meat, fish or other flesh foods should not be used. When you eat the flesh of an animal you eat the waste products of the animal's life processes, urea, uric acid, cell waste, etc., all of which are poisons. If you add to this the quantity of waste products and poisons produced in your own body it is very evident that by eating of meat foods you are putting double work on the organs of elimination. Excess quantities of starches, proteins and fats are not desirable in the natural regimen, for the reason that they may produce acids and ptomaines which are difficult to eliminate. The digestion of starchy foods begins in the mouth. Therefore it is important that they be thoroughly masticated and mixed with saliva before being swallowed. This can be accomplished much better if the starchy foods are eaten dry or nearly dry, as this promotes the flow of saliva.

The ideal breakfast should consist of raw fruits only; best, one kind of fruit at a meal. However, if it agrees with you, you may add to the raw fruit some dried, stewed or baked fruit. During the treatment of serious chronic ailments, however, the breakfast should consist of raw juicy fruits only, such as oranges, grapefruit, watermelon, cantaloup, apples, plums, pears, cherries, berries, etc. Dinner, the chief meal of the day, should be eaten after the day's work is over. It is never advisable to eat a heavy meal when it has to be immediately followed by great physical or mental exertion. Either work or digestion will suffer. The vital force employed in manual or intellectual labour cannot at the same time be utilized for digestion and assimilation of food. If circumstances are such that dinner must be eaten in the middle of the day, take a short rest and relax thoroughly, physically and mentally, from ten to fifteen minutes before eating. You should also relax for about one half hour before going back to your work. The American habit of sitting down to meals in a tense, strained condition of mind and body is to blame for much of the chronic

12

dyspepsia from which we as a nation are suffering. Dinner should be composed of the following foods: — Soup, which should not be served more than twice or three times a week. For relishes use raw vegetables and olives. Vegetable salads. One cooked leafy, juicy vegetable. Selection of potatoes or roots. For desserts take fruits or recipes of the kind given in the Lindlahr Cook Book. Health bread and butter, or rye crisp. This does not mean that you should necessarily have all the above dishes at one meal. As a matter of fact, the less variety of food at one meal the better. In order to lessen the intake of protein and starchy foods, it is a good rule to take either a potato or bread, not both, at the same meal. The noon lunch might consist of salads, vegetable relishes; alkaline fruits, such as figs, dates, raisins, prunes, etc.; cereal dishes; health bread and butter, cottage cheese or honey; also dried, stewed or baked fruits, and nuts. The principal rule to observe in the planning of meals is that one half of them should consist of juicy fruits and juicy, leafy vegetables. The other half may consist of foods of the starch, sugar, fat and protein varieties. (This is explained more fully in the table at the end of this chapter and further information about the selection, combination and preparation of foods is given in Sec. X of this volume.)

11. **Frequency of Meals.** The frequency of meals cannot be determined by hard and fast rules. Various factors must be taken into account — occupation, physical condition, circumstances in the home, etc. As a rule the two-meal plan is the best. The ideal way is to have breakfast between nine and ten o'clock in the morning and dinner between five and six in the afternoon. This allows sufficient time for thorough digestion and assimilation. In our experience, the no-breakfast plan does not agree with most people. Putting off the first meal until noon is likely to create excessive hunger and a tendency to overeat. It also brings the noonday meal and the evening meal very close together. If circumstances are such that breakfast has to be taken early in the day and dinner late in the evening, it may be found advisable to eat the raw fruit meal at noon.

12. **Hot Food and Drink.** Next to eating the wrong kinds of food or good food in abnormal combinations, there is nothing more injurious to the digestive organs, particularly the teeth, than the foolish custom of swallowing food and drink piping hot and mixing the glowing viands with ice water. Solid foods, soup, coffee and tea are served at temperatures varying from $120°$ to $160°F$. (as much as $70°$ above blood heat), or as hot as the food can be conveyed from the cooking utensils to the table. Hands or feet immersed in water of the temperature at which food is usually served would be severely scalded, yet the tender membranes of the mouth, throat, oesophagus and stomach are brought a few times daily into intimate contact with burning hot food and drink. None other of

the many foolish customs of hyper-civilization contributes so much to the early decay and destruction of the teeth and gums as scalding them with hot food and drink and then chilling suddenly with ice cold water. The sudden application of heat to the teeth will crack the enamel in similar manner as glass will crack when suddenly immersed in hot water. The destruction of the enamel is hastened by abrupt changes from excessive heat to contact with ice cold drinks or ices. Is it any wonder that decay of the teeth and pyorrhoea are almost universal in this country? While among Europeans the custom of serving food as hot as possible is as prevalent as in this country, they have not yet acquired the injurious ice water habit. The American traveller is greatly surprised when he asks in vain for ice water in the home, the railroad trains, and in the best hotels in Europe. Nature nowhere serves her wild creatures with hot food and drink; that is one of the reasons why they do not need dentists. In our institutions we make it a practice to serve the food moderately warm. At first many of the guests are strongly inclined to resent this practice, but they quickly become accustomed to the better way and then thoroughly relish the warm viands; it is all a matter of habit and we might as well indulge in the right habits as in the wrong ones which tend to create suffering for us in the long run. The injurious habit of "fire eating" accounts to a large extent not only for early decay of the teeth and for diseases of the gums, but also for acute and chronic inflammation of the stomach and, in many instances, for ulcers, and for the development of benign and malignant tumours.

13. **Drinking.** We are not in favour of excessive drinking. The "flushing of the system" fad is a mistake. The purification of the body is not a mechanical process like the flushing of a sewer with water. It is a chemical process which depends upon the proper concentration of the different secretions in the system. These secretions, the most important of which is the blood, cannot be made more effective by diluting with large amounts of water. Most of the people that come to us for treatment suffering from stubborn chronic constipation have been "flushing" for years, through mouth and rectum, using quarts and even gallons of water daily, with the result that they were getting more constipated all the time. On our dry food diet and with our treatments, the bowels begin to act normally within a short time.

Very large quantities of lime, iron, sulphur or other inorganic minerals in water that is used constantly for drinking or bathing are injurious to the system, but we do not sanction the use of distilled water under any circumstances, because it has a tendency to leach the mineral elements from blood and tissues. If the water contains vegetable or animal organic matter it should be filtered.

14

It is the customary highly spiced meat and egg diet which creates excessive, abnormal thirst. A rational, non-irritating and non-stimulating vegetarian diet furnishes the organism with fluids of the best possible kind in the form of fruit and vegetable juices, prepared in nature's own laboratory, rich in medicinal qualities and free from all objectionable constituents. Under ordinary conditions, drink from four to eight glasses of pure water at ordinary temperature in the course of the day, according to your own individual inclination; in the morning before breakfast, at night before going to bed and at intervals during the day.

14. **Drinking at Meals.** The less you drink with your meals the better. The dryness of the food furnishes the necessary stimulus to the secretion of saliva and of gastric and intestinal juices. An abundance of liquid in the digestive tract interferes with the action of the secreting glands. It dilutes the secretions and thereby weakens their digestive qualities. The juices of the stomach and the intestines cannot be made more effective by adding to them large amounts of water at mealtime. Coffee and tea or alcoholic drinks should be especially avoided at meals. The former retard digestion; the latter overstimulate temporarily the secretion of gastric and intestinal juices and this unnatural stimulation is followed by corresponding weakness and inactivity of the secreting glands in the digestive tract. Liquor taken before and during meals, therefore, encourages overeating, and when the reaction sets in, the secretions as well as the vitality are lacking in strength to digest properly the excess of food taken under the influence of unnatural stimulation. A glass of water taken from one half to one hour before meals will in most cases do away with the desire to drink at meal time. However, if there be actual thirst it must be satisfied. If you prefer a warm drink, you may take cereal coffee or warm milk or (sparingly) cocoa. Skimmed milk, buttermilk and fruit juices diluted with water are good cold drinks.

15. **Losing weight.** As before stated, the first effect of the natural regimen and of the natural methods of treatment is to promote the elimination of morbid matter from the system and this is naturally accompanied by some loss of weight. Many patients, unless they are instructed on the subject, become alarmed over this, especially since the laity as well as the old school of medicine seem to regard the increase of flesh and fat as evidence of increasing strength and better health. This, however, is another popular fallacy. To increase flesh and fat in a diseased body by stuffing and swamping it with large quantities of fat-producing foods and drink simply means increasing the disease conditions. It is the purpose of natural methods of living and of treatment first to purify cells and tissues of their encumbrances with morbid matter and disease taints. When this has been accomplished and when the blood has been built up on a natural

basis, then will come a perfectly natural gain in flesh and strength; and whatever is built up then in new tissue is certain to be solid, pure and wholesome. If all directions are carried out faithfully, there may be some loss of flesh but no corresponding loss of strength. On the contrary, in most cases there will be a decided increase of vital energy. Therefore do not dread the loss of a few pounds of flesh during the first periods of treatment. Whatever you lose is not good anyway. The old, diseased man must go before the new man can be built up in perfect health, strength and beauty.

16. **Mental Attitude.** The attitude of the mind is of great importance in following the natural regimen of living and of treatment. By our habitual thoughts we create in our brains the actual centres which make either for weakness and disease, or for health and strength (see Sec. VI). From these centres impulses or vibrations are changed into the corresponding physical conditions of health or of disease. This very important subject is treated at greater length in Vol. I, Chap. XL.

17. **Relaxation.** In our strenuous modern life the art of relaxation is known little and practised less. Perfect relaxation is of the greatest importance for the conservation of our vital energies. It allows the greatest possible inflow of vital force into the system and economizes its expenditure. Most people spend the best part of their vitality not in the amount of work they do, but in the way they do it. We must learn to be perfectly relaxed not only during the periods of rest and sleep, but also during the hours of physical and mental activity. Some people, on account of a tense nervous condition, spend more vital energy when resting and sleeping than others do while at work. In most instances, nerve exhaustion in its many different manifestations is brought about not through overwork, but through the tense, fretful, impatient, irritable, hurrying way in which the work is performed. The ability to rest, to sleep and to work in a condition of perfect relaxation and repose plays an important part not only in the ordinary daily life but especially in the natural treatment of diseases. We have therefore a special chapter on the subject of relaxation (Vol. I, Chap. XLII).

18. **Sleep.** During sleep the liberation of vital energy in the body continues as during the wakeful hours of active work, but none is expended. The body acts as a storage battery. A reserve of vital energy is thus accumulated for the work of the following day. The moment the consciousness wakens and mental activity begins the expenditure of vital force commences. It is for these reasons that nothing can take the place of sleep as a restorer of vital energy. No amount of food and drink, no tonics or stimulants can make good for lost sleep. Therefore we must learn how to derive the greatest good from deep sound sleep. This can be

learned and the habit acquired even by those who have suffered from insomnia for years. It is fortunate for insomnia patients that they sleep more than they are aware. If it were not so, they could not live. The following rules, if closely followed, will help to induce sound sleep: (a) Sleep in a well ventilated and not overheated room. (b) Never sleep in the garments worn during the day. Wear a night garment of light, porous material, so that the poisonous exhalations of the skin may easily escape; or, better still, wear none. (c) Let the covering be neither too warm or too heavy. (d) Avoid excitement or extraordinary strain just before bedtime. (e) Do not eat heavy food shortly before bedtime. However, it is a good practice to eat one kind of juicy fruit before retiring, and many nervous, wakeful people are benefited by taking a glass of milk. (f) After going to bed, practise the formulae for "Relaxation Before Sleeping" (see Vol. I, Chap. XLII).

19. **Bedtime.** Two hours before and the two hours after midnight are the most valuable for sleep of all the twenty-four hours of the day. In these four hours mental and physical vigour are at their lowest ebb and sleep is soundest and most natural. It is true, therefore, that "one hour of sleep before midnight is worth two at any other time". Actors and others whose occupations require intense mental work during midnight hours are prone to suffer from nervous disorders. Establish the habit of going to bed early. If you have extra work let it not be done during the precious midnight hours, but rather in the early morning after the organism has been refreshed and strengthened by sleep.

20. **Duration of Sleep.** Eight hours of sleep a day is considered the average amount required by the average person. However, some people require more sleep than others, especially those who are nervous or an-aemic. On the other hand too much sleep begets a tendency to laziness. Therefore no general rule can be established as to the exact amount of sleep required. This must be determined by the individual through close observation of the amount of sleep required to keep him in the best possible condition.

21. **The Noonday Nap.** If you are weak and nervous or subject in your daily work to considerable physical and mental strain, make it a practice to take a nap after the noonday meal or at any other suitable time. Retire to a quiet place where you will be undisturbed. Sit in a chair in a comfortable, relaxed position or, better still, lie down on a couch or bed. If there be sufficient time for doing so, take off shoes and loosen the clothing. Dismiss all disturbing thoughts from your mind and go through one of the formulae for relaxation given in Vol. I, Chap. XLII.

If in this manner you can rest and relax sufficiently to lose consciousness for a short while, even if it should not be for more than ten or fifteen minutes, you will rise strengthened and refreshed. Only through entire temporary loss of consciousness can perfect relaxation be attained. In order to ascertain whether you have accomplished your purpose, hold some small object, say a pencil, in your closed hand when you take your rest. If loss of consciousness and complete relaxation have taken place, you will find your hand has opened and the pencil has slipped from it. Some people claim that they feel worse after a brief nap in the daytime, but it has been my experience that by persisting in this practice the seemingly adverse effects are soon overcome. I believe that many overtired and nervous people would find this noonday nap or "psychic" nap, as it has been called, more beneficial for rest and recuperation than the taking of a walk. Neither is it true that the noonday nap keeps one from sleeping at night. Insomnia is caused by overwrought nerves. The more relaxed the brain and nervous system during the day, the deeper and more normal the sleep at night. It is the exhausted and overworked brain that has been kept at work for many hours without intermission or relaxation that either cannot go to sleep at all, or obtains at best but a disturbed, fitful, half-conscious and therefore unrefreshing sleep.([1])

([1])
    There is no doubt that sleep is something of the highest importance and that it has an unique function to perform in the restoration of vital energy. However, there is an enormous difference in the amount of sleep which different people require and some seem to require very little. It is even reported that some can live for long periods with no sleep at all and remain in good health. It may be argued that relaxation is more important than sleep for bringing about the restoration of vital energy. People who can learn to relax can restore their energy as well or better than people who sleep a lot. Moreover to relax rather than to try to sleep seems to be the best way of getting to sleep, and thorough relaxation before sleep leads to deeper and better sleep. People who suffer from insomnia should relax and rest and not get into a condition of nervousness and tension because they cannot sleep. They should rather cultivate a feeling of indifference as to whether they sleep or not and they should not take sleeping pills. In a longer or shorter time they will begin to sleep though they may go through a period of seeming to have little or no sleep. It would seem that the physiologists have much to learn about sleep, the causes and nature of which are not well understood. What is it that causes sleep, and what takes place physiologically when we go to sleep? Daniel Mackinnon, the disciple of Lindlahr, has the following to say on the subject of sleep. "Sleep implies the withdrawal of the contact of the physical with the higher mental body. The inflow of energy is reduced to a minimum. Sleep allows the emotional body to adjust itself and this gives harmony and a feeling of rest. Fatigue is a disturbance in the emotional body and the accumulation of waste and wastage of chemical material in cells and tissues. Sleep enables readjustment to take place and allows the emotional body and the cells to recover themselves."

* See page 312 Dietetics in a Nutshell.

PART II

TREATMENT OF ACUTE DISEASES

INTRODUCTION

Many people who have observed the wonderful results of natural treatment in chronic diseases of the so-called incurable types have an idea that while the natural methods are good enough to cure tuberculosis, cancer, infantile paralysis, locomotor ataxia, etc., they are not sufficient to cope with inflammatory feverish diseases. They seem to think it requires "good, strong medicine" or surgical treatment to cure acute diseases.

Some years ago we cured a lady of cancer of the lower jaw after she had undergone three operations and had been told that it was necessary to remove the entire lower jaw in order to save her life. Such treatment seemed rather heroic and drove her to a Natural Therapeutic practitioner. After six months of natural living and treatment the affected jaw was in sufficiently good condition to support a set of artificial teeth and she has been in good health ever since. I met her about a year ago on a street car, and in answer to my enquiry as to the state of her health, she replied, "I am feeling fine, but I have had a lot of trouble in the family. Since I was with you I lost one of my daughters with diphtheria. Another daughter injured her breast through a fall. This resulted in a hardening of the breast and in the formation of an open sore. The doctor who treated her claimed there was danger of cancer and on his recommendation the breast was removed; since that time my daughter has not felt well." On enquiry she admitted that diphtheria antitoxin had been administered in the diphtheria case. I asked her why in the name of common sense she had not called on us or some other Nature Cure physician for advice and treatment. "Oh well," she answered, "I did not know that you treated such cases. I thought you only cured chronic diseases like mine." Surely some people get well under natural treatment and never know what has cured them.

As a matter of fact, it is in the treatment of acute diseases that our methods show the most marvellous results. In the treatment of chronic diseases we undertake the most difficult and most thankless work of healing practice. When a child recovers from measles, the mother thinks the doctor performed a miracle, but when a patient recovers, under natural treatment, slowly and laboriously from advanced stages of cancer or tuberculosis, it scarcely arouses attention. The symptoms of acute disease are so much more terrifying and the recovery so quick and complete that it impresses the lay mind as a remarkable performance of the attending physician. It is this which keeps alive the old school system of medicine. The laity does not understand that acute disease is in itself the cure, and the doctor gets the credit for nature's healing efforts. The same is true of Christian Science. The disease which it tries to ignore and whose very existence it denies is in reality the cure. Nature does the curing with or without Science, but the healer gets the credit.

In my first volume I have described the results of the wrong, that is, suppressive, treatment of acute diseases. I shall now say a few words about the simple and uniform methods of natural treatment. If the uniformity of acute disease be a fact in nature then it follows that it must be possible to treat all acute diseases by uniform methods. That it is possible to treat all acute diseases most successfully by natural methods which anybody possessed of ordinary intelligence can apply has been demonstrated for more than seventy years by Nature Cure practitioners in Europe, and by myself during the last seventeen years in an extensive practice in this country.

One of the many advantages of natural treatment is that it may be applied right from the beginning, as soon as the first symptoms of acute febrile conditions manifest. It is not necessary to wait for a correct diagnosis of the case. The regular physician, with his "specific" treatment for the multitude of "specific" diseases which he recognizes, often has to wait several days or even weeks before the nature of the disease becomes clear to him, before he is able to diagnose the case or even to make a good guess and prescribe his specific remedy. How difficult this is was proved by the candid report of Dr. Cabot, which is now making the rounds in medical journals and other publications. Dr. Cabot, who is in charge of the Autopsy Department of the Massachusetts General Hospital, made the statement that autopsies in a thousand cases of death which occurred revealed the fact that only 53 percent of the diagnoses made before the deaths of the patients had been correct. From this it follows that in 47 percent of these cases the patients were doctored for diseases which they did not have.

The conscientious medical practitioner has to postpone actual treatment until the symptoms are well enough defined to enable him to affix the orthodox label. Meanwhile he applies so-called "expectant treatment", that is he gives a purgative or a "placebo", to make the patient and his friends believe that something is being done. But during this period of indecision and inaction very often the best opportunity for aiding nature in her healing efforts is lost, and the inflammatory processes may reach such virulence that it becomes very difficult or even impossible to keep them within constructive limits. The bonfire that was to burn up the rubbish on the premises may, if not watched and tended, assume such proportions that it damages or destroys the house. It must also be remembered that very frequently acute diseases do not present the well defined sets of symptoms which fit into the accepted medical nosology or symptomatology. On the contrary, in many instances the symptoms suggest a combination of different forms of acute diseases. If the character of the disease is ill defined and complicated, how can the physician select the proper "specific" remedy? In such circumstances the diagnosis of the case as well as the medical treatment will at best be largely guesswork. Compare with this unreliable and unsatisfactory treatment the simple and scientific, exact and efficient natural methods. The natural remedies can be applied from the start at the slightest manifestation of inflammatory and febrile symptoms. No matter what the specific nature or trend of the inflammatory process, whether it be a simple cold, or whether it take the form of measles, scarlet fever, diphtheria, smallpox, appendicitis, etc. — it makes no difference in the mode of treatment. In many instances the natural treatment will have broken the virulence of the attack or brought about a cure before the allopathic physician would be ready to apply his "specific" remedy.

The natural methods of treatment of acute diseases ensure the largest possible percentage of recoveries and at the same time do not in any way tax the system or cause undesirable after-effects which may develop into many forms of chronic invalidism. The most important of the natural remedies can be had free of cost in any home. They are Air, Fasting, Water and the right Mental Attitude. I am fully convinced that these remedies offered freely by Mother Nature are sufficient, if rightly applied, to cure any acute disease arising within the organism. If circumstances permit, however, we may advantageously add, when indicated, manipulation of the spine, massage, magnetic treatment and homoeopathic remedies.

SECTION II

FRESH AIR TREATMENT

A plentiful supply of fresh pure air is of vital importance at any time. We can live without food for several weeks and without water for several days, but we cannot live without air for more than a few minutes. Just as a fire in the furnace cannot be kept up without a good draught which supplies the necessary amount of oxygen to the flame, so the fires of life in the body cannot be maintained without an abundance of oxygen in the air we breathe. Fresh air is of vital importance at all times, but especially in acute disease because here, as we have learned, all vital processes are intensified. The system is working under high pressure. Large quantities of waste and morbid materials, the products of inflammation, have to be oxidized, that is, burned up and eliminated from the system. In this respect Nature Cure practitioners have brought about one of the greatest reforms in medical treatment — the admission of plenty of fresh air into the sickroom.

Strangely enough the importance of this most essential natural remedy is not universally recognized even by doctors. Time and again I have been called to a sickroom where "by order of the doctor" every window was closed and the room filled with pestilential odours, the poisonous exhalations of the diseased organism added to the stale air of the unventilated and often overheated room. It is not the cold draught that is to be feared in the sickroom. Cold air is most agreeable and beneficial to the body burning in fever. What is to be feared is the reinhalation and reabsorption of poisonous emanations from the lungs and skin of the diseased body. Furthermore, the ventilation of a room can be so regulated as to provide a constant and plentiful supply of fresh air without exposing its occupants to a direct draught. Where there is only one window and one door, both may be opened and a sheet or blanket hung across the opening of the door, or the single window may be opened partly from above and partly from below, which ensures the entrance of fresh, cold air at the bottom and the expulsion of the heated and vitiated air at the top. The patient may be protected by a screen, or a board may be placed across the lower part of the window in such a manner that a direct current of air upon the patient is prevented. In very cold weather, or if the conditions are not favourable to constant ventilation of the sickroom, the doors and windows may be opened wide for several minutes every few hours, while the patient's body and head are well protected. There is absolutely no danger of taking cold if these precautions are observed.

Under right conditions of room temperature, frequent exposure of the patient's nude body to air and sunlight will be found most beneficial and will often induce sleep when other means fail.   I would strongly warn against keeping the patient too warm.   This is especially dangerous in the case of young children, who cannot use their judgement or make their wishes known.   I have frequently found children in high fever smothered in heavy blankets under the mistaken impression on the part of the attendants that they had to be kept warm and protected against possible draught.   In many cases the air under the covers was actually steaming hot.   This surely does not tend to reduce the burning fever heat in the body of the patient.

SECTION III

FASTING IN ACUTE DISEASE

Total abstinence from food during acute febrile conditions is of primary importance.   In certain diseases which will be mentioned later on, especially those involving the digestive tract, fasting must be continued for several days after all fever symptoms have disappeared.   In cases of extreme weakness, and where the acute and subacute processes are long drawn out and the patient has become greatly emaciated, it may be advisable to give such easily digestible foods as soft boiled egg, milk, buttermilk, and whole grain bread with butter in combination with raw and stewed fruits, and with vegetable salads prepared with lemon juice and olive oil. There is, however, no greater fallacy than that the patient must be "sustained" and "his strength kept up" by plenty of nourishing food and drink or, worse still, by stimulants and tonics.   This is altogether wrong in itself, and besides, habit and appetite are often mistaken for hunger.

Food is prescribed by old school physicians and urged by relatives and friends of the patient under the mistaken idea that he must be strengthened in order to endure the strain of the disease.   We have learned in Volume I that we do not derive life, vital force, vitality or strength from food and drink, but that vital force, the source of our strength, flows into our bodies through the sympathetic nervous system from the source of all life, intelligence and creative power.   A common spectacle at the bedside of the sick is that of well meaning but misguided relatives and friends forcing food and drink on the patient — often, "by order of the doctor" — when his whole system rebels against it and the nauseated stomach expels the food as soon as taken. Sedatives and tonics are then resorted to in order to force the digestive organs into submission.

1. **Why Fasting Is Necessary.** Aversion to eating during acute diseases, whether they represent healing crises or disease crises, is perfectly natural, because the entire organism, including the mucous membranes of stomach and intestines, is engaged in the work of elimination, not assimilation. Nausea, slimy and foetid discharges, constipation alternating with diarrhoea, etc., indicate that the organs of digestion are throwing off disease matter and that they are not in a position to take up and assimilate food. Ordinarily, the digestive tract acts like a sponge which absorbs the elements of nutrition; but in acute diseases the process is reversed, the sponge is being squeezed and gives off large quantities of morbid matter. The processes of assimilation and digestion are at a standstill. In fact, the entire organism is in a condition of prostration, weakness and inactivity and the vital energies are concentrated on the cleaning and healing processes. Accordingly there is no demand for food. This is verified by the fact that a person fasting for a certain period, say, four weeks, during the course of a serious illness, will not lose nearly as much weight as the same person fasting four weeks in days of healthful activity.

It is for the foregoing reasons that nourishment taken during acute disease is not properly digested, assimilated and transmuted into healthy blood and tissues and instead ferments and decays, filling the system with waste matter and noxious gases. It also interferes seriously with the elimination of morbid matter through stomach and intestines by forcing these organs to take up the work of digestion and assimilation and diverts the vital forces from their combat against the disease conditions and draws upon them to remove the worse than useless food ballast from the organism. This explains why taking food during feverish diseases is usually followed by a rise in temperature and by aggravation of the other disease symptoms. As long as there are signs of inflammatory, febrile conditions and no appetite, do not be afraid to withhold food entirely, if necessary for as long as five, six or seven weeks. I have treated several virulent cases of typhoid-malaria which lasted for six weeks before the acute febrile symptoms subsided. During this time the patients did not receive any food whatsoever, not even a drop of milk. I continued the fasting during the seventh week in order to allow time for the building up of the intestinal membranes which had sloughed as a result of the inflammatory processes. Toward the end of the seventh week the patients developed natural hunger. Then the feeding commenced and they made a perfect recovery, gaining more in flesh within a few months than they had lost during the illness. In cases of gastritis, appendicitis, peritonitis, dysentery, or typhoid fever, abstinence from food is absolutely imperative.

2. **Breaking the Fast.** After fever and inflammation have entirely subsided, a few days should be allowed for the healing and restoring of the broken-down tissues before any food is taken. Many of the serious chronic after-effects of these diseases are due to too early feeding, which does not allow the healing forces of nature time to rebuild the sloughed membranes and injured organs. After a prolonged fast great care must be observed when commencing to eat. Very small quantities of light food may safely be taken at intervals of a few hours. A good plan, especially after an attack of typhoid fever or dysentery, is to break the fast by thoroughly masticating one or two tablespoonfuls of popcorn. This gives the digestive tract a good scouring and starts the peristaltic action of the bowels better than any other food. The popcorn may advantageously be followed at intervals by small amounts of raw subacid fruit. For several days or weeks after a fast, according to the severity of the "acute disease" or healing crisis, a diet consisting largely of raw fruits, such as oranges, grapefruit, apples, pears, grapes, etc., and juicy vegetables, especially lettuce, celery, cabbage slaw, watercress, young onions, tomatoes or cucumbers should be adhered to. No condiments or dressings should be used with the vegetables except lemon juice and olive oil.

SECTION IV

DRINKING IN ACUTE DISEASE

As the system needs more oxygen in febrile diseases, so it also needs more fluids. Excessive drinking, however, has a weakening effect. Increased production and accumulation of heat in the body evaporates more water and much water is needed to dilute and eliminate the morbid products of inflammation through the skin, kidneys and bowels. Therefore water should be given freely, mixed with acid and subacid fruit juices. The best of these are the juices of lemon, lime, grapefruit and orange. If the acid juices for any reason do not agree with the patient, they may be alternated with the juices of stewed prunes or figs. Grape juice contains too much sugar. It would tend to increase heat production unnecessarily. The acid and subacid fruit juices do not contain sufficient amounts of starches, fats or proteins to start the digestive processes; on the other hand they are very rich in the positive alkaline mineral elements which the system needs in order to neutralize and eliminate pathogenic substances liberated in large amounts through the inflammatory processes. The fruit juices are also natural tonics to all the vital organs and the finest antiseptics in nature. In brief, they are nature's best remedies in acute as well as in chronic diseases.

Flaxseed tea is a valuable remedy for colds, croup and catarrhal diseases. It has a soothing effect upon the raw and sore membranes of the throat, and upon the digestive and urinary organs. Take a few tablespoonfuls when needed to allay soreness in the throat and bronchi. The best way to prepare this tea is to boil a tablespoonful of flaxseed in one and a half pints of water for five minutes, then strain and add some honey and lemon juice.

Rutabagas, or Swedish turnips, furnish another splendid remedy for colds, croups and catarrhs. Take a large rutabaga, scrub clean with a vegetable brush but do not peel; then wipe dry. Remove top and scoop out centre, leaving a shell about an inch and a half in thickness. Fill the cavity with unrefined brown sugar or with pure maple sugar. Now place in a very slow oven or on top of a cookstove for eight to twelve hours, in such a way that the sugar and the juice of the rutabaga form a thick syrup. If the sugar absorbs too fast, more must be added. A teaspoonful of this syrup should be taken whenever needed to allay the irritation and soreness in the throat and bronchi.

Teas made from watercress, asparagus or juniper berries have a relaxing effect upon the urinary organs and are therefore valuable aids to promote the flow of scanty urine (see Sec. XIX. Nos. 5 and 6).

SECTION V

HYDROTHERAPY IN ACUTE DISEASES

We claim that in acute diseases water treatment will accomplish all the beneficial effects which the old school practitioners ascribe to drugs, and that it will produce the desired results much more efficiently and without any harmful side-effects or after-effects upon the system. The principal objects to be attained in the treatment of acute inflammatory diseases are:

(a) To relieve the inner congestion and consequent pain in the affected parts.

(b) To keep the temperature below the danger point by promoting heat radiation through the skin.

26

(c) To increase the activity of the organs of elimination and thus to facilitate the removal of morbid materials from the system.

(d) To increase the positive electromagnetic energies in the organism.

(e) To increase the amount of oxygen and ozone in the system and thereby to promote the oxidation and combustion of effete matter.

The above-mentioned objects can be attained most effectually by the simple cold water treatment. Whatever the acute condition may be, whether an ordinary cold or the most serious type of febrile disease, the applications described in the following pages, used singly, combined or alternatively according to individual conditions, will always be in order and sufficient to produce the best possible results.

1. **Baths and Ablutions.** Cooling sprays or, if the patient be too weak to leave the bed, cold sponge baths or ablutions, repeated whenever the temperature rises, are very effective for keeping the fever below the danger point, for relieving the congestion in the interior of the body, and for stimulating the elimination of systemic poisons through the skin. However, care must be taken not to lower the temperature too much by the excessive coldness or unduly prolonged duration of the application. It is possible to suppress inflammatory processes by means of cold water or ice bags just as easily as with poisonous antiseptics, antifever medicines and surgical operations. It is sufficient to reduce the temperature just below danger point. This will allow the inflammatory processes to run their natural course through the five progressive stages of inflammation, and this natural course will then be followed by perfect regeneration of the affected parts. In our sanitorium we use only water of ordinary temperature as it flows from the tap, never under any circumstances ice bags or ice water. The application of ice keeps the parts to which it is applied in a chilled condition. The circulation cannot react and the inflammatory processes are thus most effectually suppressed.[1]

To recapitulate: Never check or suppress a fever by means of cold baths, ablutions, wet packs, etc., but merely lower it below the danger point. For instance, if a certain type of fever has a tendency to rise to 104°F. or more, bring it down to about 102°. If the fever ordinarily runs at a lower temperature, say at 102°F., do not try to reduce it more than one or two degrees. Natural Therapeutics pays more attention to the severity of the toxic symptoms than to the height of the temperature. A person endowed with good vitality and active elimination may not suffer greatly under high degrees of temperature, while another with lower vitality and

[1]
Basil Shackleton in his book on the Grape Cure discusses a method for using small ice packs in a way which is eliminative and not suppressive. ("The Grape Cure", Basil Shackleton, Thorsons Ltd.)

defective elimination may exhibit alarming symptoms of toxicity, such as dyspnoea (laboured breathing), delirium, coma, etc., at a much lower degree of temperature. The treatment should be adjusted accordingly. If the temperature be subnormal, that is below the normal or regular body temperature (98.6°), the packs should be applied in such a manner that a warming effect is produced; that is, less wet cloths and more dry covering should be used; and the packs left on the body a longer time before they are renewed. Never lose sight of the fact that fever is in itself a healing, cleansing process which must not be checked or suppressed.

2. **Cold Tub or Spray in Fever.** As long as a fever patient is strong enough to leave the bed and sit in an ordinary bathtub, one of the most effective fever treatments is to pour cold water over the neck, head and body by means of a sprinkler (Kneipp Cure), an ordinary bathtub spray, a pitcher or a dipper. After the bath the patient must receive a brisk rub down with a rough towel which will help to produce a good reaction; or he may go back to bed without drying. In that case the warmth of the bed and the dampness of the body will act as a wet pack. This is one of the most pleasant, refreshing and efficient methods of treating any kind of fever. The effects of it are little short of miraculous.

3. **Hot Water Applications Are Injurious.** Especially is it wrong to apply hot water to seats of inflammation as, for instance, the inflamed appendix or ovaries, sprains, bruises, etc. Almost in every instance where I am called in to attend a case of acute appendicitis or peritonitis, I find hot compresses or hot water bottles, by means of which the inflamed parts are kept continually in an overheated condition. It is in this way that a simple inflammation is nurtured into an abscess and made more serious and dangerous. The hot compress or hot water bottle draws the blood away from the inflamed area to the surface temporarily; but unless the hot application is kept up continually, the blood, under the law of action and reaction, will recede from the surface into the interior, and as a result the inner congestion will become as great or greater than before. If the hot applications are continued, the heat applied tends to maintain and increase the heat in the inflamed parts. "Inflammation" means that there is already too much heat in the affected part or organ. Common sense, therefore, would dictate cooling applications instead of heating ones.

The cold packs and compresses, on the other hand, have a directly cooling effect upon the seat of inflammation, and in accordance with the law of action and reaction their second, lasting effect consists in drawing the blood from the congested and heated interior to the surface, thus relaxing the pores of the skin and promoting the radiation of heat and the elimination of impurities. Both the hot water applications and the use of ice are, therefore, to be absolutely condemned. The only rational and

28

natural treatment of inflammatory conditions is that by compresses, packs and ablutions, using water of ordinary temperature as it comes from the tap. By means of the simple cold water treatment and fasting, all fevers and inflammations can be reduced in a perfectly natural way within a short time without undue strain on the organism.

4. **The Whole Body Pack.** The whole body or sheet pack is most effective if by means of it the patient can be brought into a state of copious perspiration. The pack is then removed and the patient is given a cold sponge bath. It will be found that this treatment often produces a second profuse sweat which is very beneficial. This after sweat should also be followed by a cold sponge bath. Such a course of treatment will often be sufficient to eliminate the morbid matter which has gathered in the system, and thus prevent in a perfectly natural manner a threatening disease which otherwise might become dangerous to life. (For description see Sec. XV.)

5. **Alternating Packs.** If and when the febrile disease, whatever its name, begins to gain a stronger hold on the system, the whole sheet packs cannot be continued. In place of them we must resort to body, throat or leg packs (Sec. XV, Nos. 14, 10, 17). If the febrile disorder continues for some length of time it is best to alternate these various packs in order to draw the blood successively into the lower and upper parts of the body. If, for instance, throat and body packs are applied continuously this will have a tendency to divert the blood from the lower extremities to the upper parts of the body. This is not advisable because in all febrile diseases the blood concentrates in the affected parts and organs and is therefore withdrawn from the extremities which, as a result, become cold and clammy. The best way to counteract this tendency to congestion in the inflamed organs is to apply the wet packs alternately to the throat, chest and lower extremities. If the temperature runs exceedingly high, it is advisable to apply packs to the body and the extremities at the same time. The packs must be taken off when they become hot or dry or if for some reason they become cold and chilling. Every time a warm pack is taken off the body this must be followed by a cold rub of the parts covered by the bandages in order to produce a better reaction and to remove from the skin the morbid materials drawn to the surface by the wet packs. If the packs remain cold they must be reinforced by hot water bottles or hot bricks.

6. **The Bed-sweat Bath.** If the patient does not react to the pack, that is, if he remains cold, or if, as is sometimes the case in malaria, the fever is accompanied by chills, or if profuse perspiration is desired, hot water bottles or hot bricks wrapped in flannel should be placed along the sides and to the feet, under the outside covering (See. XIV). This form of

29

application also may be used with good results when an incipient cold or fever is to be aborted.

7. **Purpose of Wet Packs.** Wet packs may be applied to the throat, the arms, legs, shoulder joints, or any other part of the body. The number of layers of wet linen and dry covering is determined by the vitality of the patient, the height of his temperature, and the particular object of the application, which may be (a) to lower high temperature, (b) to raise temperature when this is subnormal, (c) to relieve inner congestion, (d) to promote elimination. If the object be to lower high temperature, several layers of wet linen should be wrapped around the body and covered loosely by one or two layers of the wrappings in order to prevent the bed from getting wet. The packs must be renewed as soon as they become dry or uncomfortably hot. If the object be to raise subnormal temperature, less wet linen and more dry covering must be used, and the packs left on a longer time, say from thirty minutes to two hours. If the patient does not react to the pack, hot bricks or bottles should be placed at the sides and to the feet, as explained in connection with the whole body pack. If inner congestion is to be relieved, or if the object be to promote elimination, less of the wet linen and more dry wrappings should be used.

When packs are applied, the bed may be protected by spreading an oilcloth or rubber sheeting over the mattress under the sheet. But in no case should oilcloth or rubber sheeting be used for the outer covering of the packs. This would interfere with some of the main objects of the pack treatment, especially with heat radiation. The outer covering should be warm but at the same time porous, so as to allow the escape of heat and of poisonous gases from the body.

8. **Local Compresses.** In case of local inflammation, as in appendicitis, ovaritis, colitis, etc., separate cooling compresses may be slipped under the pack and over the seat of inflammation. These local compresses may be removed and changed when hot and dry without disturbing the larger pack.

In all fevers accompanied by high temperature, it is advisable to place an extra cooling compress at the nape of the neck (the region of the medulla and the back brain), because here are located the brain centres which regulate the inner temperature of the body (thermotaxic centres), and the cooling of these brain centres produces a cooling effect upon the entire organism.

9. **Epsom Salt Treatment.** In serious acute cases beneficial effects of hydrotherapy treatment may be augmented or intensified by applications of Epsom salt solution. Epsom salt solution instead of plain water is used in the various applications (Sec. XVII).

10. **Enemas.** While ordinarily we do not favour the giving of injections

or enemas unless they are absolutely necessary, we apply them freely in feverish diseases in order to remove from the rectum and lower colon any accumulations of morbid matter, and thus prevent their reabsorption into the system.   In cases of exceptionally stubborn constipation, an injection of a few ounces of warm olive oil may be given.   Allow this to remain in the colon about thirty minutes in order to soften the contents of the rectum, and follow with an injection of warm water.

11. **How Cold Packs Promote Heat Radiation.**   Many people are under the impression that the packs reduce the fever temperature so quickly because they are put on cold.   But this is not so, because, unless the reaction be bad, the packs become warm after a few minutes' contact with the body.   The prompt reduction of temperature takes place because of increased heat radiation.   The coldness of the pack may lower the surface temperature slightly; but it is the moist warmth forming under the pack on the surface of the body that draws the blood from the congested interior into the skin, relaxes and opens its minute blood vessels and pores, and in that way facilitates the escape of heat from the body.   In febrile conditions the pores and capillary blood vessels of the skin are tense and contracted.   Therefore the heat cannot escape, the skin is hot and dry, and the interior of the body remains overheated.   When the skin relaxes and the patient begins to perspire freely, we say the fever "is broken".   The moist warmth under the wet pack produces this relaxation of the skin in a perfectly natural manner.   By means of these simple packs followed by cold ablutions, the temperature of the patient can be kept at any point desired without the use of poisonous anti-fever medicines, serums and antitoxins which lower the temperature by benumbing and paralysing heart action, respiration and the red and white blood corpuscles, and thus generally lowering the vital activities of the organism.

12. **How Cold Packs Relieve Inner Congestion.**   In all inflammatory febrile diseases the blood is congested in the inflamed parts and organs. This produces the four cardinal symptoms of inflammation: redness, swelling, heat and pain.   If the congestion be too great, the pain becomes excessive, and the inflammatory processes cannot run their course to the best advantage.   It is therefore of great importance to relieve the local blood pressure in the affected parts, and this can be accomplished most effectively by means of the wet packs. As before stated, they draw blood into the surface of the body and in that way relieve inner congestion wherever it may exist, whether it be in the brain, as in meningitis, in the lungs, as in pneumonia, or in the inflamed appendix.   In several cases where a child was in the most dangerous stage of diphtheria, where the membranes in throat and nasal passages were already choking the young patient, the wet packs applied to the whole body from neck to feet relieved

31

the congestion in the throat so quickly that within half an hour after the first application the patient breathed easily and soon made a perfect recovery. The effectiveness of these simple water applications in reducing congestion, heat and pain is little short of marvellous.

13. **How Cold Packs Promote Elimination.** By far the largest number of deaths in febrile diseases result from the accumulation in the system of poisonous substances, which paralyse or destroy vital centres and organs. Therefore it is necessary to eliminate the morbid products of inflammation from the organism as quickly as possible. This also is accomplished most effectively and thoroughly by the application of wet packs. As they draw the blood into the surface and relax the minute blood vessels in the skin, the morbid materials in the blood are eliminated through the pores of the skin and absorbed by the packs. That this is actually so is verified by the yellowish or brownish discolouration of the wet wrappings and by their offensive odour.

14. **Cold Water Enemas Dangerous.** One of the main causes of constipation in febrile diseases is the inner congestion and fever heat. Through the cooling and relaxing effect of the packs upon the intestines this inner fever heat is reduced, and the natural movement of the bowels greatly facilitated. If constipation should persist in spite of the packs and cooling compresses, injections of tepid water (about blood heat) should be given every day or every other day in order to prevent the reabsorption of poisonous products from the lower colon. But never give injections of cold water with the idea of reducing fever in that way. This is very dangerous and may cause fatal collapse.

15. **Electromagnetic Effect of Cold Water.** One of the most important but least understood effects of hydropathic treatment is its influence upon the electromagnetic energies in the human body. I have never found any allusions to this aspect of the cold water treatment in any books on hydrotherapy which have come to my notice. The sudden application of cold water or cold air to the surface of the nude body and the inhalation of cold air into the lungs have the effect of increasing the amount of electromagnetic energy in the system. This can be verified by the following experiment: Insert one of the plates of an electrometer (sensitive galvanometer) into the stomach of a person who has remained some time in a warm room. Now let this person inhale suddenly fresh, cold outside air. At once the galvanometer will register a larger amount of electromagnetic energy. The same effect will be produced by the application of a quick, cold spray to the warm body. It is the sudden lowering of temperature on the surface of the body or in the lungs, and the resulting contrast between the heat within and the cold outside, that causes the increased manifestation of electromagnetic energy in the system. This, together with the

acceleration of the entire circulation, undoubtedly accounts for the tonic effect of cold water applications such as cold packs, ablutions, sprays, sitz baths, barefoot walking, etc., and for the wonderfully bracing influence of fresh cold outside air. In our Nature Cure work we find all the way through that the continued application of warmth has a debilitating effect upon the organism, and that only by the opposing influences of alternating heat and cold, including seasonal climatic variations, can we produce the natural stimulation which awakens the dormant vital energies in the body of the chronic.

16. **Increase of Oxygen and Ozone.** The liberation of electromagnetic currents through cold water applications has other very important effects upon the system besides that of stimulation. Electricity splits up molecules of water into hydrogen, oxygen and ozone. We have an example of this in the thunderstorm. The powerful electric discharges which we call "lightning" separate or split the watery vapours of the air into these elements. It is the increase of oxygen and ozone in the air that purifies and sweetens the atmosphere after the storm. In acute as well as in chronic disease, large amounts of oxygen and ozone are required to burn up the morbid materials and to purify the system. Certain combinations of these elements are among the most powerful antiseptics and germicides. Likewise, the electric currents produced by cold packs, ablutions and other cold water applications split up the molecules of water in the tissues of the body into their component parts. In this way large amounts of oxygen and ozone are liberated, and these elements assist to a considerable extent in the oxidation and neutralization of waste materials and disease products.

The following experiment proves that sudden changes of temperature create electric currents in metals: When two cylinders of dissimilar metals are welded together, and one of the metals is suddenly chilled or heated, electric currents are produced which will continue to flow until both metals are at the same temperature. Another application of this principle is furnished by the oxydonor. If both poles of this little instrument are exposed to the same temperature, there is no manifestation of electricity; but if one of the poles be attached to the warm body and the other immersed in cold water or exposed to cold air, the liberation of electromagnetic currents begins at once. These electric currents set free oxygen and ozone, which in their turn support the oxidation and neutralization of systemic poisons. According to my experience, however, the cold water applications are more effective in this respect than the oxydonor.

SECTION VI

THE RIGHT MENTAL ATTITUDE IN ACUTE DISEASE

We have learned that in the process of inflammation a battle is going on between the healing forces of the body on the one hand and the disease taints on the other — that the millions of little cells are struggling to throw off their hostile invaders, the morbid encumbrances and systemic poisons. The battle is real in every respect, as real as a combat between armies of living soldiers. In this conflict, going on in all acute inflammatory diseases, mind plays the same role as the commander of an army. The great general needs courage, equanimity and presence of mind most in the stress of the battle. So the mind, the commander of the vast armies of cells battling in acute disease for the health of the body, must have absolute faith in the superiority of nature's healing forces. If the mind becomes frightened by the inflammatory and febrile symptoms, and pictures to itself in darkest colours their dreadful consequences, these confused and distracted thought vibrations are conveyed instantaneously to the millions of little soldiers fighting in the affected parts and organs. They also become confused and panic-stricken. The excitement of fear in the mind still more accelerates heart action and respiration, intensifies the local congestion, and greatly increases the morbid accumulations in the system. In the first volume of this series we have dealt more particularly with the deteriorating influence of fear, anxiety, anger, irritability, impatience, etc., and have explained how these and all other destructive emotions actually poison the secretions of the body.

In acute disease we cannot afford to add to the poisonous elements in the organism, because the danger of a fatal ending lies largely in the paralysis of vital centres by the morbid and poisonous products associated with inflammation. Everything depends upon the maintenance of the greatest possible inflow of vital force; and there is nothing that impedes the inflow, distribution and normal activity of the vital energies like fear. A person overcome by sudden fright is actually benumbed and paralysed, unable to think and act intelligently.

These truths may be expressed in another way. The victory of the healing forces in acute disease depends upon an abundant supply of the positive electromagnetic energies. In the first volume of this series we have learned that "health is positive, disease negative". The positive mental attitude of faith and equanimity creates positive electromagnetic energies in the body, thus infusing the system with increased vigour and healing power, while the negative, fearful and worrying attitude of mind creates in the system the negative conditions of weakness, lowered resistance and actual paralysis. In the chapter dealing with the effects of cold water treatment we learned that the electric currents created in the organism split up the molecules of water in the tissues into their component elements (hydrogen and oxygen), thus liberating large amounts of oxygen and ozone; and that these, in turn, support the processes of combustion and oxidation in the system and burn up waste and morbid matter. However, the electromagnetic forces are not only increased and intensified by positive foods, exercise, cold water treatment, air baths, etc., but also by the positive attitude of mind and will.

The positive mind and will are to the body what the magneto is to the motor car. As the electric sparks from the magneto ignite the petrol, thus generating the power which drives the machine, so the positive vibrations, generated by a confident and determined will, create in the body the positive electromagnetic currents which incite and stimulate all vital activities. Common experience teaches us that the concentration of the will on the thing to be accomplished greatly heightens and increases all physical, mental and moral powers. Therefore the victory in acute diseases is conditioned by absolute faith, confidence and serenity of mind on the part of the patient. The more he exercises these harmonizing and invigorating qualities of mind and soul, the more favourable are the conditions for victory of the millions of cells in their struggle against disease. The blood and nerve currents are less impeded and disturbed, and flow more normally. The local congestion is relieved, and this favours the natural course of the inflammatory processes. Therefore, instead of being overcome with fear and anxiety, as most people are in such circumstances, do not become alarmed, nor convey alarm to the millions of little cells battling in the inflamed parts. Speak to them like a commander addressing his troops: "We understand the laws of disease and cure, we know that these inflammatory and febrile symptoms are the result of nature's healing efforts, we have perfect confidence in her wisdom and the efficiency of her healing forces. This fever is merely a good house cleaning, a healing crisis. We are eliminating morbid matter and poisons which were endangering health and life. We rejoice over the purification and regeneration now taking place and benefiting the whole body. Fear not. Attend to your work quietly and serenely. Let us open ourselves wide to the inflow of life from the source of all life in the innermost parts of our being. The life in us is the life of God. We are strengthened and made whole by the divine life and power which animate the universe." The serenity of your mind, backed by absolute trust in the law and by the power of a strong will, infuses the cells and tissues with new life and vigour, enabling them to turn the "acute disease" into a beneficial, cleansing and healing crisis.

In the following we give a similar formula for treating chronic constipa-

35

tion. Say to the cells in the liver, the pancreas and the intestinal tract: "I am not going to force you any longer with drugs and enemas to do your duty. From now on you must do the work on your own initiative. Your secretions will become more abundant. Every day at — o'clock the bowels will move freely and easily." At the appointed time make the effort, whether you are successful or not, and do not resort to the enema until it becomes an absolute necessity. If you combine with the mental and physical effort a natural diet, cold sitz baths, massage and neurotherapy treatment, you will have need of the enema at increasingly longer intervals.

Be careful, however, not to employ your intelligence and your will power to suppress acute inflammatory and febrile processes and symptoms. This can be accomplished by the power of the will as well as by ice bags and poisonous drugs, and its effect would be to turn nature's acute cleansing efforts into chronic disease.

What has been said about the patient is true also of his friends and relatives. Disease is negative. The sick person is exceedingly sensitive to his surroundings. He is easily influenced by all depressing, discordant and jarring conditions. He catches the expressions of fear and anxiety in the looks, the words, the gestures and actions of his attendants, relatives and friends, and these intensify his own depression and gloomy forebodings. This applies especially to the influence exerted by the mother upon her ailing infant. There exists a most intimate sympathetic and telepathic connection between mother and child. The child is affected not only by the outward expression of the mother's fear and anxiety, but likewise by the hidden doubt and despair in the mother's mind and soul.

Usually the first thing that confronts me when I am called to the sickbed of a child is the frantic and almost hysterical mental condition of the mother, and to begin with I have to explain to her the destructive influence of her behaviour. I ask her: "Would you willingly give some deadly poison to your child?" "Certainly not," she says, to which I reply: "Do you realize that you are doing this very thing? That your fear and worry vibrations actually poison and paralyse the vital energies in the body of your child and most seriously interfere with nature's healing processes? Instead of helping the disease forces to destroy your child, assist the healing forces to save it by maintaining an attitude of absolute faith, serenity, calmness and cheerfulness. Then your looks, your voice, your touch will convey to your child the positive magnetic vibrations of health and strength. Your very presence will radiate healing power." Then I explain how faith, calmness and cheerfulness on her part will soothe and harmonize the discordant disease vibrations in the child's body. Herein lies the *modus operandi* or working basis of all successful mental and metaphysical treatment.

36

SECTION VII

HOW WE MET THE TEST

The case of my son, here described, shows in strong contrast the allopathic and natural methods of treatment, and proves that the simple, natural methods are fully sufficient to meet the demands of the most violent types of acute disease.

The accident happened on May 8th, 1914. As on my way home, I stepped from the street car to the sidewalk I saw a throng surrounding a man who was carrying in his arms the seemingly lifeless body of a boy. A lad ran up to me saying, "Doctor, that is Otto. He was run over by a motor car." I followed the man across the street into a drug store where he laid the boy on a bench. I knelt beside the unconscious form and examined for signs of life. The heart beat feebly; respiration was hardly perceptible. I had the boy carried to our home, which was nearby, and then called in several allopathic physicians of good repute, not with the idea of securing their advice as to treatment but on account of the legal aspects of the case. Other physicians living in the neighbourhood who knew the boy came in voluntarily and made friendly suggestions. The little patient remained unconscious for eighteen hours. Pulse and respiration at times were so feeble that the end seemed near. Enquiries brought out the facts concerning the accident. The boy had been playing with others on the sidewalk. He had run across the street to pick up a stray ball, when a car shot round the corner at a speed of over fifteen miles an hour, struck him and threw him to the ground. The machine ran over his prostrate body lengthwise without touching him. This was the fortunate part of the accident. Had he fallen in any other position he would have been crushed by the wheels. As it was he suffered no injuries other than those to the head caused by the blow from the machine on the back of the head and the violent thrust to the roadway.

Treatment. On examination we found a large swelling in the back of the head in the median line, at the junction of cerebrum and cerebellum. It was impossible to ascertain whether there was a fracture of the skull without removing the swelling. This was recommended by the other physicians, whose unanimous opinion it was that a blood clot had formed and that this, together with the shock, had brought about the unconscious condition. All recommended trephining — that is, cutting out a piece of skull in order to relieve internal pressure and provide drainage. As for medical treatment, they recommended stimulants, such as strychnine, digitalis, etc., to revive the dormant functions. The danger of giving stimulants in such cases is that in the reaction and depression following the

37

primary stimulation, the spark of life may be extinguished altogether. Instead of the drugs we applied cold salt water rubs and gently stimulating manipulative and magnetic treatment. As for trephining and drainage I feared that along with the debris of the injury there might pass away parts of the brain matter itself.

After a lapse of eighteen hours the patient partially revived. In this semiconscious condition he began to shout at the top of his voice, continually repeating three words, "Help, Murder, Police." During this hysterical or delirious stage, which lasted for several days without interruption by day or night, the visiting physicians recommended sedatives and hypnotics, such as bromides, morphine, hyoscine; also ice packs to the brain. We refrained from applying these brain and nerve paralysing agents, but continued the natural treatment — the wet packs (alternating body and leg packs), followed by cold ablutions to relieve the congestion in the brain, accompanied by relaxing and inhibitive manipulation of the brain and nerve centres, and soothing mental and magnetic treatment. During this stage the suggestive and magnetic treatment proved the most effective. Though violently noisy, the patient was in a trancelike condition. In order to reach his inner consciousness I had to give suggestions for relaxation, rest and peace in a loud tone of voice close to his ears. This would be followed by short periods of comparative rest and quiet. He would then respond to the soothing and relaxing effects of magnetic treatment.

On the ninth day the delirious condition developed into cerebral meningitis. The decomposing blood clot in the brain had by this time caused active inflammation accompanied by high temperature and the typical convulsions. Every twenty or thirty minutes the little body was bent backwards, only the back of the head and the heels touching the bed (opisthotonos). During this stage the doctors recommended ice packs to the brain and powerful antipyretics, such as opium, morphine, iodide of potassium, ergot, belladonna and bromide of potassium. They also urged that the spinal column be punctured, some of the fluid withdrawn and the meningococcal serum be injected. In place of drugs and serums we administered the ordinary natural treatment for inflammatory feverish diseases, consisting of fasting, wet packs followed by cold ablutions, manipulative and magnetic treatments. On the sixth day after its inception the inflammation in the brain subsided, the temperature fell to subnormal. On the following day we discovered that the boy was completely paralysed and totally blind. While he was in this condition the allopathic physicians recommended the use of powerful stimulants and plenty of nourishing food, i.e. strong soups, meat, soft boiled eggs, etc.

Six weeks after the beginning of the paralytic condition I tested his eyes one morning by waving a pencil before them. In answer to my question whether he could see anything he replied that he saw something moving in front of him. From that time on the eyesight as well as the paralytic condition showed continuous improvement. For several months both eyes had only central vision. The right eye improved much more quickly than the left. The sight of the left eye remained very defective for about nine months. Then he developed a vigorous case of chicken pox. After this had run its course in the natural way, the sight of the left eye improved greatly. The chicken pox had evidently acted as a true healing crisis. In another two months his sight and general condition had improved so remarkably that he could go to school and pursue his studies without much difficulty. Today he looks the proverbial "picture of health" and is indeed in splendid condition, both physically and mentally.

Taking it all in all, this was as difficult a case to manage as I have met with in my medical practice, but the simple natural treatment and manipulative adjustments proved sufficient to bring about the best possible results. In this case, as is true in many others, the greatest difficulty was to maintain an attitude of "masterful inactivity" — to be able to look on patiently and allow nature to have her way in and through the most serious reactions. As a rule the friends of the patient want "something done" continually and "regular medicine" complies with their demands. When nature pulls right, the doctor pulls left. Every serious symptom is counteracted. When the patient is in a comatose condition, the doctor tries to stimulate him into premature consciousness; when there is furious delirium, the brain and nervous system are paralysed into inactivity. Those not conversant with the philosophy of Natural Therapeutics fail to realize that nature, through all these varying conditions, is doing the best possible under the circumstances. Herein Natural Therapeutics differs most radically from the old school philosophy and practice. We believe that the wisdom which created this wonderful human body, and maintains it with marvellous regularity and precision through the complexities of vital processes, knows also how to cure it. The young man just released from medical college is of a different opinion. He believes that nature creates disease, but does not know how to cure; that it requires his superior wisdom to correct nature in her foolish ways, and that the medicines in his little poison satchel are able and necessary to correct nature's mistakes. If he has sufficient innate intelligence, not altogether perverted through the hypnotic influence of the schools and "authorities", he will know better after a few years of experimentation.

Comparison of the Methods of Allopathy and of Natural Therapeutics

In the following diagram I place on the one side the various kinds of medical treatment which the little patient would have received under the care of allopathic physicians, and on the other side the simple natural methods which were actually applied under the Natural Therapeutic system. Compare, think and decide for yourself which is the more rational.

Allopathic	Natural Therapeutics

First Stage

Unconscious, due to shock and actual injury to back brain

1. Trephining of the skull.	1. Neurotherapy, massage and magnetic treatment.
2. Stimulants and antiseptics, such as alcohol, strychnine, digitalis, urotropine.	2. Quick, cold water rubs at intervals of from thirty to sixty minutes.

Second Stage

Furious maniacal delirium

3. Ice caps to the brain.	3. Inhibitive neurotherapy.
4. Sedatives and hypnotics, such as morphine injections, hyoscine, chloroform, sulphonal, etc.	4. Wet packs and cold ablutions.
	5. Magnetic and mental treatment.
5. Forced feeding.	6. No food.

Third Stage

Cerebral inflammation (brain fever)

6. Antipyretics; opium, Hypodermic injections of morphine, iodide of potassium in large doses, ergot, belladonna, bromide of potassium.	7. The regular natural fever treatment given in all inflammatory feverish diseases.
7. Ice caps to the brain.	8. Absolute fasting; for thirst, diluted fruit juices.
8. Tapping the spinal column, withdrawing some of the spinal fluid, and injecting the meningococcal serum.	9. Wet packs, followed by cold ablutions, inhibitive and corrective manipulation.
9. Strong, nourishing food — milk and broth.	10. Mental and magnetic treatment.

Fourth Stage

Paralysis and blindness

10. Powerful stimulants and alteratives, such as strychnine, arsenic, etc.
11. Forced feeding.

11. Beginning of careful feeding.
12. Quick cold salt rubs; gently stimulating massage and Swedish movements.
13. Mental and magnetic treatment.
14. Correcting spinal and other bony lesions through neurotherapy.

Fifth Stage

Recuperative stage

12. Stimulants, alteratives, as in previous stage.

15. Continuation of natural treatment as in previous stage.

Just think what the poor little body would have had to endure and how it would have been saturated with the most virulent poisons on earth, had the patient undergone the allopathic treatment. Under which form of treatment would nature have the best chance to work out the problem in her own way — under the allopathic treatment, which would have counteracted every move she made, or under the natural treatment which did not check or counteract nature in any way but cooperated with her and assisted her to the best advantage at every stage of development? The outcome has surely justified the natural treatment in this case as in many thousands of others.

As a further illustration of the efficacy of the natural treatment at the onset or in the initial stages of acute disease, the following bit of personal experience may be interesting. Some twenty years ago, while I was studying natural methods of healing in Germany, I paid a visit to some friends in a neighbouring village. I found the housewife in great anxiety about her husband. She told me that the day before he had been taken with pneumonia, and that two physicians had pronounced the case a very serious one. In her imagination she saw herself already a widow, with a mortgaged farm and several small children on her hands. The patient was in a high fever, exhibiting all the symptoms of croupous pneumonia. Carried away by my enthusiasm for Nature Cure, I explained to the friends the difference between natural and medical treatment. They both insisted that I should give him the water treatment. After giving the general explanation as to ventilation and fasting, I prepared a couch for the whole sheet pack, placed the patient on it, and wrapped the wet sheets and a few dry blankets around his body. Within a few minutes he started to perspire profusely. He endured this about thirty minutes. Then I uncovered him and gave him, while standing in a washtub, a thorough, cold ablution. I put him to bed without drying, well covered with blankets. Immediately he developed a good after-perspiration. This continued for three-quarters of an hour. Next I gave him another cold ablution and thorough rubbing down with a rough towel. After this he was placed in a bed with fresh dry sheets, and allowed to rest.

This happened in the afternoon. Next morning about ten o'clock, I went to visit my patient and found him working in the meadow. The family doctor, who called early in the morning, was greatly surprised to find the bird had flown. I remember this incident well, because it was my first experience of treating a serious case of acute disease. Since that time I have aided in aborting many a serious acute case by similar treatment. This quick recovery was not the result of suppression but was brought about through vigorous elimination of pathogenic matter all over the cutaneous surface of the body, thereby relieving the pathogenic congestion in the lungs in a perfectly natural manner.

SECTION VIII

PRACTICAL APPLICATION OF NATURAL TREATMENT IN ANY GIVEN CASE OF COLD, INFLUENZA, PNEUMONIA OR OTHER ACUTE DISEASE

Upon the first appearance of symptoms — such as acute nasal catarrh, headache, backache, general malaise, fever, chills, sore throat, etc. — the patient should be put to bed, and active treatment begun at once. From the very beginning every precaution should be taken to conserve the energy of the patient, since acute feverish processes are very weakening. In nearly every case of the recent (1918) epidemic the heart was seriously affected, hence extreme caution must be used during convalescence not to overdo in any way. Work or exercise while they affect the heart unduly must be avoided, and should be resumed cautiously when the patient grows stronger.

1. **Enemas.** In case the bowels are not moving freely, a warm water enema should be given in order to remove accumulated faecal matter, and to prevent reabsorption and additional systemic poisoning. The water introduced into the bowels should be about body temperature and this may be determined nearly enough by testing with the elbow. If necessary, the enema may be repeated every two or three days, until the bowels move naturally. If the fasting be continued more than a week, the enemas may be given at longer intervals. In case the bowels have been in a constipated condition prior to the illness, an enema may precede the first pack.

2. **Packs.** The first application should be a whole body pack. The patient may at the same time be given a hot lemonade, without sugar, which will aid in bringing about free perspiration. The patient should remain in the pack as long as he can stand it — perhaps twenty to thirty minutes. The removal of the pack should be followed by a quick, cold water ablution, which may be taken in a bath tub, or while standing in a washtub in a warm room. The body should be quickly washed with cold water, from the feet up, and then dried with a rough towel. Or, in case of considerable fever the patient may return to bed without drying, in which case the moisture on the skin and the bed covering acts like a pack and produces further heat radiation, and sometimes a second perspiration. In the latter case, after another good sweat the body should again be sponged with cold water, and the patient allowed to rest. As already stated, in many cases the application of a whole body pack, with hot lemonade, followed by a good night's rest, is sufficient to break up a cold or fever and to ward off some serious disease. Sometimes it happens that notwithstanding early treatment the fever continues and develops into some serious disease, but these patients are often of low vitality and usually have been suffering from chronic ailments. This goes to prove our claim that one of the predisposing conditions to infectious diseases, as well as feverish disease of any kind, is low vitality.([1])

If the fever persists after the first whole body pack, and the patient be

([1])
There appears to be something somewhat paradoxical or contradictory in what Lindlahr has to say about the genesis of acute conditions. While on the one hand he here maintains that lowered vitality is a predisposing cause of infectious and feverish diseases, on the other hand he states elsewhere that healing crises and acute reactions are generally a manifestation of there being sufficient vitality and energy to produce a crisis. If one must choose, this latter point of view would seem to be the more convincing and more consistent with the idea that the body does not generally undertake a serious acute reaction unless it has the strength to carry it through. Moreover, it must be remembered that the heavy colds and fevers which occur in winter and which mostly involve the respiratory apparatus must largely be due to a lowering of elimination through the skin, thus throwing an additional burden on the other eliminative organs, especially the respiratory tract and kidneys. This produces a rise in toxicity in the body and it is in cases of this kind that one could hope for a complete and quick cure by the application of the whole body pack.

not too weak, the application may be repeated. If the symptoms become more distressing, and the patient grows weaker and more sensitive to handling, partial packs must be applied instead of the whole body pack. Those best suited are the throat, Scotch (or shoulder) pack, and the trunk or leg packs.

3. **Alternating Packs.** If the fever runs steadily at high temperature the packs should be applied continuously, or with brief intermissions. It is best to alternate the body, throat, shoulder and leg packs, and apply one or two at a time in order to equalize the circulation and to draw the blood away from the congested parts. For instance, at one time apply the throat and leg packs, next throat and trunk packs, another time shoulder and leg packs. If the fever remains high, and the symptoms distressing, all these may be applied at one time.

4. **Renewal of the Packs.** The packs should be removed when they become hot and dry, because in that case they increase the inner heat instead of diminishing it. If the patient develops chills and the packs remain cold, hot water bottles or hot bricks wrapped in flannel may be applied outside the packs in order to bring about reaction and, if possible, perspiration.

5. **Chills.** The impression prevails that cold water applications are not to be given in case of chills. This, however, is a mistake. The thermometer will show that the chills are accompanied by high temperature within the body. It is the inner heat and congestion which causes the outer chill. Anything that will relieve this will break the chill, and the best applications to draw the blood from the interior into the surface are the cold, wet packs, if necessary reinforced for a time by hot water bottles.

6. **After the pack has been removed,** the body must immediately be thoroughly rubbed down with cold water in order to remove the systemic poisons drawn to the surface. That the wet packs actually promote the elimination of morbid matter through the skin is proved by the yellow and brown discolouration of the wet bandages and by their offensive odour.

7. **In case of great weakness,** care must be taken not to expose the body unduly. It should be uncovered, sponged, dried, and re-covered quickly, part by part. In order to save the vitality of the patient, only those parts of the body covered by the packs need be washed off with cold water. If the patient feels weak and chilly after the application, from twenty to sixty minutes may be allowed to elapse before the next pack is applied.

8. **Care must be taken not to reduce the temperature too rapidly;** all that is necessary is to keep it below the danger point. It must be remembered that it is possible to suppress inflammation and fever by the excessive application of cold water, as well as by ice and drugs.

9. **Danger Point.** The question will be asked, "What constitutes the danger point?" Since we look upon inflammation and fever as constructive in nature, not destructive, we do not fear temperature as does the "old school" physician and laity. Furthermore, in one case life may be in danger at 102° or 103°F., while in another, 106° or 107° may be below the danger point. We should be actuated in the frequency of cold water applications by the urgency of the symptoms rather than by the height of the temperature. In pneumonia, for instance, the following are serious symptoms, requiring more careful and persistent treatment: increasing congestion in the lungs, symptoms of consolidation, laboured breathing, bloody sputum and delirium. Extreme weakness and subnormal temperature require packs warmed by hot water bottles, gentle stimulation by manipulative treatment, mild stimulants in the form of fruit juices, hot lemonade sweetened with a little brown sugar or honey, etc. Hot water bottles or other hot applications applied directly to the inflamed parts, as well as the use of ice, in the treatment of inflammation and fever, are positively dangerous. The former increase the heat instead of diminishing it; the ice bags or packs chill the parts and suppress the inflammatory processes. Both practices may result in the formation of abscesses and in serious, chronic after-effects. In a general way we may say that it is sufficient to lower the temperature one or two degrees below the high level peculiar to the disease.

10. **As the temperature declines** during the stages of absorption and reconstruction the packs and ablutions may be applied at longer intervals. When the temperature sinks to near the normal two or three packs and ablutions may be applied at longer intervals. When the temperature sinks to near the normal, two or three packs in twenty-four hours may be sufficient to bring about complete absorption of the morbid waste — the debris of the battle — and to promote elimination through the skin, bowels, kidneys and lungs.

11. **Excessive pain in the head** should not be treated by local wet packs. This would have a tendency to draw blood to the head, and cause greater congestion. The packs applied to the body will draw the blood from the head and the spinal cord, and thus relieve the headache and backache. However, the forehead, the temples and face may be bathed with cold water at frequent intervals, without drying. The evaporation of the cold water will be cooling and refreshing.

12. **In cases of mild fever** and low temperature it may be fully sufficient to take at intervals a cold ablution, and lie down under the bed covers without drying. The cool moisture on the body and the warm bed covering will have practically the same effect as a full body pack. If this produces perspiration, so much the better; it should be followed by

another cold ablution. In many instances this simple treatment will be found to be sufficient to abort an oncoming fever, and to ward off serious disease.

13. **Cold Water Treatment during Menstruation.** There should be no fear of applying cold water treatment during menstruation when high fever rages in the body. I have found in many instances that this has not a suppressive effect upon the flow. To delay the water treatment might allow the inflammatory processes to become so destructive as to make it impossible to control them. The water treatment at best reduces the temperature only a few degrees, which cannot interfere with the menstrual process but rather allows it to run a more normal course.

14. **The number of wet wrappings** and of dry coverings is governed by the amount of heat in the body, the room temperature and the reactionary powers of the patient. The higher the body temperature, the colder the room and the better the vitality of the patient, the more wet bandages may be wrapped around the body. The throat will warm up the bandages quicker than the trunk, and the trunk quicker than the legs. This is due to the fact that large streams of hot, pure blood pour continually through the throat, near the surface, and because the trunk radiates more heat than the lower extremities. In high fever the throat may react to four, five or six wet wrappings, the body to three or four, while one or two may be sufficient for the lower extremities or arms. In very violent fever the dry covering may be omitted entirely, and instead of changing the packs at frequent intervals, which may be very annoying and weakening to the patient, the wet bandages may be moistened by pouring cold water over them.

Whenever cold water treatment is applied to a patient in bed, the mattress should be covered by a rubber or oilcloth sheet. Under no circumstances should the wet bandages be covered by rubber or oilcloth wrappings. This would have a tendency to prevent heat radiation and to retain the poisonous exhalations of the body.

15. **Cleansing of the Packs.** When treating high and persistent fever, two or three complete pack outfits should be at hand. As soon as one is removed from the body the different wrappings should be thoroughly washed — particularly the wet bandages — and allowed to dry in the open air. There is no better disinfectant and germ killer than air and light.

16. **Manipulative Treatment.** The importance of neurotherapy treatment for the prevention as well as the cure of inflammatory febrile diseases has been very evident in the influenza and pneumonia cases treated by us during the 1918 epidemic. Those of our workers and patients who showed premonitory or, in several cases, well advanced symptoms recuperated immediately after receiving thorough manipulative treatment.

In all cases of advanced stages of influenza and pneumonia the manipulative work brought great relief, and facilitated and hastened the normal development of the inflammatory processes. It was very instructive to observe that those who succumbed to the infection were affected primarily, and most seriously throughout the course of the disease, in those parts and organs that were or had been affected by chronic ailments, and which therefore offered least resistance to infection and to the progress of the disease. One of these patients, for instance, suffered from the beginning and all through the attack with the most excruciating backache, which at one time had been a serious chronic affection. Another, who several years ago had incipient tuberculosis, was affected most seriously in the lungs, in the form of a violent attack of pneumonia. Still another, who for many years had suffered from chronic rheumatism and had been cured by natural treatment, was tortured during the attack of influenza by aches and pains all over the body, particularly in the joints. In many instances these sufferers exhibited a strained and painful condition of the muscular structures on either the left or the right side of the neck and in the upper region of the back. In several cases the tension was so pronounced that it drew the head over to the affected side. This condition was promptly relieved by administering tonic manipulative treatment, followed by relaxing movements, and completed with thorough inhibition along the course of the hypersensitive nerves. Every case, in accord with its predominating symptoms, exhibited certain specific lesions which were corrected by neurotherapy treatment. By means of manipulative treatment we attain all the good results that are attributed to drug treatment, without its destructive side- and after-effects.

The most important of the therapeutic effects of manipulative treatment are: (1) stimulating effects upon the circulation of the vital fluids and nerve currents, locally or generally; (2) relaxation and inhibition of hyperactive or acute and subacute inflammatory processes; (3) the softening and relaxation of tense and contracted muscles, ligaments and other connective tissues; (4) the loosening of stiffened spinal and other joints; (5) the correction of luxations, subluxations and dislocations of spinal vertebrae and of other bony structures.

SECTION IX

SUMMARY

Of Natural Methods in the Treatment of Acute Diseases

I. Fresh Air

A plentiful supply of pure air in the sick room.
Frequent exposure of the nude body to air and sunlight.
Patient must not be kept too warm.
Rest and relaxation are important.

II. Fasting

In acute febrile conditions and during healing crises no food whatever.
Only enough water to quench thirst, preferably mixed with acid fruit juices.
In diseases affecting the digestive organs fasting must be prolonged several days beyond the cessation of febrile symptoms.
Great care must be observed when breaking fast.

III. Water Treatment

Wet packs and cooling sprays or sponge baths whenever temperature rises.
Fever and inflammation must not be *suppressed* by excessive cold water applications, but kept below the danger point.
Neither ice nor hot applications should be used.
Wet packs followed by cold ablutions for elimination of systemic poisons.
Separate compresses over seat of inflammation, also at nape of neck.
Kind and duration of pack to be determined by condition of patient and object to be attained.
Injections of tepid water to relieve constipation when necessary.

IV. Medicaments

No poisonous drugs, no medicines or applications which may check or suppress the feverish inflammatory processes.
Homoeopathic medicines and herb decoctions when indicated. (Chap. XXV, Vol. I.)

48

V. Manipulative Treatment

Neurotherapy, massage or magnetic treatment when indicated and available.

VI. Mental Attitude

Courage, serenity and presence of mind important factors.

Fear and anxiety intensify disease conditions, poison the secretions of the body and inhibit the action of the healing forces.

Do not suppress acute inflammatory and feverish processes by the power of the will.

The right mental and emotional attitude of relatives and friends exerts a powerful influence upon the patient.

The methods described in the preceding sections should be used in the treatment of the following as well as all other acute febrile diseases.

Acute Diseases

Ague
Appendicitis
Asiatic cholera
Asthma
Boils
Bright's disease
Bronchitis
Bubonic plague
Burns and scalds, *see also* First Aid
Carbuncles
Chicken pox
Cholera infantum
Cholera morbus
Colds
Colic
Congestion of kidneys
Congestion of liver
Coughs
Convulsions, *see also* First Aid
Croup
Cystitis

Delirium tremens, *see also* First Aid
Diarrhoea or purging
Diphtheria
Dysentery
Endocarditis, acute
Enteritis, acute
Erysipelas
Eyes, inflammation of all kinds
Furuncles (boils)
Gastritis
German measles
Glaucoma
Gout, acute
Gonorrhoea
Grippe
Haemorrhages, *see also* First Aid
Hay fever
Heat prostration, *see also* First Aid
Hives

Hydrophobia
Hysteria, *see also* First Aid
Influenza
Insect bites, *see also* First Aid
Intestinal toxaemia or ptomaine poisoning
Iritis (Inflammation of the iris)
Ivy poisoning, *see also* First Aid
Jaundice
Laryngitis
Lumbago
Lungs, all acute diseases of
Malarial fever
Mastoiditis
Measles
Meningitis, cerebral and cerebro-spinal

Mental diseases, all
 kinds
Mouth breathing
Mumps
Nephritis, acute
Orchitis
 (inflammation of
 testes)
Otitis (inflammation
 of middle ear)
Pericarditis
Phlebitis
 (inflammation of
 veins)
Pink eye (disease of
 conjunctiva)
Pleurisy

Polypus
Pneumonia, all forms
Purulent
 conjunctivitis
Quinsy
Renal hyperaemia
Rheumatism, acute
 articular
Rheumatism, acute
 sciatic
Rheumatism, acute
 gonorrhoeal
Rhinitis
Scarlet fever
Smallpox
Sunstroke, *see also*
 First Aid

Syphilis
Tetanus (lockjaw)
Tonsillitis
Toothache
Tuberculosis of the
 lungs, acute
Typhoid fever
Typhus fever (spotted
 fever
Uraemia
Vaccination, effects of
Varioloid
Whooping cough
Winter cholera
Yellow fever

PART III

TREATMENT OF CHRONIC DISEASES

INTRODUCTION

Acute diseases represent nature's efforts to purify and regenerate the human organism by means of inflammatory feverish processes, while in the chronic condition the system is not capable of arousing itself to such acute reactions. It must be prepared to become aroused through natural methods of living and treatment, as has been explained in Vol. I.

Natural treatment of acute diseases tends to relieve inner congestion, to facilitate the radiation of heat and elimination of morbid matter and systemic poisons from the body. In this way it eases and palliates the feverish processes and keeps them below the danger point without in any way checking or suppressing them. While our methods of treating acute diseases have a sedative effect, our treatment of chronic diseases is calculated to stimulate, that is, to arouse the sluggish organism to greater activity in order to produce the acute reaction or healing crisis. If the unity of disease, as demonstrated in Vol. I, be a fact in nature, it must be possible to treat all chronic as well as all acute diseases by uniform methods, and the natural methods must correspond to the primary causes of disease.

These natural methods may be divided into two groups: (a) those which the patient can apply himself, provided he has been properly instructed in their correct selection, combination and application; (b) those which must be applied by or under the direction of a competent Natural Therapeutic physician.

To the first group belong diet, fasting, bathing and other water applications, correct breathing, general physical exercise, psychological exercise, corrective gymnastics, air and sun baths, mental therapeutics. To the second group belong special applications of the methods mentioned under the first group, and in addition to these, hydrotherapy, Swedish movements, neurotherapy, orificial dilation, medical treatment in the form of homoeopathic remedies, non-poisonous herb extracts, and, most important of all, the right management of healing crises which develop under the natural treatment of chronic diseases.

The treatment outlined in the following sections applies to all forms of disease listed previously after they have entered upon the chronic stages. In addition to these, we may classify as chronic diseases the following:

Abscesses of liver
Acne
Adenoids
Addison's disease
Amyloid kidney (a
  form of Bright's
  disease)
Anaemia (primary
  and secondary)
Aneurysm
Angina pectoris
Apoplexy
Arteriosclerosis
Arthritis deformans
Atrophy of bones
Barber's itch
Bed wetting
Caculi (stones, all
  kinds)
Carcinoma (cancer)
Caries of the bones
Chorea
Cirrhosis of liver
Comedones
  (blackheads)
Constipation
Congenital
  malformation of hip
  joint
Dandruff
Debility
Deformity of spine or
  other bony
  structures

Diabetes (functional
  or organic)
Dropsy
Dyspepsia
Eczema, all kinds
Emphysema of the
  lungs
Enlarged prostate
Enteritis
Epilepsy
Erysipelas
Fatty degeneration of
  liver
Fatty degeneration of
  heart
Goitre
Gall-stones
Gastric and duodenal
  ulcers
Heart disease (all
  kinds)
Haemorrhoids (piles)
Hernia (rupture)
Herpes (shingles)
Hoarseness
Hookworm
Hydrothorax
Hyperaemia of liver
Hypochondria
Impotence
Impetigo (chafing)
Infantile paralysis
Inflammation of
  bones (periostitis,

osteomylitis)
Insanity, many forms
Insomnia
Interstitial nephritis
Leukaemia
Locomotor ataxia
Lungs, all diseases of
Lupus
Masturbation
Necrosis of bones
Nephritis, chronic
  (Bright's disease)
Nervous debility
Neuralgia
Neuritis
Night losses
Obesity
Oedema of the lungs
Paralysis of all kinds
Passive hyperaemia
Prolapsus of the
  rectum
Prostatitis
Pseudo-angina
  pectoris
Rectal diseases
Rachitis
Rickets (rachitis)
Rheumatism, all
  forms
Sarcoma
Scabies
Scrofula
Sleeping sickness

52

Suprarenal calculus	Tuberculae enteritis	Varicose veins
Tapeworm	Tumours, all kinds	Worms, all kinds
Trichina spiralis	Ulcers, chronic	Writer's cramp
Tinea tricophytina (ringworm)	Varicocele	Wry neck

SECTION X

IMPORTANCE OF NATURAL DIET

The ordinary meat-potato-white bread-coffee and pie diet customary in the American home, restaurant or hotel is bound to create, sooner or later, disease conditions in the system. This combination of foods creates in the body large amounts of poisonous acids, alkaloids and ptomaines, and does not contain enough of the alkaline mineral elements on which depend the purification of the system from morbid matter and poisons.

The foods which are generally considered most nutritious — meat, eggs, dried peas, beans, lentils and cereals — are the greatest danger foods because they are exceedingly rich in acid-producing starches, fats and proteins, and are deficient in acid binding and eliminating alkaline elements. These purifying elements can be secured in sufficient amounts only in fruits and vegetables which run low in starches, fats and proteins, but contain large amounts of the mineral salts of iron, lime, potassium, sodium, magnesium and silicon. Among the thousands of young people reared in this country whom I have had the occasion to examine by diagnosis from the iris, I have found very few who did not suffer to some extent from digestive troubles. It is a fact that the American people, notwithstanding all the natural advantages which they enjoy, suffer more from indigestion, malassimilation, and from the multitude of diseases growing out of these primary causes, than any other people on earth. The reason for this is that from the cradle up all the laws and principles governing right eating and drinking are continually violated. The child is allowed to eat and drink what it pleases, and since indulgence in unnatural food and drink creates abnormal appetite, he soons learns to crave those things which are most detrimental to health. As he becomes accustomed to meats, strong spices and condiments, pastry, coffee and tea, he loses all relish for fruits and vegetables, especially the latter. Piping hot soups and meats are washed down with ice water and mixed with ice cream, which only too often is a mixture of skimmed milk, glue, chemical colouring and artificial flavouring compounds. These unwholesome food combinations are supplemented by large quantities of white sugar and adulterated candies, all of which are very injurious to the system. Is it any wonder that the prosperous and well fed American people suffer almost universally from early decay of the teeth, digestive troubles, chronic constipation, haemorrhoids, nervous dyspepsia, appendicitis, rheumatism, cancer, tuberculosis and a host of other diseases directly caused by food and drink poisoning?

Among the peasantry of European countries the meaning of the words "dyspepsia" and "dentist" is hardly known. A dentist can make a living only in the largest cities; the country people live closer to nature than our overfed but mineral-starved Americans. In Europe, on account of the high cost of flesh foods, meat is used very sparingly. White sugar, coffee, tea and pastries are holiday luxuries. Ice water is not found even in the homes of the wealthiest people nor in the best hotels. The peasantry and middle-class people in northern European countries live largely on whole grain bread, potatoes, vegetables and dairy products. When they come to this country they are the picture of health and robust strength, but they eagerly adopt American customs of living, believing that meat, white bread and coffee three times a day constitute "high living". The natural result is that in a few years most of them lose their red cheeks and become dyspeptic and nervous like their new compatriots. I have frequently noticed the gradual lowering of the health standard in descendants of immigrants. In many families you will find the grandfather and grandmother who came from the "old sod" hale and hearty in their old age; the second generation, at middle age, dyspeptic and nervous; and the grandchildren anaemic, wearing glasses at a tender age and affected by all sorts of chronic ailments. Statistics show that in our largest cities, where surroundings and habits of living are most unnatural, the fourth city-bred generation dies out unless regenerated by the inflow of fresh, healthy blood of immigrants from northern Europe, and of the sturdy young people who crowd in from the farming communities to be swallowed up by the insatiable maw of the great city.(¹)

1. **Proteins.** The belief prevails that in order to make rich blood one must eat large amounts of meat and eggs. The science of natural dietetics, however, teaches that the richness of the blood depends not so much

(¹)
It is doubtful whether the robust peasant healthiness to which Lindlahr refers is now found to the same extent in the countries of Western Europe as it was in his day. The use of processed, refined and mass produced foods has spread to the country so that country people grow and prepare their own food less than they formerly did. Also it is probable that the quality and food value of much of the produce has declined under modern methods of cultivation.

on sugars, fats and proteins, as on the positive mineral elements. Almost any ordinary food mixture will provide enough of the former elements of nutrition, but it is much more difficult to provide sufficient amounts of the mineral salts. In order to feed the blood with all the elements it needs in the right proportions and in that way to maintain it in a normal healthy condition, one half of the diet should consist of fruits and vegetables, and the other half should be made up of starches, sugars, fats and proteins. Meats, if used at all, should be eaten very sparingly. Multitudes of enthusiastic vegetarians have proved that it is better to do without meat altogether. Eggs also should be used sparingly, at an average of not more than four a week.

2. **Coffee and Tea.** Coffee and tea have no place in the natural diet. They contain powerful nerve stimulants. I believe that their influence on the system, in the long run, is worse than that of weak alcoholic drinks.

3. **White Flour.** White bread and pastry should be avoided altogether or used very sparingly. Bread and other cereal products should be prepared from whole grain only. Nothing should be taken away from the grain in the milling process. As a result of the agitation against white flour by Nature Cure people, Graham bread, entire wheat health breads and whole grain cereal foods are coming more and more into favour with the public. In this respect the stringent war regulations which by many were considered a great hardship were in reality a blessing in disguise. In order to comply with the popular demand for white flour, the hulls and life germs containing the mineral salts, vitamins and valuable ferments, as well as some of the gluten which is equal in nutritious value to the high priced steak, are "refined" out of the flour and go into the bran. Our domestic animals wax fat and strong on the bran and life germs (shorts), while their masters, living on impoverished white flour products, grow constipated, dyspeptic and nervous. The excessive use of meat, white bread, coffee and white sugar is undoubtedly the most common cause of constipation and the resulting autointoxication.

4. **Vinegar and Condiments Injurious.** Green vegetables are most beneficial when eaten raw with a dressing of lemon juice and olive oil. Avoid the use of vinegar. It is a product of fermentation and a powerful preservative which retards digestion as well as fermentation, both processes being very much the same in character. Lemon juice, being a live vegetable product, rich in vitamins, promotes digestion. Do not use pepper, salt or sugar on fruits and vegetables at the table. They may be used very sparingly in cooking. Strong spices and condiments are more or less irritating to the mucous linings of the intestinal tract. They gradually benumb the nerves of taste. At first they stimulate the diges-

tive organs, but, like all other stimulants, produce in time weakness and atrophy. Fruits and vegetables are rich in all the mineral salts in the live, organic form, and therefore the addition of inorganic mineral table salt is not only superfluous but positively harmful.([1])

The juicy fruits and green leafy vegetables are not improved by cooking. The only foods which are made more digestible by cooking are grains, rice, potatoes and the legumes. Here cooking serves to break up and separate the hard starch granules and to make them more pervious to penetration by the digestive juices.

5. **How to Cook Vegetables — Steaming.** After the vegetables are thoroughly washed and prepared place them in a cooking vessel, adding only enough boiling water to keep them from burning, cover the vessel closely with the lid, and let them steam slowly in their own juices. The leafy vegetables (spinach, Swiss chard, beet tops, etc.) contain enough water for their own steaming. If placed in a vessel over a slow fire enough juice will gather in a few moments to prevent burning. Cook all vegetables only as long as is required to make them soft enough for easy mastication. Do not throw away a drop of the water in which vegetables have thus been cooked. Use whatever is left for the making of soups and sauces.

The following methods of cooking the savoury vegetables are highly recommended, as they leave in the vegetable after cooking all the tenderness and delicacy of flavour of the raw article.

(a) *Cabbage.* Have the water slightly salted and actively boiling when ready to toss in the finely chopped cabbage. This stops the boiling. Watch carefully for the first signs of bubbling again and immediately turn down the flame or set the vessel where the contents cannot possibly boil. The vessel must not be covered. The cabbage will gradually settle to the bottom and appear as if not cooking, but will be thoroughly done in about twenty-five minutes if the vegetable is fresh. When done it should be instantly removed from the fire, drained and served with butter and white sauce. The flavour is in the volatile oil within the cells, and this oil is thrown off into the air if the cabbage is cooked above the boiling point. Boiling also toughens the woody fibre. If cooked as above there will be no odour and the cabbage will have the same green and white colour as before cooking.

(b) *Cauliflower* should be cooked in the same manner, first separating the flowerets.

([1])
Vinegar (acetic acid) is known to induce anaemia, weak heart, haemorrhages, wasting and debility. Fortunately, with Cider Vinegar other by-products help to counter the acetic acid, and the easily assimilated potassium helps to replace that which is boiled out of vegetables in our society and thrown away. About 50 percent of patients are definitely better for taking it.

(c) *Onions* should be cooked in the same manner except that they may be allowed to boil gently.

(d) *Turnips* and vegetables of a like nature, such as rutabaga and kohlrabi, should be cut in small cubes and cooked in much the same manner, uncovered, in boiling, slightly salted water. These vegetables may be allowed to boil very gently until transparent, and should be removed and drained as soon as the pieces can be pierced with a fork. They should retain their natural colour and flavour. Serve with butter or white sauce. Cooked in this manner, below the boiling point, almost none of the mineral salts of the vegetables are leached into the water, which has, therefore, little value, but it may be used as a foundation for soups.

If the vegetables, as is usual, are boiled hard and for a long time in a large quantity of water, then drained or, what is worse still, pressed out, they have lost their nutritive and medicinal value. The mineral salts have vanished down the sink pipes, the remains are insipid and indigestible and have to be soaked in soup stock and seasoned with strong condiments and spices to make them at all palatable. The natural flavours of the vegetables are the most delicious.

6. In order to ensure the full benefits of mouth digestion, the starchy foods should be thoroughly masticated and mixed with saliva. The drinking water must be of natural temperature as it comes from well or hydrant. Food and drink should never be taken hot or icy cold. This foolish habit will, in time, ruin the best stomach and the finest set of teeth. Do not eat when overtired or emotionally excited. Do not eat the heavy meal of the day between working hours. These are just a few of the more important rules which, if strictly followed, will soon improve the digestion and ensure better elimination and freer movement of the bowels.

In many instances, however, even the best combination of food and drink will not overcome indigestion and malnutrition, because, through long continued abuse, the digestive organs have become so diseased and atrophied that they cannot properly digest and assimilate even the best of food materials. In such cases the digestive organs must be made more active and alive by the natural methods of sanatorium treatment, such as hydrotherapy, massage, neurotherapy, deep breathing, curative exercises, Swedish movements, air and sun baths, homoeopathic remedies and last but not least, by the right mental and emotional attitude.

7. **A General Vegetarian Regimen. Sample Menus.** Breakfast should consist of acid and subacid fruits only; or berries only; or raw vegetable relishes only; or of a mixture of both fruits and relishes — for those who have a good digestion. If, however, for some reason it is better to take the raw food meal at noon or in the evening, the daily regimen must be adjusted accordingly. For instance, if the raw food is taken at noon, the

luncheon foods may be taken in the morning. I find this advisable in cases where people leave early in the morning for work and would otherwise become hungry and faint before noon. In our sanatorium regimen we find the raw breakfast most beneficial.

Breakfast No. 1. Raw acid and subacid fruits, such as orange, grapefruit, apple, grapes, berries, peaches, pears, apricots, cherries, plums, watermelon, cantaloup, etc.

Breakfast No. 2. Raw vegetables relishes or a vegetable salad.

Breakfast No. 3. Raw fruit, in combination with stewed prunes, apple sauce, rhubarb, baked apple, etc.

Luncheon is served at noontime and consists of cereal foods, health bread, rye crisp with butter, cottage cheese, peanut butter or honey. To balance the starchy and protein food we serve vegetable relishes, vegetable salads and sweet alkaline fruits such as figs, dates or raisins. This does not mean that many of these foods should be taken at the same time; on the contrary, the more limited the variety representing the various groups, the better is the effect on the system. The weaker the digestive organs, the more care must be taken in the selection and combination of foods. In all chronic disease it is of great importance to limit the intake of starchy foods to a minimum, therefore no more than one kind should be taken at a meal. For instance, if bread or rye crisp is taken, potatoes and cereal should be excluded, and vice versa.([1])

Luncheon No. 1. Steamed wheat with honey and milk; celery or lettuce salad.

Luncheon No. 2. Health bread or crisp with butter or peanut butter; sliced tomatoes or cucumbers; radishes or young onions.

Luncheon No. 3. Shredded wheat biscuit, honey, milk; berries, figs or dates.

Luncheon No. 4. Baked potato, a vegetable salad, stewed fruit, raisins, figs or dates.

Luncheon No. 5. A raw vegetable relish, a cooked vegetable, baked or boiled potato, alkaline fruits, berries, nuts.

Luncheon No. 6. Vegetable salad, soft boiled or poached eggs, health bread or rye crisp, raw or stewed fruit or berries.

Nuts, figs, dates or raisins may be taken in moderate quantities with any luncheon combination.

Dinner No. 1. *Relish* — cucumbers; *Salad* — raw carrot salad; *Veg-*

([1])
Figs, dates and raisins are splendid foods but are now often so processed as to be harmful. Dates, for example, are often washed in a detergent, then treated with an anti-mould, anti-rotting liquid and then finally put in a liquid to give them a shiny, luscious appearance. The more you pay for such things the less healthy they are to eat.

etables — beets and greens, new peas, steamed potatoes; *Dessert* — strawberries.

Dinner No. 2. *Relish* — celery, ripe olives; *Salad* — pineapple salad; *Vegetables* — buttered cabbage, macaroni and tomatoes; *Dessert* — raisins.

Dinner No. 3. *Relish* — radishes, ripe olives; *Salad* — fruit salad; *Vegetables* — vegetable roast and brown gravy, spinach, mashed potatoes; *Dessert* — ice cream.

Dinner No. 4. *Relish* — raw asparagus or cauliflower; *Salad* — tomato salad; *Soup* — vegetable soup; *Vegetables* — carrots and peas, baked potatoes; *Dessert* — fruit, tapioca and cream.

Dinner No. 5. *Relish* — green onions; *Salad* — Waldorf Astoria; *Vegetables* — asparagus, vegetable stew, baked potatoes; *Dessert* — rhubarb puddings.

8. Raw Food Diet. Sample Menus. A. This diet consists of raw foods, fruits, berries and juicy leafy vegetables. Vegetables may be taken with dressing of lime or lemon juice and olive or other vegetable oil. No starchy foods or vegetables such as bananas, potatoes or cereals must be included. **B.** This diet takes in all fruits, berries, vegetables, nuts and cereals that can be relished in the raw state. It also includes all raw dairy products, honey and raw or soft boiled eggs. The foods may be selected and combined for the various meals according to individual taste and requirements.

Breakfast No. 1. Vegetable relishes or vegetable salads.

Breakfast No. 2. One or two kinds of raw fruits or berries with or without milk or cream.

Luncheon No. 1. Dates, figs, raisins or currants with crushed cereals or "vitamine" or nuts.

Luncheon No. 2. Bananas, apples, nuts or "vitamine" with milk or honey.

Luncheon No. 3. Combination salad of grated beets or carrots, sweet corn, asparagus or cauliflower; nuts or bananas with any kind of vegetable salad.

To any of these may be added milk, buttermilk, sumik, "vitamine", raw eggs or honey.

"Vitamine". This is a very nutritious and palatable combination of cereals, nuts, and raisins or currants. On a hand grain mill crush wheat and rye, mix one pound of this with a quarter pound of crushed nuts or whole pine nuts. To this mixture add one quarter pound of seedless raisins or currents. One may also add *ad libitum* chopped dates, figs or prunes. It is best not to mix the "vitamine" with milk or cream, as this would tend to prevent thorough mastication. Milk or other drink may be taken separately as required.

9. Dry Diet. Our dry diet is a modification of the Schroth Cure much in vogue in European sanitoria. Under the latter regimen patients are fed on dry toasted bread with moderate doses of light wine. No other drink is given until excessive thirst forces it. The diet is accompanied by eliminative hydropathic applications such as wet packs, bed sweat baths, etc. While this has proved very effective in the treatment of the most stubborn chronic diseases, the fruit diet is to be preferred for the following reasons: The dry diet promotes elimination because it draws the fluids from the tissues and with these the pathogenic materials encumbering the system. But why use for this purpose food like toasted bread, when the large amount of starches and proteins it contains tend to create more pathogenic materials? Why not use in its place dried fruits which are themselves rich in the eliminative mineral elements and which serve as well the purpose of dehydrating the tissues? The thickening of the blood and lymph streams with pathogenic materials has a depressing effect upon brain and heart. This undesirable condition Scroth tried to overcome by giving light wine, but alcoholic stimulation is always followed by corresponding depression and therefore nothing can be gained by it. The dry diet, for obvious reasons, usually produces profuse mucoid elimination all through the system. It frequently hastens the development of healing crises. As a rule patients endure the dry food diet from one to two or three days only. It should then be followed by a raw food regimen.

10. **Milk Diet.** Milk is the only perfect, complete or standard food combination in nature. This is evident from the fact that it contains all the elements of nutrition which the newborn infant body needs, not only for its vital activities but also for the building of its rapidly multiplying cells and tissues. It is for this reason that Dr. Lahmann, one of the pioneers of Nature Cure, selected the chemical composition of milk as a standard, or yard stick, by which to measure all other normal food combinations. The analysis of cow's milk and human milk* shows that there is very little difference between the two. As a matter of fact, cow's milk is to be preferred as a standard because it contains more positive mineral elements than human milk. This is due to the fact that cattle, especially those on pasture, consume more of natural foods fresh from the soil and rich in mineral salts. This is the reason why calves do not suffer from rachitic diseases as do infants fed by anaemic, mineral-starved mothers.

This praise of milk as natural food frequently provokes the question, why then not live on milk entirely? To this I reply that while milk is the natural food for the newborn and growing infant it is not so well adapted

---

*See page 313 for Quantitative and Qualitative Analysis of Milk.

to the adult. The digestive apparatus of the infant is especially adapted to the digestion of milk, while that of the adult requires more solid and bulky food. The advent of the teeth indicates that nature intends to change from fluid to solid food. The liver is especially concerned in the digestion of milk. This organ is comparatively three times larger in the infant than in the adult. The digestive juice of the stomach in the infant is alkaline; it is acid in the adult. Therefore milk in the stomach of the infant curds; in the stomach of the adult it curdles. The stomach and upper parts of the intestines in the infant form almost a straight tube, and the contents of the former are easily discharged, while in the deep curvature of the adult stomach the milk easily stagnates. The more relaxed and atrophic the stomach, the worse for the digestion and discharge of milk. Furthermore, the digestive processes and peristaltic action in the young child are much more active than in the adult. This explains why not everybody can use milk as a food or medicine — why in many instances it causes biliousness, fermentation and constipation. Patients have come to us from institutions where everybody is subjected to the sweet milk diet. Under long continued forced milk feeding they had become so constipated that the bowels could not be made to move by any means whatsoever. They were literally pasted together with colloid materials. It required several weeks of careful management and treatment to bring about a natural movement of the bowels. Milk causes constipation because it contains large amounts of soft, pulpy, cheesy matter, which tends to coagulation and slime formation. On the other hand, it does not contain sufficient tough cellulose matter which stimulates the peristaltic action of the bowels and acts at the same time as a most efficient scourer and cleanser. It is for this reason that we frequently find it advisable to give fruits and leafy vegetables with the milk diet. In cases where it is easily digested a straight sweet milk diet often proves very beneficial. We prescribe it frequently with splendid results. As a rule, however, it is better to take fruit or leafy vegetables with the milk.

A great deal of chronic disease is caused by starch and protein poisoning, i.e. autointoxication, due to the pathogenic materials such as acids, ptomaines, alkaloids and xanthines, resulting from starch and protein digestion. Since milk contains no starch at all, only low percentages of proteins and fats, and considerable amounts of minerals salts, it will be seen that a straight milk diet means a mild form of protein and starch starvation, which favours the elimination of pathogenic products. However, a study of the comparative analyses of milk, fruits and vegetables will show that juicy fruits and juicy, leafy vegetables are much lower in proteins and fats than is milk, and much richer in mineral salts. Furthermore, the tough, bulky cellulose wastes of fruits and vegetables acts as good scouring material for the stomach and bowels. This is the reason why in most instances we prefer a fruit and vegetable diet to the milk diet.([1])

The prevalent idea that acid fruit juices do not behave well when taken with sweet milk is another popular fallacy. The only food material I know of with which fruit acids do not agree very well is starch, and milk does not contain starch. The digestion of protein materials in the milk requires an acid medium and the sugar or glucose in the milk is already predigested, therefore I do not know of anything in milk that is incompatible with fruit acids. Practical experience also proves this to be true. As a matter of fact, I have met with many confirmed dyspeptics who could not digest milk unless they took acid fruit juices with it.

There is one method of forced milk feeding which is particularly revolting to me. It is patterned after the Weir–Mitchell rest-cure and stuffing treatment. The patient is put to bed and prohibited from making the slightest exertion. He is then given one, two or three tumblerfuls of milk every half hour, according to his capacity. The most remarkable results in the way of flesh and energy building are claimed for this stuffing treatment. It is especially intended for patients who are extremely weak and emaciated. Often they gain a pound or more each day. One advocate of the milk diet describes its beneficial effects as follows:

"Within two hours the action of the heart will have greatly accelerated, and within twelve to twenty-four hours there will be a gain of about six beats to the minute. The pulse will be full and bounding, the skin flushed and moist, and the capillary circulation quick and active. The natural increase in the circulation results from the increased amount of blood material assimilated by the stomach and intestines."

In the first place I do not consider the forced circulation a "natural" result. It is in reality caused, not by the "increased amount of blood", but by the enormously increased amounts of water in the blood and tissues. This to some extent accounts for the increase in weight. Another reason for the sudden increase in weight is the abnormal fat formation. Large amounts of water in the tissues of the body deaden the processes of oxidation and favour fat formation, but this is an unhealthy process. A lymphatic or watery condition of the system is one of the principal causes of obesity. But suppose new flesh and fat cells are

([1])
It should be noted that Lindlahr was definitely hostile to the high protein kind of diet which is frequently advocated even by those who believe in cutting down the starchy foods. It should be remembered that milk, which is designed by nature to be the sole food of small children, is not what is considered a high protein food even though children are growing and may therefore be regarded as requiring more protein than those who are not.

formed under the "masting" process, which, however, is hardly possible in so short a time; this would simply mean increasing disease in the system. To put flesh and fat on a diseased body means an increase of diseased cells and tissues. The new or "daughter" cells are formed by division of the "mother" cells. The daughter cells are therefore of exactly the same material as the mother cells. In other words, if the protoplasm in the mother cells is abnormal or diseased it will be the same in the daughter cells. It is for this reason that under natural treatment we first endeavour to purify the blood and tissues of all abnormal products through natural diet and treatment. This usually entails some loss of weight, which we welcome as a sure indication of elimination and regeneration. After these stages of elimination and purification, with their healing crises, have been safely passed, then come the periods of regeneration and upbuilding of new blood and tissues. What is thus gained will be pure and wholesome. Therefore we favour the various forms of milk diet during the last regenerative or upbuilding stages of treatment. I make these statements backed by much experience in our institutional practice. We have treated many patients who had undergone the stuffing (masting) milk cure treatment for many months at a time, but the results had been only partly beneficial, and these in many instances were far outbalanced by detrimental after-effects.

A gentleman who has become one of the most efficient members of our staff suffered for twenty years from a bad form of arthritic rheumatism. Among many other things he had taken for eight months the forced Milk Cure, but without receiving any appreciable benefit. Under our strict raw food diet and neurotherapy treatment he experienced marked improvement from the start. During the sixth month he passed through a remarkable healing crisis in the form of malarial fever. Such a fever had been "cured" with quinine twenty years before. From this suppression dated the beginning of his chronic "rheumatism". The healing crisis was treated in the natural way, and from that time on he improved more rapidly than ever and regained mobility of the ankylosed joints. Another young man who is now under our treatment had suffered for years from extreme emaciation and nervous weakness, due to indigestion and malassimilation. He also tried the forced milk treatment (forced milk feeding while lying in bed), but to no avail. He finally had to abandon it on account of the aggravation of all his symptoms. He is now gaining under natural diet and treatment, which had to change the abnormal condition of his ductless glands before he could gain by the milk or any other diet. The swamping of the system with enormous quantities of milk in this case had only aggravated the abnormal condition of these wonderful organs by increasing colloid obstruction and the percentage of leucocytes.

63

(a) *Straight Milk Diet.* When the system, through natural diet and treatment, has been duly prepared for the upbuilding process, then the straight milk diet may be applied to good advantage. Under this regimen the patient receives no other food but sweet milk. It is taken every hour or half hour, in quantities ranging from one to two glasses (one half to one pint). The milk should always be sipped slowly. Masticating is of no particular benefit, as it contains no starch. Those who enthusiastically advocate prolonged mastication of milk forget that the ferment (ptyalin) of the saliva acts on starch only. On the other hand, it is certainly not advisable to take the milk down in great gulps. It is important that it should mix gradually and thoroughly with the gastric juice, which acts upon the protein matter in the milk. If large quantities of milk create revulsion or unpleasant results, acid fruit juices, or better still the meat of acid fruits such as lemon, grapefruit, lime or orange, will give relief and create better tolerance for the milk. If one finds it impossible to take large quantities of milk every hour, from the start, smaller quantities may be taken at intervals. For instance, one half pint every hour the first day, one pint every hour the second day, one pint every half hour the third day. The quantity of milk to be consumed per day depends upon the size and weight of the patient. It may range from three quarts per day for a person weighing from ninety to one hundred pounds and suffering from indigestion and malassimilation, to eight or ten quarts for a person of large size and weight and endowed with fairly good digestive capacity.

(b) *Milk Diet for Fleshy People.* Those who suffer from an over-abundance of fat and flesh must take milk only in moderate quantities, say, from two to five quarts of sweet skim milk daily. The cream, in such cases, would only tend to perpetuate and increase fat formation. In many cases of obesity a straight skim milk or buttermilk diet is a splendid remedy for reducing fat. As I said before, the milk diet means a mild form of starch and protein starvation. On the other hand, it increases the activity of the kidneys and flushes the capillaries. In such cases the sweet skim milk may be reinforced by acid fruits taken either with the milk or between the milk feedings.

(c) *Buttermilk Diet.* We find that with many people buttermilk agrees much better than whole milk or skim milk. Others cannot tolerate it at all. The buttermilk may be taken at intervals similar to those prescribed for sweet milk, but not in excessive quantities. I find by experience that on an average one half or one third of the sweet milk quantity is sufficient for the buttermilk. Buttermilk is especially beneficial in cases of low acidity of the stomach and is a tonic for an atrophic condition of the intestines. Quite often it can only be determined by some experimentation whether sweet milk or buttermilk diet is more beneficial in a given case.([1])

(d) *Sour Milk, Clabber or Sumik Milk.* Sour milk may be prepared in various ways, either by exposing whole or skim milk to warm air, or by enclosing unskimmed milk in an air-tight jar or bottle. It is allowed to remain in ordinary living room temperature of from 60° to 70°F. until the milk has become clabber. The clabber is produced by lactic acid fermentation under proper conditions. However, strictest cleanliness must be observed in the preparation of the sour milk, or germs of putrefaction may enter and create a dangerous product. The longer it is allowed to stand in a warm temperature the more acid it becomes. After being properly soured, or clabbered, it should be thoroughly stirred or aerated with an egg beater until it assumes the consistency of thick cream. This is called sumik. With some patients it agrees splendidly, while others cannot tolerate it. Sumik may be taken at intervals and in quantities the same as sweet milk or buttermilk.

(e) *Natural Milk Diet.* Under this regimen, whole or skim milk, buttermilk, sumik or clabber may be taken at intervals and in quantities in accordance with the desire and capacity of the patient. In many instances this will prove the best of all methods. The patient should be encouraged to take milk as frequently and in as large quantities as he can easily tolerate. With the various milk regimens, water should be taken only when distinctly desired. Ordinary milk contains more water than the system requires.

(f) *Milk and Acid Fruit Diet.* Many people who become bilious and constipated on a straight milk diet, or who develop quickly a revulsion to milk, will tolerate milk and digest it much better if they take it with acid or subacid fruits, such as limes, lemons, grapefruit, oranges or berries. They should be allowed to partake of fruit as often as desired but should be cautioned not to take any more fruit than necessary to counteract the unpleasant effects of the milk.

(g) *Milk and Fruit Diet.* While many patients can take acid fruits to good advantage with the milk, I have often found it of greater benefit to give sweet alkaline fruits, such as figs, dates, prunes, raisins, dried currants, etc., with the milk, and acid or subacid fruits between the milk feedings. The following mixed fruit and milk diet has proved beneficial

[1] Buttermilk diet does correct the intestinal flora. However, this and all milk diets in which large quantities are used for long periods can have very deleterious effects on account of the excessive calcium they contain. For example, in parts of Africa, tribal brides, specially fatted up on fourteen pints of milk daily for three months, develop teeth which stick out like rabbits' teeth. Milk diets also tend to upset the thyroid and cause a lot of phlegm and "chestiness".

to many patients who for some reason or another cannot take the straight milk diet:

Breakfast. One to three pints of milk sipped slowly. With the milk take any of the sweetish alkaline fruits, such as melons, pears, prunes, dates, figs, raisins, or raw vegetable relishes such as celery, raw cabbage, watercress, green onions, carrots, etc.

At ten a.m. One of the following fruits: Grapefruit, oranges, peaches, apples, apricots, berries, grapes or any other acid or subacid fruit.

Luncheon. The same as breakfast.

At three p.m. The same as at ten a.m.

Supper: The same as breakfast.

An orange or apple may be taken on retiring.

11. **The Exclusive Meat Diet.** Through theoretical research as well as through actual experience in an extensive institutional practice, I have become convinced that in the great majority of diseases a well balanced vegetarian diet is essential to improvement and cure. However, there are exceptions to this, as to any other rule. In the treatment of certain negative physical and psychical conditions, when the vitality is below par, when the digestive organs have grown so weak that they cannot properly digest and assimilate the ordinary vegetable foods, we found it advantageous to put these patients, temporarily, on a partial meat diet.

Then again, there is a certain type of dyspeptic patient who, on account of abnormal conditions of the digestive organs, cannot digest and assimilate starchy foods. In these cases even small amounts of starches cause fermentation, gas formation and many other distressing symptoms. Usually these people are so weak that they cannot subsist on an exclusive fruit and vegetable diet. Both fruits and vegetables cause more or less distress in the way of indigestion and gas formation. In such cases we have found various forms of meat diet of temporary benefit.

There are several kinds of meat regimen which have thus proved beneficial in some instances.

(a) *Salisbury Exclusive Meat Diet.* Dr. Salisbury claimed that consumption (tuberculosis) is caused by fermentation of food in the stomach, and that the cure consists in excluding those foods which ferment and confining the diet to the most nutritious as well as the most easily assimilated food, beef being the best. Broiled round steak, ground or chopped small, is preferred, as being the most nutritious and having the least waste in the form of fat, bone or any undesirable tissues. Seven mouthfuls of the beef is given to one of toasted whole wheat bread or boiled rice. I would recommend the exclusive Salisbury meat regimen only in exceptional cases of incipient or advanced tuberculosis or in other cases which exhibit positive intolerance of starchy and vegetable foods. A meat diet may prove beneficial also in cases of abnormal psychism caused by negative physical and mental conditions. In such cases the meat diet has a tendency to fortify the animal magnetism of the psyche and thus to break contact with conditions on the spiritual plane. Even in most of these cases a vegetarian diet including the dairy products will bring all the good results without the danger of uric acid poisoning which is always present under an exclusive meat diet. I have seen many people cure themselves through the Salisbury method from carbonic acid poisoning due to an excessive starch diet, only to develop serious forms of uric acid poisoning, such as rheumatism, heart disease, high blood pressure, etc.

(b) *Combination Meat and Vegetable Diet.* *Breakfast.* Acid and subacid fruits.

Dinner. A small portion of broiled Salisbury steak, rare broiled beefsteak, mutton, rare roast beef, or roast mutton, with raw vegetable relishes, salads and one cooked leafy (not starchy) vegetable.

Supper. A raw or soft boiled egg three times a week, together with a baked or boiled potato and vegetable relishes or salads. On other evenings a slice or two of health bread or a dish of cereal, together with vegetable relishes, salads, olives, figs, dates or raisins.

(c) *Modified Combination Meat and Vegetable Diet.* Under this regimen starchy foods are restricted to a minimum. A small portion of meat is allowed three or four times a week. Suitable foods besides meat are acid and subacid fruits, especially for breakfast, raw vegetable relishes and salads, cottage cheese, cooked vegetables, olives, dates, figs, raisins, nuts in moderate quantities; eggs (raw, soft boiled or poached) in moderate quantities — not more than four a week; cereals, bread and potatoes, if used at all, in very moderate quantities only, but not in combination with meat or acid fruits.

(d) *Hot Water Drinking.* Advocates of the Salisbury diet and others advise the drinking of hot water as a preserver of health and as a therapeutic agency in the treatment of chronic disease, but the claims made on its behalf are directly contrary to the teachings of orthodox physiology and food chemistry as well as the Natural Therapeutic philosophy. It is, however, evident why the Salisbury meat diet requires enormous quantities of hot water to counteract its bad effects upon the system. The ingestion of such large masses of meat, unbalanced by mineral salt foods, would cause excessive accumulation of colloids, alkaloids of putrefaction, and other pathogenic materials, if these were not washed out of the system by correspondingly large amounts of hot water. Excessive thirst, which occurs in such cases, is caused by the increased oxidation of morbid products. Thirst disappears almost entirely under a well balanced vegetarian diet. This explains why an exclusive meat diet necessitates the hot water flushing.

SECTION XI

FASTING([1])

One of the most common complaints of the sick is that they have "lost their appetite". They seem to imagine that this is a terrible affliction. Quite the reverse is true, however. In the majority of cases nature takes away the appetite because a fast is needed. They do not know that the greatest blessing to them would be to "lose their appetite" long enough to find their hunger. Loss of appetite is simply an indication that the system is overcharged with pathogenic matter and that nature is trying to stop the eating long enough to give these clogging, benumbing or irritating accumulations a chance to escape from the system, or it may be that the digestive organs are too weak to take care of large quantities of food. However, the laity for ages has been encouraged by the medical profession in the idea that to lose the appetite and miss a few meals is a great calamity; that this must be prevented by taking powerful stimulants in the form of appetizers and tonics. These serve to create a false and artificial appetite and cause the sufferer to stuff the weak stomach with more food, while that taken in previous meals is fermenting and putrefying, filling the system with noxious poisons.

Many people are learning the trick of curing their colds, headaches, nervous spells and other acute troubles, by missing a few meals or taking a short fast. It is the quickest, simplest and most efficient method of relieving the overloaded, food poisoned system. We would be surprised if we knew how little food is actually required to keep the human organism in good condition. The majority of people are food poisoned — even those who believe they are eating moderately. Cornaro, the great Italian Nature Cure apostle, who lived in Venice in the fifteenth century, proved these facts which humanity at large has not digested and taken advantage of even at this late day. At forty he was dying from chronic diseases resulting from overeating, drinking and riotous living generally. Being gifted by nature with some intelligence and will power, he essayed to cure himself by reversing his habits of living, i.e., by reducing the daily allowance of food and drink to a minimum. For nearly forty years his daily allowance of solid food was not more than twelve ounces. Then he yielded to the urgings of his relatives and friends, who believed that he was starving himself, and took a few more ounces of food than his former quota. The result was that he immediately began to feel most miserable, both physically and mentally, and his former good health and energy did

([1])
See also Vol. I, "Philosophy of Natural Therapeutics".

not return until he reduced his daily allowance to the old accustomed twelve ounces. After the age of eighty he wrote several books on matters of health, and particularly his own experiences. His most ambitious work, which is even now in print and widely read, he finished when he was over one hundred years old. The history of this man and his experiences with moderate living and fasting should be taught in every school in the land.

1. **The Physiology of Fasting.** Fasting is undoubtedly one of the most potent and incidentally the cheapest of all natural remedies. The reason why it is not more universally applied is that the laity at large, as well as the medical profession, are under the impression that the interruption of eating even for a brief period will greatly reduce the vitality of the individual. This popular fallacy is caused by the belief that food and drink are the only source of strength. In other parts of these writings I have shown that this is not so — that the life force which is the real source of our vitality or strength is entirely independent of our material bodies (physical and spiritual) and of food, drink, medicines, tonics and stimulants; that this life force flows into us from the source of all life, intelligence and creative force in the universe; from that which we variously call God, Nature, Universal Intelligence, the Oversoul, the Will to Live, and by many other names. If people fully realized this fact they would not be in such great fear of missing a few meals or of undergoing a more or less prolonged fast.([1])

Fasting as a remedy is fully in harmony with our philosphy of the causes of disease. If disease is created through abnormal composition of blood and lymph and through accumulation of morbid matter in the system, it stands to reason that fasting will help to eliminate from the system waste matter and morbid accumulations. The most difficult feature about fasting is the breaking of the eating habit. Therefore the first three or four days of fasting are always the hardest. They are usually accompanied by craving for food, nervous disturbances, mental depression, headaches, sleeplessness, etc. We must remember that eating is the oldest and most firmly established of all habits. Therefore it is not easily broken. After the habit is broken, which usually requires two or three days, fasting becomes easier day by day. One reasons for this is that about the third or fourth day the mucous membranes of the intestines begin to eliminate morbid matter. The processes of assimilation have come to a standstill. The membranous linings of the stomach and intestines, which ordinarily act as sponges for the absorption of food materials, are now throwing off effete matter from the system. The sponge is being squeezed. This is

([1])
See also "Philosphy of Natural Therapeutics" and "Nature Cure Cook Book".

indicated by the foetid breath and coated tongue which reflect the foul condition of the digestive organs. These are not fit to digest or assimilate food; therefore hunger ceases. The system now has to draw for food upon its reserve stores. The waste and morbid materials are stirred up and eliminated first.

When we consider that the digestive canal from mouth to anus is about twenty-six feet long and lined all through with eliminating cellular and glandular structures, then we can better appreciate the purifying effect of a protracted fast. One need not fear the weakening effects of fasting, since of late years it has been proved in thousands of cases that fasts of even forty, fifty and sixty days' duration have no perceptible weakening effect upon the system, unless the patient be greatly weakened and emaciated by disease at the beginning of the fast. One of our patients recently finished a forty-nine day fast. At the end he felt actually stronger than he did at the beginning. Up to the last day he took long walks. At the same time the chronic troubles which were caused by drug poisoning and surgical operations wer greatly alleviated. The foregoing explains why short fasts of from one to three days have not a decided curative effect. It takes that much time to start the eliminative processes in the linings of the intestines. As soon as food is taken these processes are interrupted and reversed. I would consider seven days a short curative fast. Shorter fasts may be taken, however, in order that one may become accustomed to the practice.

In this, as well as in many other things, much depends upon the right mental attitude. If one fears the effects of fasting and believes that it is going to weaken him, this causes mental and nervous depression which is bound to react disastrously upon his system. If, on the other hand, one becomes thoroughly convinced that rational fasting cannot injure the system, that whether eating or abstaining from food the life force will flow into the body just as abundantly, then the fasting will greatly facilitate the elimination of waste and pathogenic matter and there will be no mental apprehension and no nervous uneasiness to affect the system and to interfere with the grand house-cleaning. Many of our patients have undergone protracted fasts, but I do not remember a single instance in which any one of them has been injured through the practice. We carefully observe the physical and mental condition of the patient from day to day and interrupt the fast when such action is indicated.

2. **Danger Signals in Fasting.** These are rapid and prolonged loss of weight approaching the danger line; serious and prolonged mental depression, and the appearance of psychical symptoms such as clairvoyance and clairaudience, which indicate abnormal psychism due to an extremely negative physical and mental condition. Also the fast should be interrupted when the patient shows great fear and apprehension of its weaken-

ing effects, as the destructive effects of anxiety and worry might overbalance the benefits to be derived from the fast. In such cases it is better to postpone a protracted fast to a time when the mental and emotional conditions are more positive.

3. **How Long Should One Fast?** I never prescribe the length of a fast beforehand. Even when I am convinced that a prolonged fast of two, three or four weeks is indicated, I would not inform the patient to this effect. I usually tell him that we shall extend or shorten the fast according to the effects it produces; that we may continue it for a few days or for a week or more, according to changing conditions. This assures the patient that the fast is not going to be continued beyond his powers of endurance. It is much easier for him to fast from day to day than to look forward to a long fixed period. The practice of fasting until the tongue becomes clean, the breath sweet and natural hunger returns is a rather dangerous one. I have found in many cases that the symptoms of the foul condition of the digestive tract would not disappear after four or five weeks of fasting nor would there be the slightest manifestation of hunger, and in several such cases it seemed doubtful whether breath and tongue would clear up before the patient was ready for the undertaker. It is much safer to break the fast before the desired results have been fully obtained and to repeat it after a period of recuperation. The digestive organs may be in such a diseased condition that it is impossible for them to become normal through one prolonged fast.

Several patients have come under our care who had protracted the fast too long while waiting for the cleaning up. One of these patients is with us now, just recuperating from a complete collapse caused by excessive fasting. When she finally tried to eat, her digestive organs were so weak that they could not take care of any food whatsoever. She was brought to our institution on a stretcher, emaciated to the proverbial "skin and bones". It required considerable careful management and treatment to revive the paralysed organs. In such cases only very small quantites of easily digestible food, such as white of egg, milk, sumik or buttermilk, must be given. With this we give subacid or sweet fruit juices. Careful massage and neurotherapy are required to revive the benumbed organs. Magnetic treatment also is of great value in accomplishing this.[1]

[1]
While loss of appetite may not generally be a cause for alarm and may in fact indicate that the patient needs to fast and would benefit by doing so, there are undoubtedly cases of anorexia in which efforts should be made from the start to get the patient to eat. The trouble may be largely psychological but, as Lindlahr points out, it is probable that the system is clogged with pathogenic matter and that the digestive organs are in a very weakened condition. This means that the emunctories must be made to function well and food of an easily digestible and eliminative kind given in small quantities until the digestion and appetite improve.

4. **Preparation for Fasting.** Most writers on fasting maintain that one can stop eating and start on a prolonged fast at any time without preparation. This, however, is not always advisable. It may be all right in certain cases which are not affected by serious chronic diseases. But where the organs of elimination are in an atrophic condition, and where the system suffers from mineral starvation and is overloaded with pathogenic matter, it is much safer to prepare the system for the fast through a low protein diet rich in positive mineral elements, or, better still, through a raw food diet and through thorough systematic natural treatment. Large amounts of negative pathogenic materials eliminated from the tissues and thrown into the circulation as the result of fasting must be neutralized by the positive alkaline mineral elements and eliminated from the system. These neutralizing and purifying elements can be introduced into the system only through a fruit and vegetable diet, low in starches and protein matter and rich in the positive alkaline mineral elements. When the natural diet and treatment have purified the system sufficiently for the manifestation of a healing crisis, then the physiological and psychological moment for fasting has arrived. Then the system is not in condition for the digestion and assimilation of food. Therefore fasting becomes imperative. The whole body, including the linings of the stomach and bowels, is engaged in the work of elimination; this results in loss of appetite, revulsion to eating, coated tongue, foul breath, mental and nervous disturbances, all of which would only be aggravated by eating. In order to prevent reabsorption of morbid excretions, enemas and treatment for constipation are indicated before and during a fast.

5. **Healing Crises Suppressed by Eating.** I have often observed that good healing crises such as diarrhoeas, acute catarrh or febrile conditions were suppressed by eating. This is easily explained by the fact that healing crises are processes of elimination, while eating promotes the processes of assimilation. This is especially true of diarrhoea, which is one of the most efficient forms of acute elimination or healing crisis. Forced absorption of food will frequently check the morbid discharges. Furthermore, it is dangerous to give food in cases of well established violent diarrhoea because it only irritates the raw surfaces in the intestines and keeps them in an inflamed condition. The food is not absorbed, but only serves to prolong the purging, dysentery or bloody flux unnecessarily, and thus may cause perforation of the bowels and even death. Not a morsel of food should pass the lips until the intestines have stopped moving and have had time to heal and to rebuild the sloughed membranes. Therefore fasting should be continued all the way from one day to a week after the cessation of purging, according to the severity and duration of the acute attack. For example, after a diarrhoea lasting one or two days

no food should be taken for twenty-four hours. After a diarrhoea lasting four or five days fasting should continue for three days or longer. After eight days or more of violent purging, no food should be taken for at least seven days.

One of the most remarkable healing crises I ever observed came in the form of a diarrhoea which lasted four weeks. During this time the patient did not receive any food whatsoever, nothing but water mixed with acid fruit juices. The discharges were of a black, watery nature. The patient assured me that during this entire four weeks' period he did not sleep one wink. Still he did not suffer particularly in the daytime. He had sufficient energy to accomplish his usual amount of work. While this may seem incredible, and while it is possible that the man may have slept more than he was aware, we have witnessed many similar instances of remarkable endurance during healing crises. The man had suffered all his life from chronic enteritis (inflammation of the bowels). The eyes showed several itch spots in the intestinal area, indicating that the under-lying cause of the trouble was suppressed itch. He remembered that such eruptions had been suppressed several times in his youth. This vigorous healing crisis eliminated the disease taint from his system, and he has enjoyed good health ever since.

6. **Fruit Juices in Fasting.** In the majority of cases we prefer to give to those who are undergoing prolonged fasts moderate quantities of diluted acid and subacid fruit juices. In this I take issue with some of the best authorities on fasting. I cannot understand why acid and subacid fruit juices should in any way interfere with the good effects of a fast. They do not contain food elements which promote the processes of digestion. On the other hand, they are rich in mineral salts which are necessary to neutralize the negative pathogenic substances with which the circulation is flooded during the fast. Besides having this neutralizing and eliminating effect, they are splendid tonics and antiseptics and are rich in vitamins, or, as I have called them, the life elements which sustain and stimulate the vital activities. Fasting, therefore, is much easier to endure and more pleasant when the diluted fruit juices are taken. The juices should not be taken pure or in large quantities because in this form they may excite the digestive processes. There is no danger of this, however, when they are taken in dilute form; for instance, the juice of half an orange or half a lemon to a tumbler of cold water. The water should be of natural temperature as it comes from the tap. Ice water should not be used in any circumstances.

7. **Hot Water Drinking.** In some cases where the stomach and intestines are in a very foul and slimy condition hot water drinking proves very beneficial. From one to two glasses of water, as hot as can be swallowed without injuring the tender membranes of the mouth and throat, may be

taken three times a day. I do not advise the continuance of hot water drinking longer than necessary to wash out the morbid accumulations in the digestive tract. This must be supplemented also by copious enemas every second or third day. The diluted fruit juices may be taken between the hot water flushings. I would advise the hot water regimen only in extreme cases where something of a radical nature has to be done to clear the digestive tract of its foetid accumulations.

8. **Exercises while Fasting.** The idea prevails that during a prolonged fast one should have complete rest. This, however, is a serious mistake. There is no reason why one should not take the usual amount of exercise or accomplish the accustomed daily tasks, provided, of course, these do not strain the physical and mental energies to the point of exhaustion. As a matter of fact many of our patients feel stronger and display more endurance after the first week of fasting than during the first few days. This is easily explained by the fact that during the fast the system eliminates large amounts of clogging pathogenic matter. This allows freer circulation of the blood and nerve currents and a more unobstructed flow of vital energy.

9. **Symptoms and Acute Reactions Caused by Fasting.**

(a) *Gas Formation.* A common symptom exhibited on starting a fast is excessive gas production accompanied by rumblings in the bowels and collicky pains. This is caused by the stirring up and disintegration of deposits of old faecal matter in the intestines, and by the elimination of pathogenic materials from the system. Usually the bowels soon stop moving when no food is taken. In such cases warm water enemas should be taken to flush the colon. The accumulations in the lower intestine during a fast are of a particularly poisonous nature, and should be removed in order to prevent absorption.

(b) *Temperature.* In many instances the temperature rises during the first day of the fast and sometimes a slight febrile condition prevails during the entire period or subsides after a few weeks. In other cases we observe a lowering of the temperature below the normal. All these and similar reactions are not of a serious nature, and nothing should be done to interfere with them. They become dangerous only by suppression.

(c) *Cotton Mouth.* Another unpleasant but perfectly natural symptom is the gathering in the mouth of thick and sticky viscous accumulations of saliva. This condition has been called "cotton mouth" by the laity. In other cases the mouth feels dry and burning hot. These symptoms are of course signs of greatly increased combustion of morbid materials and their elimination through the membranes of the mouth and throat. Similar conditions exist in the stomach and intestines.

(d) *Bilious Vomiting.* In some cases where the liver has been enlarged

74

and engorged with morbid accumulations, bile discharges in large quantities into the intestine and from there regurgitates into the stomach, causing bilious vomiting of an extremely offensive character. This symptom also is more terrifying than dangerous. It is a rather unpleasant but nevertheless effective way of house-cleaning.

People who have taken a great deal of calomel or mercury in other forms often develop violent vomiting while fasting. This may continue for a week or more. If they are robust enough to stand the ordeal it is well to let the crisis run its course, but if they are in a very weakened condition it may be advisable to interrupt the fast for the time being. In such cases it is best to give white of egg to soothe the inflamed lining of the stomach. It must be remembered tht in these mercurial patients the liver and stomach are particularly affected and that these organs try to throw off the mercurial poison through vomiting. I have frequently perceived distinctly the peculiar metallic and mercurial odour of the breath and of the bilious discharges.

(e) *Offensive Perspiration.* Another unpleasant symptom frequently observed in a long fast is a very offensive odour of perspiration, which indicates vigorous elimination of pathogenic materials through the skin. Frequent quick cold rubs will promote this form of elimination and at the same time remove the offensive excretions and thus prevent their re-absorption. In some cases it may become necessary to employ warm water and soap to remove the offensive elimination.

10. **Fear of Fasting Unfounded.** The majority of those who undergo their first long fast are most pleasantly surprised to find that the terrors of starvation existing only in people's minds. It has happened that people stranded on barren islands or lost in desert places or entombed in mines, even where they had water, have died apparently from starvation in the course of a week or two. It is now fully proved by thousands who have fasted for long periods ranging from forty to ninety days that death in such cases is not due to actual starvation. The real cause must be fear and apprehension — proving again that the things we fear we materialize. We cannot reiterate too often that fear is a perversion of the great law of faith. It is faith in evil. By submitting to fear we give evil power over us. The most necessary requirements, therefore, for a successful fast is the profound conviction that it cannot harm us in any way, but that it will prove of great benefit, physically, mentally and morally, because it not only purifies the body but strengthens will power and self control.

11. **Fasting Regimen.** Before, during and after a therapeutic fast, everything must be done to keep elimination active, in order to prevent the reabsorption of the toxins which are being stirred up and liberated. Fasting involves rapid breaking down of the tissues. This creates great

quantities of worn-out cell materials and other morbid substances. Unless these poison producing accumulations are promptly eliminated, they will be reabsorbed into the system and cause autointoxication. To prevent this, bowels, kidneys and skin must be kept in active condition. The diet, for several days before and after a fast, should consist largely of uncooked fruits and vegetables, and the different methods of natural stimulative treatment should be systematically applied.

During a fast, every bit of vitality must be economized; therefore the passive treatments are to be preferred to active exercise, although a certain amount of exercise (especially walking) daily in the open air, accompanied by deep breathing, should not be neglected. While fasting, intestinal evacuation usually ceases, especially where there is a natural tendency to sluggishness of the bowels. Enemas are therefore in order and during prolonged fasts may be taken every few days. By "prolonged" fasts I mean fasts which last from one to four weeks; "short" fasts being those of one, two or three days' duration.

Moderate drinking is beneficial during a fast as well as at other times; but excessive consumption of water, the so-called "flushing of the system", is very injurious. Under ordinary conditions from five to eight glasses of water a day are sufficient; the quantity consumed must be regulated by the desire of the patient. Those who are fasting should mix their drinking water with the juice of acid fruits, preferably lemon, lime, orange or grapefruit. These juices act as eliminators and are fine natural antiseptics. Never use distilled water, whether during a fast or at any other time. Deprived of its own mineral constituents, distilled water "leeches" the mineral elements and organic salts out of the tissues of the body and thereby intensifies dysaemic conditions.

While fasting, the right mental attitude is all-important. Unless you can do it with perfect equanimity, without fear or misgiving, do not fast at all. Destructive mental conditions may more than offset the beneficial effects of the fast. To recapitulate: never undertake a prolonged fast unless you have been properly prepared by natural diet and treatment, and never without the guidance of a competent adviser.

(a) *The Regular Fast.* Under this regimen no food is taken, but sufficient water to quench the thirst. In some cases it may be advantageous to increase the quantity of drinking water in order to dilute the pathogenic materials in the circulation and thus facilitate their elimination through the skin and kidneys. Thirst, therefore, is a safe indicator of the amount of fluid needed.

(b) *The Dry Fast.* This means total abstinence from food and drink. Most people cannot endure this radical fast more than two or three days. It is a very powerful agent for promoting elimination. When no fluids are taken, the tissues are drawn upon for the elimination of waste materials. It has been found that such fluid starvation, which is directly contrary to the popular idea of flushing, is a powerful method of promoting elimination of morbid matter and disease taints, especially from the systems of individuals who are obese or whose tissues are "waterlogged".

(c) *The Seven Day Fast.* If no adverse symptoms interfere, we frequently prescribe short fasts of seven days. This in the great majority of cases cannot produce any harmful or weakening results, and, understanding the laws of periodicity, we prefer a seven day period. If developments are favourable to a prolongation of the fast we endeavour to extend it to the fourteenth, twenty-first, twenty-eighth or subsequent seven day periods.

(d) *The Long Fast.* Long fasts may extend from one to seven or more weeks, according to individual indications and the vitality of the patient. As already explained, we never fix a definite period for the fast beforehand but extend it from time to time according to conditions. We add small quantities of acid fruit juices to the drinking water as long as it agrees with the patient. If a revulsion to it develops, the water may be taken pure. After the bowels stop moving naturally enemas must be taken from time to time. Indications for breaking the fast have been described above.

12. **Breaking the Fast.** The great benefit derived from a fast may be lost and may be followed by harmful after-effects if it is not broken in the right way. In fact, the best effects of a fast depend upon the dietic management after it is broken; and the longer it is, the more care must be taken in breaking it. The greatest danger lies in eating too frequently and too much at a time. After a long fast the digestive organs are in a condition of complete inactivity and to overload them suddenly with a large amount of food may provoke acute attacks of indigestion and produce many other kinds of serious disturbances. The organs must be trained into normal activity gradually, beginning with very small quantities of light food. I have frequently found it very good to break the fast with a few tablespoonfuls of freshly toasted popcorn, unsalted and unbuttered. This is a splendid scour for the membranous linings of the stomach and bowels, and its tough particles stimulate the peristaltic action of the intestines. The popcorn may be followed within an hour by some mild fruit juice, preferably lemon, lime, orange or grapefruit. Not more than the juice of half a grapefruit or of one orange should be taken at a time. The quantity of undiluted juice may be gradually increased on the second day to three or four half tumblerfuls. On the third day the meat of acid or subacid fruits may be taken instead of the juice alone. After the third day the fruit diet may be supplemented and combined with raw vegetable relishes and salads. If a person is sensitive to the mixing of acid fruits

77

with vegetables, they should be taken at separate meals. To this raw food diet may be added small quantities of nuts or a ripe banana. The raw food diet may be continued from a few days to many weeks, according to the individual conditions of the patient, or it may be followed, whenever it seems advisable, by the regular vegetarian diet. On the other hand it may be advisable to follow the fruit diet by a straight or modified milk diet. This is especially indicated where milk agrees with the patient and where it is desirable to give animal food in order to overcome a negative mental and physical condition and to build flesh more rapidly.

No hard and fast rules can be established concerning any of these regimens or practices. One must be guided by conditions and requirements. It is dangerous for people to experiment along these lines without the guidance of a competent and experienced natural therapist. If the fast is broken in the right way it will be found that lost weight is regained very quickly. In many instances people gain much more, after a prolonged fast, than they weighed before. Moreover, the new blood and tissues will be purer and healthier than the old, effete tissues which have been eliminated through strict diet, natural treatment and fasting.([1])

SECTION XII

HYDROTHERAPY OR WATER TREATMENT

INTRODUCTION

While in our treatment of acute diseases we use wet packs and cold ablutions to promote the radiation of heat and thereby to reduce the fever temperature, our aim in the treatment of chronic diseases is to arouse the

([1])
Lindlahr's attitude towards fasting as a therapeutic procedure is broadly speaking that it should not be used except in acute feverish diseases or when the body has clearly undertaken a strong elimination by way of skin, bowels or mucous membranes. It is no doubt true that this is a sound rule, but there seem to be circumstances in which a more or less prolonged fast may be beneficial and time saving at the beginning of an effort to cope with a chronic condition or to bring about a general cleansing and rejuvenation of the body. It has the effect of giving the digestive organs a complete rest and of knocking the body out of a rut of inertia. On the other hand there is reason to think that in most cases if not in all better results may be obtained by doing the "Grape Cure" than by absolute fasting. It appears that grapes and grape juice throw so little strain on the digestive system and are so non-toxic and assimilable that their use makes an exception to the general rule that the body cannot assimilate and eliminate, tear down and build up at the same time. The successful use of the Grape Cure in cases in which the body was too weak to sustain a long fast or to benefit by it is discussed in the books on the Grape Cure by Brandt and Shackleton.

system to acute eliminative effort.   In other words, while in acute disease our hydropathic treatment is sedative, in chronic diseases it is stimulative.

The Good Effects of Cold Water Applications

1. **Stimulation of the Circulation.**   As before stated, cold water applied to the surface of the body arouses and stimulates the circulation all over the system.   Blood counts before and after a cold application show a very marked increase in the number of red corpuscles.   This does not mean that the cold water has in a moment created new blood cells, but it means that the blood has been stirred up and sent hurrying through the system, that the lazy cells which were lying inactive in the sluggish and stagnant blood stream and in the clogged and obstructed tissues are aroused to increased activity.   Undoubtedly, the invigorating and stimulating influence of cold sprays, ablutions, sitz baths, barefoot walking in the dewy grass or on wet stones and of all other cold water applications depends largely upon their electro-magnetic effects upon the system.   (See Chap. XXXIV, Vol. 1.)

2. **Elimination of Impurities.**   As the cold water drives the blood with increased force through the system, it flushes the capillaries in the tissues and cleanses them from the accumulation of pathogen which is one of the primary causes of acute and chronic diseases.   As the blood rushes back to the surface it suffuses the skin, opens and relaxes the pores and the minute blood vessels or capillaries, and thus unloads its impurities through the cuticle.

3. **Why We Favour Cold Water.**   Some advocates of natural methods still favour warm or hot applications in the form of hot water baths, various kinds of steam or sweat baths, electric light baths, hot compresses, fomentations, etc.   However, the great majority of Nature Cure practitioners have come to abandon hot applications almost entirely because of their weakening and enervating after-effects and because in many instances they have not only failed to produce the expected results but have aggravated the disease conditions.

We can explain the different effects of hot and cold water as well as of all other therapeutic agents upon the system by the law of action and reaction.   Applied to physics this law reads: "Action and reaction are equal but opposite."   I have adapted the law of action and reaction to therapeutics in a somewhat circumscribed way, as follows: Every therapeutic agent affecting the human organism has a first, temporary, and a second, permanent effect.   The second, lasting effect is contrary to the first, transient effect.   The first, temporary effect of warmth above the body temperature, whether it be applied in the form of hot air, water, steam or light, is to draw the blood into the surface. Immediately after such an application the skin will be red and hot. The second and lasting effect, however, is that the blood recedes into the interior of the body and leaves the skin in a bloodless and enervated condition, subject to chills and predisposed to "catching cold". On the other hand, the first transient effect of cold water applications upon the body as a whole, or upon any particular part, is to chill the surface and send the blood scurrying inward, leaving the skin in a chilled, bloodless condition. The lack of blood and sensation of cold are at once telegraphed over the afferent nerves to headquarters in the brain and from there the command goes forth to the nerve centres regulating the circulation: "Send blood to the surface." As a result the circulation is stirred up and accelerated throughout the system and blood rushes with force into the depleted skin, flushing the surface of the body with warm blood and restoring to it the rosy colour of health. This is the second effect. In other words, the well applied cold water treatment is followed by a good reaction, and this is accompanied by many permanent beneficial results. The drawing and eliminating first effect of hot applications, of sweat baths, etc., is at best only temporary, lasting but a few minutes, and is always followed by a weakening reaction, while the drawing and eliminating action of cold water applications, being the second, lasting effect, exerts an enduring, invigorating and tonic influence upon the skin which enables it to throw off morbid matter not merely for ten or fifteen minutes, as in the sweat bath under the influence of excessive heat, but continually by day and night.

4. **The Danger of Prolonged or Excessively Cold Applications.** As I have pointed out, only water of ordinary temperature as it comes from the tap should generally be used in hydropathic applications. It is positively dangerous to apply ice bags to an inflamed organ or to use icy water for packs and ablutions in febrile conditions. Likewise, ice or icy water should not be used in the hydropathic treatment of chronic diseases. Excessive cold is as suppressive in its effects upon the organism as are poisonous antiseptics and antifever medicines. The baths, sprays, douches, etc., should not be kept up for too long. The duration of the cold applications must be regulated to the individual condition of the patient and by his power of reaction. It should be borne in mind that it is the short, quick application that produces the stimulating, electromagnetic effects upon the system.

SECTION XIII

COLD WATER APPLICATIONS

1. **Outdoor Bathing and Swimming.** This is very beneficial to those who are strong enough to secure reaction. It should never be extended too long. Twenty minutes is sufficient even for a young and vigorous person. There must be no feeling of chilliness or exhaustion afterwards. This would be a sign of overdoing. If the reaction is good there should follow a feeling of comfort and warmth, especially of the feet and hands. There will be a good appetite and the sleep will be sound and refreshing. Ocean bathing is more tonic than inland bathing because the salts in the sea water have a positive electromagnetic effect upon the body.

2. **Foot Bath.** Stand in cold water reaching up to the ankles for one to two minutes, according to the summer or winter temperature of the water. Dry the feet with a coarse towel and rub them vigorously with the hands, or walk about briskly for a few minutes. Repeat if necessary.

3. **Leg Bath.** Stand in water up to calves or knees in the same manner.

4. **Barefoot Walking.** Walk barefoot in wet grass or on wet stone pavements several times a day, from ten to twenty minutes at a time, or less in case of weakness. The early morning dew upon the grass is especially beneficial; later in the day wet the grass or pavement with a hose. After barefoot walking, dry and rub the feet thoroughly and take a short, brisk walk in shoes and stockings.

5. **Indoor Water Treading.** Stand in a bathtub or large foot-tub containing about two inches of water, step and splash vigorously for several minutes, then dry and rub the feet, and increase the circulation by walking around the room a few times.

6. **Foot Spray.** Turn the full force of water from a hose first on one foot, then on the other. Let the stream play alternately on the upper part of the feet and on the soles. The coldness and force of the water will draw the blood to the feet. These applications are excellent as a means of stimulating and equalizing the circulation, and a "sure cure" for cold and clammy feet, as well as for excessive perspiration of the feet. In this connection, we warn our readers most strongly against the use of drying powders or antiseptic washes to suppress foot-sweat. Serious nervous disorders have been traced to this practice.

7. **Partial Ablutions.** Partial ablutions with cold water are very useful in many instances, especially in local inflammation or where local congestion is to be relieved. The "kalte Guss" forms an important feature of the Kneipp system of water cure. Sprays or showers may be administered to the head, arms, chest, back, thighs, knees or wherever indicated, with a

81

dipper or a sprinkler attached to a tap. The water should be of natural temperature and the "Guss" of short duration.

8. **Limb Bath.** Take up cold water in the hollow of the hands from a running tap or bucket of water, rub arms and legs briskly for a few minutes.

9. **Upper and Lower Body Baths.** Stand in an empty tub and take water from a tap or bucket in the hollow of the hands and rub briskly the upper or lower half of the body for a few minutes.

10. **Hip Bath.** Sit in a large basin or in a bathtub in enough water to cover the hips completely, the legs resting on the floor or against the side of the tub. While taking the hip bath, knead and rub the abdomen. Dry with a coarse towel, then rub and pat the skin with the hands for a few minutes.

11. **The Morning Cold Rub.** The essentials for a cold rub, and in fact for every cold water treatment, are warmth of the body before the application, coolness of the water (natural temperature), rapidity of action, and friction or exercise to stimulate the circulation. No cold water treatment should be taken when the body is in a chilled condition.

(a) Directly from the warmth of the bed, or after sun bath and exercise have produced a pleasant glow, go the the bathroom, sit in the empty tub with the stopper in place, turn on the cold water, and as it flows into the tub, catch it in the hollow of the hands and wash first the limbs, then the abdomen, then the chest and back. Throw the water all over the body and rub the skin with the hands like you wash your face. Do this quickly but thoroughly. The entire procedure need not take up more than a few minutes. By the time the bath is finished, there may be from two to four inches of water in the tub. Use a towel or brush for the back if you cannot reach it otherwise. As long as there is a good reaction, the cold rub may be taken in an unheated bathroom even in cold weather.

After the bath, dry the body quickly with a coarse towel and finish by rubbing with the hands until the skin is dry and smooth and you are aglow with the exercise, or expose the wet body to the fresh air before an open window and rub with the hands until dry and warm. A bath taken in this manner combines the beneficial effects of cold water, air, exercise, and the magnetic friction of the hands on the body (life on life). No lifeless instrument or mechanical appliance can equal the dexterity, warmth and magnetism of the human hand. The bath must be so conducted that it is followed by a feeling of warmth and comfort. Some persons will be benefited by additional exercises or, better still, a brisk walk in the open air, while others will get better results by returning to the warmth of the bed.

There is no better means for stimulating the general circulation and for increasing the eliminative activities of the system than this cold morning rub at the beginning of the day after the night's rest. If kept up regularly, its good effects will soon become apparent. This method of taking the morning bath is to be preferred to the plunge into a tub filled with cold water. While persons with very strong constitutions may experience no ill effects, to those who are weak and do not react readily, the "cold plunge" might prove a severe shock and strain upon the system.

(b) When a bathtub is not available, take the morning rub in the following manner: Stand in an empty washtub. In front of you in the tub place a basin or bucket filled with cold water. Wet the hands or a towel and wash the body, part by part, from the feet upward; then dry and rub with the hands as before directed.

12. **The Evening Sitz Bath.** The sitz bath is best taken in the regular tub made for the purpose, but an ordinary bathtub or a washtub or pan may be used with equally good effect. Pour into the vessel a few inches of water at natural temperature as it comes from the tap, and sit in the water until a good reaction takes place — that is until the first sensation of cold is followed by a feeling of warmth. This may take from a few seconds to a few minutes, according to the temperature of the water and the individual powers of reaction. Dry with a coarse towel, rub and pat the skin with the hands, then, in order to establish a good reaction, practise deep breathing for a few minutes, alternating with the internal massage exercise described in Sec. XXI.

The morning rub is stimulating in its effects; the evening sitz bath is quieting and relaxing. The latter is therefore specially beneficial if taken just before going to bed. The cold water draws the blood from brain and spinal cord, and thereby ensures better rest and sleep. It cools and relaxes the abdominal organs, sphincters and orifices, stimulates gently and naturally the action of the bowels and the urinary tract, and is equally effective in chronic constipation and in affections of the kidneys or bladder.

13. **The Head Bath.** Loss or discolouration of the hair is generally due to the lack of hair-building elements in the blood, or to sluggish circulation of the scalp and a diseased condition of the hair follicles. Nothing more effectually stimulates the flow of blood to brain and scalp or promotes the elimination of waste matter and poisons from these parts than the head bath, together with scalp massage.

Under no circumstances use hair tonics, dandruff or eczema cures or hair dyes. All such preparations contain poisons in the form of strong antiseptics and germicides. Dandruff is a form of elimination and should not be suppressed. When the scalp is in good condition, it will disappear of its own accord. The diagnosis from the iris of the eye reveals the fact that glycerin, quinine, resorcin and other poisonous antiseptics and stimulants absorbed from dandruff cures and deposited in the brain are, in many cases, the real cause of chronic headaches, neuralgia, dizziness, roaring in the ears, loss of hearing and sight, mental depression, irritability and even insanity. Cold water is an absolutely safe and at the same time a most effective means to promote the growth of hair, as many of our patients can testify.

If the hair is short, the head should be washed thoroughly with cold water each time the face is washed. While doing this the scalp should be vigorously pinched, kneaded and massaged with the finger tips. When feasible, turn the stream from a tap or hose on the head. This will add the good effect of friction to the coldness of the water. Where the hair is too long for such frequent washing, daily cold water treatment may be applied by dipping the finger tips in cold water and rubbing it into the scalp, progressively covering the whole surface and vigorously massaging. Frequent washing of the hair in cold water, without soap, and drying in the air will obviate the necessity of washing often with soap. When it becomes necessary to use soap for cleansing purposes (and it should be used no oftener than absolutely necessary), use only pure Castile soap and tepid, never hot, water, rinsing thoroughly in warm and then cold water. If plenty of cold water is used in finishing, the scalp thoroughly rubbed and the hair dried in the open air, there will be no danger of "catching cold" if one is living according to the natural regimen. Avoid the use of commercial shampoos.([1])

SECTION XIV

WARM AND HOT WATER APPLICATIONS

1. **Tepid Baths.** Tepid baths vary in heat from 70° to 90°F. Many find them refreshing, but those who have become used to the effect of cold bathing find them rather enervating and weakening.

([1])
    It should be noted that baldness and an unhealthy condition of the hair are commonly associated with an imbalance of the endocrine system and may be due to this as much as to circulatory trouble or disease conditions of the scalp. In such cases it may, therefore, be indicated that some form of endocrinotherapy such as that of Dr. Jules Samuels is required. It should also be noted that Lindlahr believed that hair should be cut only during the first quarter of the moon and that this promotes the health and growth of the hair.

2. **Tepid Sitz Bath.** The tepid sitz bath is taken in the same way as the cold sitz bath but with the water somewhat warmer, say from 60° to 70°F. Such a lukewarm sitz bath is often indicated where there is retention of urine from a heated or inflamed condition of the urethra or bladder. It soothes and relaxes these structures and allows the urine to flow. If the temperature of the body is much above the normal the sitz bath should be taken in water of natural temperature, as it comes from the tap. In all cases of fevers, where the patient is able to arise from the bed and take the cold sitz bath, it will prove of great benefit. While in the bath the patient should lave the abdominal parts with the cold water.

3. **Warm and Hot Baths.** It is only on rare occasions that we recommend bathing at high temperature. Continually indulged in, it weakens the circulation, enervates the superficial nervous system and leads to atrophy of the cuticle. The effect of warm and hot bathing on the skin shows in the eyes through the heavy dark scurf rim in the outer border of the iris.

4. **Turkish, Russian and Electric Light Baths.** For reasons before mentioned the natural healer never uses these or other forms of sweating processes unless it is as a temporary application for the breaking of a cold or incipient fever as described under Sweating in Bed. While it is true that vigorous perspiration draws blood to the surface and promotes elimination of waste matter, such perspiration should be induced in a natural way, not through heating the body artificially. The best perspiration is that induced through walking or other exercise in warm weather, or through wet packs in bed, which we shall describe hereafter. Sweating, if it can be produced without overheating the body unduly, is of especial value in dropsical conditions and in cases of advanced diabetes and Bright's disease. It is also very beneficial in all forms of chronic rheumatism.

5. **Sweating in Bed.** This is best accomplished by means of the cold whole body pack, if necessary, assisted by hot water bottles or hot drinks. The sheet can be wrung out in warm water instead of cold if the temperature of the body is subnormal. The procedure to be used is fully explained in Sec. XV. The removal of the pack must be followed immediately by a quick cold rub, standing up in the bathtub or in a washtub; or if the patient is too weak for this, by a cold friction rub in bed. The cold rub is frequently followed by a fine after-sweat, which may continue from ten to thirty minutes, according to the vitality of the patient. After this another cold bath or cold rub should be given. The patient is then allowed rest. One or two such bed sweat baths or whole body packs are usually sufficient to break up a bad cold or incipient febrile disease. If it should not succeed in breaking up the congestion and aborting the fever, it will surely cause it to run a much easier course. This is accomplished in a

perfectly natural manner through increased heat radiation and forced elimination of morbid matter through the skin. Perspiration will be greatly facilitated by drinking either cool or warm water, or hot lemonade. In extreme cases, where the patient does not react to a whole body pack and is in danger of chilling, perspiration can be induced by giving hot lemonade or a small cup of hot coffee with lemon juice. If the patient is too weak to endure the rather heroic but very effective whole body pack treatment, partial packs such as trunk, throat and leg packs may be applied, reinforced by hot water bottles or hot bricks. These are more easily applied and endured. (For description of the partial packs see Sec. XV, Nos. 9 to 19.)

In an extensive practice, extending over a period of eighteen years, I have always found the sweating in bed perferable to the use of artificial apparatus, which is always more or less dangerous and more exhausting and injurious to the skin than the simple hot or cold wet packs, which have a powerful "drawing" effect upon the circulation and at the same time relax the pores of the skin.([1])

Sweating for the cure of disease is very much in favour among the Indians. While living in the Rocky Mountains I frequently had occasion to observe the Turkish bath contrivance of the Indians. The sweating treatment is given (no matter what the disease may be) by placing the patient under a wickerwork frame covered almost airtight with skins. Before the patient enters the low, boxlike hut, several pails or tin pans have been set into holes in the ground. These are filled with boiling water and from time to time hot stones from a nearby fire are dropped into the hot water to keep up the production of steam. When the patient has perspired to the limit of his endurance he is taken out and plunged into a nearby creek or lake, or in the winter time he is rubbed down quickly with snow. I relate this not because I approve of the steam bath but to draw attention to the fact that the natural instinct and good sense of the Indian has hit upon elimination as a therapeutic measure.

6. **Sweating by Exercise.** The most beneficial perspiration is that induced by brisk walking or other exercise. This should be followed by a quick cold bath, spray or rub. The warmer the body, within natural limits, the quicker the reaction from the cold water applications.

7. **Hot Compresses and Fomentations.** To prepare a fomentation take

([1])
It would seem that there are circumstances and cases in which pyretic baths, in which some degree of artificial fever is produced, can be of great value. They can be used rapidly to revivify and reactivate skin which has become dead and inactive and is too clogged to respond. It appears that the synapses involved react better with heat. The same may be said of Turkish and Finnish baths. After such procedures a cold shower or rub down should, of course, be taken.

a piece of flannel and fold it from six to ten times and form it into a roll. Dip this into water as hot as the patient can stand it. The temperature should range from blood heat to about 110°F., according to the endurance of the patient. Wring out the roll, unroll it quickly and lay it on the part which is to be treated. This may be the chest or abdomen, or the whole front or back, or it may be an inflamed arm, leg or joint. The hot compress should be covered and held in place by a cloth around the body or the limb, pinned down with safety pins.

We use hot fomentations or compresses only when the temperature is subnormal, and when the patient's vitality is so low that he cannot react to a cold pack or cold ablutions. It is a good sign if the body temperature rises as the result of the hot pack or compress. It means that the system, as the result of the tonic application, is arousing itself to acute febrile reaction, which we always welcome as nature's purifying, healing effort.

These procedures should be supplemented if possible by expert manipulative treatment.

SECTION XV

WET BANDAGES AND WET PACKS

1. **Wet Bandages.** Old muslin, linen sheeting, or soft, well worn towelling are the best materials for bandages and packs. Bandages are used mostly for extracting internal heat, for relieving internal congestion, and for promoting elimination of morbid matter through the skin. Cold water is best suited for these purposes, but where the patient is very sensitive to cold, or the temperature subnormal, the chill may be taken off or tepid water may be used. The bandages are soaked in the water, then lightly wrung out and applied to the body where desired.

2. **Wet Packs.** The wet pack consists of the wet bandage before described plus a covering of dry flannel or woollen material, or of heavy towelling. The dry covering must overlap the upper and lower borders of the wet bandage about one half an inch. The dry covering serves to bring about a warm reaction and preserves the moisture in the bandage, and therefore the drawing effect of the pack is more powerful than that of the plain bandage.

The dry flannel, woollen or cotton covering may consist of from one to three or even four layers wrapped round the wet bandage. The outer end of the dry covering is pinned down and held in place by safety pins. The number of wet and dry wrappings depends upon the heat of the body and the vitality and power of reaction of the patient. The higher the fever heat and the more vigorous the body, as in childhood and youth, the more wet wrappings and the less dry covering is required. The lower the fever and the lower the vitality and power of reaction of the patient, the less wet wrappings and the more dry, warm covering is required. In chronic cases, with low or subnormal temperature, where packs are indicated to relieve inner congestion and pain, to induce sleep or to promote elimination, one wrapping of wet material is fully sufficient, and this must be covered with two or three wrappings of dry, warm material, in order to bring about the necessary reaction.

3. **Vinegar Bandages and Compresses.** Some hydrotherapists recommend an addition of vinegar or Epsom salts to the water from which the bandages or compresses are wrung out — about one half vinegar and one half water, or one tablespoon of Epsom salt to one quart of water. (See article on Epsom salt treatment below.)

4. **Potato Compress.** A compress made of grated raw potato, applied between pieces of thin linen or cotton cloth, is especially recommended in all forms of inflammation of the eye. It must be renewed before it becomes hot and dry.

5. **How Often Should the Wet Packs Be Renewed.** This depends upon the severity of the fever, height of the temperature, and upon the vitality of the patient. In an ordinary cold it may be sufficient to apply a throat and short body pack in the evening and to leave it on all night, to be followed in the morning by a good cold rub and cold water sniffing. The more pronounced the fever and the higher the temperature, the oftener the wet bandages must be renewed. In fevers such as diphtheria, smallpox, typhoid, cerebrospinal meningitis, etc., the packs must be taken off and replaced by fresh ones as soon as they are hot and dry. In such cases it is advisable to have on hand several sets of bandages. Those which come from the body must be thoroughly washed, rinsed in cold water and hung up to dry in the fresh air and sunshine. In serious and prolonged cases of inflammatory feverish disease it is advisable to alternate between throat, trunk and leg packs. For instance, at one time put on throat and trunk pack, then apply leg packs only, then again throat, and so on. This tends to equalize the circulation.

6. **Ablution After Pack.** Every time a bandage or pack has served its purpose and is taken from the body, the parts covered by it must be rubbed with a rough towel dipped in cold water. This serves several important purposes: first, to cleanse the skin of the morbid matter and poisons which the bandage or pack has drawn to the surface; second, to

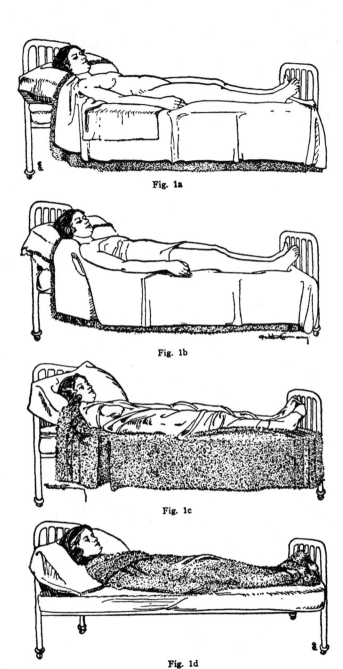

Fig. 1a

Fig. 1b

Fig. 1c

Fig. 1d

89

secure a better reaction; third, to promote heat radiation; fourth, to increase the electromagnetic energies of the body.

7. **Whole Body Pack.** Spread on a bed or couch two or three blankets, according to the season of the year, the warmth of the room and the heat of the patient's body. Over the blankets spread a bed sheet which has been wrung out in cold water; over this spread the muslin strip of a trunk pack wrung out in cold water. Wrap this strip about the trunk; then wrap the wet sheet quickly around the body of the patient, tucking it in between the legs and also between the body and the arms. Then pick up the top blanket and tuck it in around the body, folding the ends over the feet and around the neck; then pick up the second and third blankets and do likewise, pinning in place with safety pins. When finished, the patient and the pack look very much like an Egyptian mummy. (Figs 1a, b, c, d.)

The patient should react and begin to perspire, or at least to feel comfortably warm, within five or ten minutes. If he remains cold too long, put along each side of the body two or three hot water bottles, or bricks heated in an oven and wrapped in flannel, then cover the whole over with a few more blankets. The patient should be allowed to remain in the whole body pack and perspire as long as he can stand it. This may be from ten to thirty minutes or more, but should not be extended too long as this might exhaust the patient unduly. The removal of the pack must be followed by a quick cold rub, standing up in the bathtub or in a washtub; or, if the patient is too weak for this by a cold friction rub in bed.

8. **Head Bandages.** These bandages are much in favour for relieving headaches and earaches. A towel or strip of muslin or linen cloth is wrung out of tepid or cold water and wrapped round the head or over the ears in order to draw the blood to the surface and relieve inner congestion. This, however, is a doubtful proceeding for treating headaches or pains in the head, because all wet bandages have a tendency to draw the blood to the part where they are applied. In this case, though the head bandage may draw the blood to the surface of the skull, at the same time it has a tendency to draw the blood from other parts of the body to the head, thereby increasing congestion. For this reason I always advise using the body, leg or throat pack to draw the blood away from the head. Besides these packs cover a greater surface of the body and therefore have greater power to relieve the inner congestion in the head, as well as anywhere else in the body. At the same time, head, face and neck may be frequently washed or sponged with cold water. The evaporation of the water on the hot surface has a very cooling, refreshing and also electrifying effect.

9. **Throat Bandage and Pack.** A thin piece of linen, muslin, towelling or soft cotton from two to four inches wide, according to the length of the neck, wrung out of cold water and wrapped from two to four or six times

90

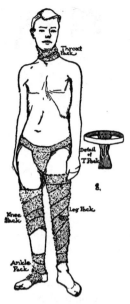

Fig. 2

around the throat is a splendid application in cases or sore and inflamed throat, tonsils and glands of the throat and neck. It also has a very cooling effect on the circulation in general, because the blood passes through the neck, back and forth through the large arteries and veins which supply the head and brain. Here large masses of blood course nearer the surface than anywhere else in the body, and therefore it is the best place for extracting heat from the blood through cold water bandages, packs and compresses. The throat pack consists of a throat bandage plus a covering of dry flannel or woollen material. (Fig. 2.)

10. **Chest Bandage and Pack.** This is of great benefit when the lungs are affected by acute bronchial catarrh or pneumonia. The cold wet strip of muslin must be wide enough to cover the chest from the armpits to the border of the small ribs, and must be long enough to go round the body from one to four times, according to the amount of heat in the body, and the vitality of the patient and his power of reaction. The chest pack consists of the chest bandage plus a covering of dry flannel or woollen material.

11. **Trunk Bandage and Pack.** The trunk bandage is applied in the same way as the chest bandage, the only difference being that it extends from under the armpits to the upper border of the hip bone or to the pubis. The full length, from armpit to pubis, must be applied in cases of

91

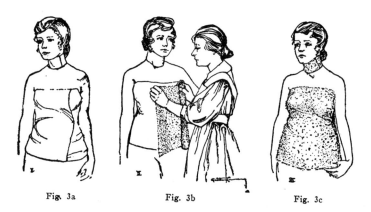

Fig. 3a   Fig. 3b   Fig. 3c

the inflammation of the bladder, appendix or ovaries. When any one of the organs is severely inflamed extra cold compresses may be placed in under the body pack and over the inflamed organ. This compress should consist of from two to six or even eight layers of muslin or towelling, and may be from six to twelve inches square, according to the size of the inflamed area and according to the heat of the parts. All bandages must be removed and renewed when hot and dry. The extra cold compresses may also be applied under the chest or body pack, to inflamed areas in the lungs, liver and stomach. The trunk pack consists of the trunk bandage plus a covering of dry flannel or woollen material. (Figs 3a, b, c.)

12. **Eye Compress.** The cold wet compress is very beneficial for relieving congestion and inflammation in the eyes. For this purpose a small compress made of several layers of muslin or linen is dipped in cold water and applied over the eyes. The compress is held in place by a dry bandage. Better than the water compress in cases of serious inflammation of the eyes is a poultice made of grated raw potatoes. The grated potato is wrapped in linen or muslin cloth and placed over the affected eye. The poultice is kept in place in the same way as the water compress. This treatment has proved very beneficial in cases of glaucoma and gonorrheal inflammation.

13. **Ankle, Knee and Hand Packs.** These are applied in the same way as all other wet packs, and are indicated in all local inflammation in the ankles, feet, toes, hands, wrists and arms. They are especially valuable in relieving inflammation is cases of inflammatory rheumatism. The results of the wet pack and general cold water treatment in the most violent cases of inflammatory rheumatism are little short of miraculous. (Fig. 2, p.91.)

14. **Leg Pack.** This may be applied from the hip to the knee or from the knee to the ankle, or may cover the whole extremity from the hip to the toes. The method of application is the same as in all other packs.(Fig. 2.)

92

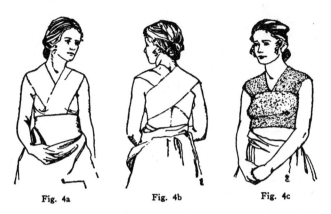

Fig. 4a   Fig. 4b   Fig. 4c

15. **T Pack.** This consists of a narrow strip of muslin, adjusted as a belt about the abdomen just above the hip bone, to the back of which is attached a bandage, cut a little narrower in the centre. The wet bandage with its flannel covering is drawn forward between the legs and fastened to the belt in front with safety pins. This pack is especially valuable in inflammations in the rectum and genito-urinary organs. In cases of high temperature, extra cold compresses may be inserted inside the pack.

16. **Shoulder or Scotch Pack.** This pack requires a bandage and flannel covering, six and eight inches wide respectively, and two and a quarter yards long. The one who applies the pack stands in front of the patient and holds equal portions of the strip of muslin or flannel in each hand. The strip is placed around the body under the armpits of the patient, the ends crossed in the back and brought up over the shoulders to the front, crossing again over the chest. After the shoulder pack itself has been applied it may be surrounded on the body by the chest or trunk pack. This pack is very valuable where the upper lobes of the lungs are affected by acute bronchial catarrh or pneumonia. (Figs 4a, b, c.)

SECTION XVI

MUD AND CLAY TREATMENT

Certain localities in Europe and in this country have attained considerable fame by the so-called mud bath treatment. We tried this form of treatment for several years in one of our institutions but with indifferent

93

success. The effect of the treatment is very much the same as that of the wet packs described in Sec. XV. The effect of the wet pack, poultice or compress is very much the same whether the material used be mud, clay, water, cottage cheese, flaxseed or any other mild acting substance. The beneficial results are brought about because the cool moisture in and under the packs or poultices relaxes the pores of the skin, draws the blood into the surface, relieves inner congestion and pain, and promotes heat radiation and elimination of morbid matter. I have found that on the whole the water applications produce fully as good results as mud, clay or other materials; besides it has the advantage of being more cleanly and more easily applied. However, it is true that in many cases of chronic inflammation resulting either from internal disease, bruises or sprains, clay packs have proved of great benefit. The one advantage I have found in them is that this substance retains moisture and coolness much longer than a water pack or compress. They are, therefore, of special benefit in cases of subacute and chronic inflammations, of persistent soreness, and for all night packs and bandages.

1. **Clay Packs.** The best way to apply clay packs is the following: Take yellow or, still better, blue potter's clay, macerate in warm water until it is reduced to a smooth paste. When cold spread this with a wooden paddle or broad knife over a strip of cloth wide enough and long enough to cover the part to be treated, then surround the clay bandage with a few wrappings of towelling, flannel or other protecting material. The clay packs may remain in place until they become hot and dry.

2. **Mud or Clay Baths.** The mud or clay baths are applied in a manner similar to that of the clay packs but on a larger scale — to the entire body from neck to feet. The mud or clay must first be macerated and sifted so as to remove all pebbles, twigs or other foreign materials. The siftings are then mixed with hot water and reduced to a smooth paste. Mud or clay does not heat on the body as readily as a water pack, therefore it is best to heat the clay to 70°F. before before it is applied. The warm paste is spread on a sheet and this is wrapped around the body. One or two blankets, according to the warmth of the room and the reactionary power of the patient, are then wrapped around the mud pack. The mud bath is applied like the full sheet pack described under Sec. XV, No. 7, the only difference being that the sheet, instead of being wrung out in water, is covered with a layer of mud or clay as described under Clay Packs. Care must be taken that the mud or clay used for such treatments is free from impurities. It should not be taken from localities contaminated by human refuse. The mud or clay bath is followed by a cleansing warm spray and rub, and finished with a quick tonic spray.

While it is true that many people suffering from rheumatism and kindred acid diseases have found temporary relief by patronizing the popular mud bath resorts, it is also true that these "cures" are not permanent. The reason is that in these places practically no attention is paid to diet. The patrons live on the ordinary hotel and restaurant food which produces hyperacidity almost as fast as the mud baths reduce it. Neither do such patients receive the benefits of hydropathic, manipulative and other natural methods. The result is that after resuming at home their accustomed mode of living, the "cured" patients soon again experience the old rheumatic aches and pains and other symptoms of hyperacidity. Many of our patients suffering from such ailments had time and again tried the various mud cures but experienced only temporary relief. It required the strict pure food diet, hydropathic and manipulative treatment, sun and air baths and the outdoor life to produce real and permanent cures.

SECTION XVII

EPSOM SALT TREATMENT

I have received numerous enquiries from readers of my writings, some of them practising physicians, asking why I have neglected to mention Epsom salt treatment, which has proved so efficacious for the cure of acute and chronic diseases. I have had ample opportunity to observe the good and bad effects of Epsom salt upon the system, and will briefly state the result of my experience.

The use of Epsom salt (magnesium sulphate), internally and externally, is in harmony with natural therapeutics in so far as the alkaline magnesium tends to neutralize and to eliminate pathogenic substances, such as carbon and nitrogen compounds, from the system. While Epsom salt taken internally as a laxative, or externally in the form of baths, packs and compresses, is a powerful neutralizer and eliminator of acids, ptomaines and xanthines, we must not overlook the fact that the inorganic minerals it contains have a strong tendency to accumulate in the system and to form deposits which may in time become as harmful as the morbid materials which the salts are meant to eliminate from the system. Some time ago, one of our house physicians attended an autopsy performed on a woman who had died from chronic rheumatism and heart disease. It was found that the woman's heart muscle contained deposits of magnesium salts and of carbonate of sodium, which she had taken through many years as a cure for acidosis and rheumatism. These alkaline mineral elements when taken in the inorganic form show plainly in the iris. Before I became acquainted with the natural laws of living and of treatment, I had for several years taken large quantities of sodium bicarbonate and magnesium sulphate to neutralize hyperacidity of the stomach and of the system in general. The presence of the minerals in my system was revealed in the eyes by a broad white ring in the outer rim of the iris. Since I have ceased taking the minerals and have lived on eliminative foods, the ring in the iris has almost entirely disappeared (see Iridiagnosis, Vol. VI). I have seen the signs of sodium, iron, potassium, calcium and magnesium in the eyes of people who had used these minerals in the form of medicines, or who had absorbed them in alkaline drinking water.

In our work we do not employ these doubtful agents which may in the long run work more harm than good, because we have other means and methods to accomplish the same results in a less harmful and more natural way. A well balanced vegetarian diet, as described above, will prevent excessive formation of pathogenic substances in the system. The best way to eliminate these morbid materials, after they have created disease conditions, is to take in sufficient amounts of the positive alkaline mineral elements in the foods classified under Group 5 (see Food Table). These mineral elements when taken in the live organic form are the best neutralizers and eliminators, and they will not accumulate and form deposits in the system even when taken in excess. In addition to the alkaline diet we use hydrotherapy, neurotherapy and other methods of natural treatment to eliminate negative, pathogenic encumbrances from the system. I do not mean to intimate, however, that I condemn the use of Epsom salt in all circumstances. On the contrary, we quite frequently make use of it in the form of external applications in order to attain quick results in acute and emergency cases. Epsom salt baths, packs and compresses are very useful in cases of acute inflammatory rheumatism, gout, pneumonia, Bright's disease, appendicitis, ptomaine poisoning and in all other feverish diseases, but in no circumstance would I use or recommend the salt for long continued treatment.

The therapeutic action of magnesium sulphate, or common Epsom salt, consists in stimulating the eliminative activity of the skin, its pores and glandular structures. The result is also obtained in a lesser degree by ordinary table salt and by sea salt.[1] All the positive alkaline salts applied to the skin in the form of packs, sponges, baths, etc., have a

[1]
Sea salt, owing to its many trace elements, is much to be preferred for baths and packs to ordinary table salt.

powerful electromagnetic effect upon the system. They arouse electro-magnetic activity between the positive alkaline salts on the surface and the negative cell constituents in the body. Physiologists claim that minerals are not absorbed through the skin unless mixed with fats in the form of unguents or emulsions. The records in the iris prove that mercury, iodine, lead, zinc, silver, etc., are absorbed through the skin and then locate in the system in localities for which they exhibit a special affinity. If the Epsom salt is not absorbed the external application can have no acid neutralizing effect within the system. If it is absorbed it is bound to assist in the formation of earthy deposits. This is sure to be the result if the salt is taken internally for any length of time.

The Epsom salt may be applied to the skin in warm or cold solutions, in the form of local applications in wet packs and compresses, as a general sponge bath, whole body bath or as a sitz or hip bath. The solution should contain from one to two ounces of magnesium sulphate to one quart of water. The bandages or compresses may be soaked in the solution and applied in the ordinary way. One of the most beneficial applications consists in sponging the entire body with the solution for from five to ten minutes and going to bed without drying. This draws the blood into the cuticle, makes the skin more alive and active, opens the pores and draws the pathogenic matter to the surface. It acts as a powerful stimulant to the glandular structures of the skin, promotes elimination and relieves the poisoned and overburdened heart and other vital organs. In similar manner it relieves the heart-regulating centre in the medulla and thereby reduces the temperature in febrile conditions. Undoubtedly a great part of the beneficial effect is due to the action of the water itself in the ablutions and compresses. The Epsom salt solution may be applied also in the form of cooling hip and sitz baths, or in the ordinary bath. In all cases the salt will heighten the tonic effect of the water. One reason why I do not recommend the continued use of the salt in such applications is because we find that the cold water alone, used continuously in the form of tonic applications, is powerful enough for the requirements of the various regimens in health and disease. In acute febrile conditions, however, when rapid neutralization and elimination of pathogenic substance is imperative, tonic applications of sea salt and Epsom salt will be found very beneficial.

SECTION XVIII

ENEMATA, KLYSMAS OR COLONIC FLUSHING

Injections of warm water into the rectum are taken in order to relieve the constipated intestines of accumulated faecal matter and thus to prevent the reabsorption of morbid matter and systemic poisons. The necessity for enemata is a sure sign that the person who needs them has not been living the natural life. If he had, he would not be constipated. We make use of enemata only in the treatment of acute diseases, during fasting and in stubborn cases of chronic constipation, in the beginning of the treatment. We look upon enemata as a necessary evil, or "crutch", to be used only until, through natural living and treatment, the intestines have become more alive and active. Enemata taken habitually have a weakening effect upon the intestines. As the saying goes they make them "more lazy". The reason for this is obvious. Dryness of the faecal matter is the stimulus for the secretion of mucous fluids by the membranous linings of the bowels. When the intestines are constantly flooded with water through the rectum, the stimulus to secretion is lacking and the cellular linings and glandular structures of the intestines become more inactive. Any function of the organism which we do not use atrophies. Continued flooding with warm water has a very relaxing effect upon the intestines. The tone of the muscular tissues is lowered from day to day and the intestines become distended, forming pockets for the retention of putrefying faecal matter. Like drugs and laxatives, the "internal bath" in the long run creates the very conditions which it is supposed to cure, namely, greater inactivity and atrophy.

The only way to restore the natural activity of the bowels in cases of chronic constipation is through natural diet, fasting when indicated, and through the various forms of massage and neurotherapy. Careful scientific manipulation of the spinal nerve centres and of the abdomen is the most efficient method for infusing the atonic organs with new life and vigour. It is impossible to cure many stubborn, chronic cases of constipation without massage and spinal treatment. Skilful manipulation of the abdomen mechanically propels the impacted faeces onward towards the outlet and at the same time stimulates and strengthens the muscles of the intestines themselves. The passive manipulative treatment is especially valuable in cases where constipation is partly due to sedentary habits of life.

1. For the passive treatment the patient should lie on the back, the knees slightly drawn up. The upper part of the body should be somewhat

elevated. The manipulator takes his position on the right side of the patient and begins to knead the colon with the flattened finger tips in circular motion on the left side, in the region of the sigmoid flexure (in the left groin). He then gradually works upward along the descending colon, shoving the faecal matter always towards the rectum; then from left to right along the transverse colon; then downward along the ascending colon. Many instructors advise the opposite procedure. They commence the kneading in the right inguinal region (right groin) and work upward along the ascending colon, then along the transverse and downward along the descending colon. This procedure, however, has a tendency to pile up the contents of the large intestine long before they reach the outlet. It may cause serious impactions and obstructions. To me it seems more rational to commence the loosening of the faecal matter near the outlet and work continually toward it. (See illustration.)

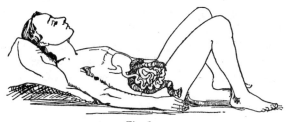

Fig. 5

2. The abdominal massage exercise (Sec. XXI, No. 10) and also the exercises in bed and on the back (Sec. XXI, Nos. 17, 18, 19) will prove of great benefit, and in many cases are absolutely indispensable.

3. In cases of spasm of the sphincter muscle and the rectum, relaxation can be induced by rectal dilatation, using various kinds of dilators, or by pressing the finger tips along both sides of the coccyx from one to three minutes at a time, two or three times a day. (See coccygeal treatment, Sec. XXVIII, Nos. 16, 17.)

4. **Temperature of Enemata.** The water for enemata or for internal douches should never be cold, as many books and certain doctors advise. This is very dangerous. The sudden internal chilling may produce depression of vital activities, collapse and even death. A year ago I was called to attend a boy eight years old. I found him in the advanced stages of cerebro-spinal meningitis. The physician who was in attendance told me she kept the fever down easily by giving three or four cold enemata every day. This probably helped to turn the gastro-enteric fever with which the illness started into cerebro-spinal meningitis. I prescribed pack treatment and fasting instead of the cold enemata and "stuffing". The

young patient made a perfect recovery. The water used for enemata or internal douches should be about blood temperature, from 90° to 100°F. If no thermometer is at hand, test the temperature by dipping the bare elbow into the water. The heat of the water should be just endurable to the sensitive tip of the elbow. For vigorous persons and in high fevers the temperature of the enema may be as low as 85°F. The lower the vitality and temperature of the patient the warmer must be the water. In cases of subnormal temperature, collapse and suspended animation, hot enemata of from 100° to 110°F. act as powerful tonics. The tonic effects are increased if the water contains about one teaspoonful of salt to a pint (normal salt solution).

5. **Application of Enemata.** Enemata should never be taken in the sitting position or while lying on the right or left side. When attempting to take an enema in either of these positions the rubber mouthpiece of the syringe strikes the sigmoid flexure and the tube coils up. The best positions for taking enemata are lying on the back, and the knee–chest position. The former is more suitable for bedfast patients too weak to assume the knee–chest position. The patient should lie on the bed or a couch or board with the knee raised. The head must lie lower than the feet. This can be attained by raising the lower end of the bed, couch or board. (Fig. 5.)

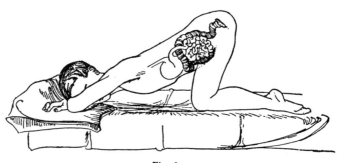

Fig. 6

6. **Knee–Chest Position.** Fig. 6 illustrates why the knee–chest position is the best of all, provided a person is strong enough to assume it. This position offers the least resistance to the passage of the warm water through the sigmoid flexure, descending colon and transverse colon. Under favourable conditions the water may descend even into the ascending colon. Care should be taken to dip the hard rubber nozzle of the tube into olive oil and the tube should not be inserted until all air has been expelled and until the water flows from the nozzle at the proper temperature. In cases where old, hard incrustations have to be softened, a little

100

Castile soap may be dissolved in the water. The water should be retained in the intestines for five or ten minutes in order to allow the hardened faecal matter and incrustations to soften. (Fig. 6.)

7. **Directions for Colon Flushing.** Apparatus necessary: a douche bag or can with rubber hose, and a flexible rubber tube about twenty-six inches long. The latter is fitted to the end of the rubber hose by means of a hard rubber connection. Fill the bag with about two quarts of warm soapy water (the soap used should be super-fatty soap free from all alkali, or, better, a good quality of Castile soap). Lubricate the colon tube with olive oil. After allowing the water to flow until it comes from the tube at the right temperature, stop the flow and insert about two or three inches of the tube into the rectum. Release the clip on the hose and allow the water to flow. Then slowly and carefully work the tube, pushing it in two or three inches more and withdrawing it about half that distance. Continue this until the greater part of the tube is within the colon. If any obstruction is met with while the tube is being inserted, withdraw the tube and allow the patient to evacuate the contents of the rectum and then begin over again. Should the accumulation of too much water in some particular part of the colon cause pain, shut off the flow by pinching the tube, have the patient take a full breath, draw in the abdomen and hold it so until the pain passes, after which again allow the water to flow.([1])

Some difficulty may at first be experienced by the patient in following out this method. However, no disappointment should be felt if the results are not satisfactory from the first or second trial. The can should be placed only two or three feet above the level of the anus. No force is necessary. Should any distress be felt during the operation, it should be abandoned for the time and taken up again the next night. Continue these colon flushings for two or three nights in succession. The last night, instead of using soapy water, use one level teaspoonful of salt to a pint of water. If there is a feeling of too great relaxation in the rectum, or a feeling of irritation, the patient should apply cold cloths to the rectum or take an after injection of from one half to a full cupful of cool water, inserting the tube only about two inches. After the patient has become somewhat experienced in the use of colonic flushings, he should endeavour to retain the water from ten to fifteen minutes, while lying on the back and massaging the abdomen.

8. **Enemata in Acute Diseases.** In all acute, inflammatory, febrile diseases we give enemata in the beginning daily, and after that at longer

([1])
The Studa Chair method of colonic flushing would appear to have great advantages over other methods as it tends to encourage the peristaltic movements of the bowel and to tone up the musculature. However, the necessary apparatus for this method is now difficult or impossible to obtain, at least in England.

intervals, according to the nature of the case and the vitality of the patient. Fasting in acute disease and increased heat in the abdominal organs usually produce constipation. We overcome this difficulty by enemata. This empties the lower intestines of morbid accumulations and prevents reabsorption of poisonous excretions. The bowels should be emptied as nearly as possible during the early stages of a fever, as long as the vitality is unimpaired.

9. **Enemata While Fasting.** While fasting the bowels usually cease moving, though I have seen remarkable exceptions where the bowels kept moving for a few weeks, though no food was taken. If they cease to move soon after the fast is begun, it is best to give enemata in order to evacuate the intestines and prevent reabsorption of morbid and poisonous excretions.

SECTION XIX

MISCELLANEOUS TREATMENTS

1. **Treatment for Retention of Urine.** Retention of urine may be due to many different causes, and treatment must vary accordingly. It occurs frequently as the result of inflammation of the kidneys, bladder or urethra. These inflammations may be caused by:

(a) Toxic conditions created by almost any form of acute disease especially by acute or chronic gonorrhoea.
(b) Certain drug poisons.
(c) Toxic condition of the system resulting from hyperacidity or from large amounts of ptomaines, alkaloids, xanthines and other systemic poisons excreted through the kidneys.
(d) Mechanical obstructions.
(e) Spastic or paralytic contraction.
(f) Inactivity of the kidneys.

The best and most efficient remedies in all such cases are cold bandages, compresses, packs, and cold hip and sitz baths. When the urinary organs are in a state of high inflammation the patient may remain in the hip or sitz bath for an hour or more at a time. While the bath must be cooling, care should be taken not to chill the parts. The temperature must vary according to the condition of the patient and his power of reaction. The greater the internal heat, the colder may be the water and the oftener it must be renewed. Although the water in the bath is cold at the start, it will quickly warm up to the body heat of the patient, and when it loses its coolness fresh cold water should be added.

102

In all cases where retention of urine is due to acute inflammatory conditions, neurotherapy must be relaxing and inhibitory. This will relieve the tension of the nerves and blood vessels and promote the excretion of the urine from the kidneys and its discharge from the bladder. Our coccygeal inhibition is of special value for this purpose. This consists in placing the thumbs on the right and left of the coccyx and exerting deep steady pressure for from three to five minutes (Sec. XXVIII, No. 17).

If the patient is too weak to use a sitz bath or an ordinary bathtub, cold compresses, bandages and packs will be the best substitutes. The packs and compresses must be changed when they become hot or dry, and should always be followed by a quick cold rub with a rough towel dipped in cold water. In cases of great weakness or collapse, where the skin is cold and pale and the pulse weak, hot enemata of normal salt solution have a vivifying effect. In such cases a brisk cold rub should be given all over the body immediately after the hot enema. If suppression or retention of urine is caused by weakness and prostration the hot enemata are the best means of stimulating the urinary organs to renewed activity. The temperature of these hot enemata may range from 100° to 115°F., according to the endurance of the patient. Warm enemata are usually followed by a more copious flow of urine, indicating that they have a relaxing effect upon the kidneys and bladder. In cases of weakness, prostration and atrophy of the urinary organs, tonic neurotherapy treatment is always of great value.

2. **The Treatment for Retention of Urine due to Mechanical Obstruction.** Obstruction to the passage of urine may be caused by stones, large clots of blood, or by profuse excretion of mucous matter. In such cases the warm and even hot sitz bath may be of good service on account of its relaxing effect upon the tissues of the urinary organs. The passage of solid substance through the ureters and the urethra may be greatly facilitated by gentle downward stroking and manipulative treatment, also through relaxing neurotherapy (coccygeal) treatment (Sec. XXVIII, No. 17). For mechanical dilatation of the rectum, prostate and urethra, see "Orificial Treatment", Sec. XXVIII, Nos. 8-12.

3. **Treatment for the Retention of Urine due to Spastic and Paralytic Conditions.** This occurs frequently after the use of irritating diuretics and in the wake of hysteria or hypochondria. In all such cases lukewarm but cooling sitz baths will be beneficial. The most important treatment in such cases consists in inhibition of the nerve centres by neurotherapy. In such cases, also, mechanical and manipulative dilatation of rectum and urethra as described under "Orificial Treatment", Sec. XXVIII, is indicated and often highly beneficial.

4. Treatment of Retention of Urine due to Inactivity of the Kidneys. This condition may be due to chronic nephritis or of a clogging of the kidneys through long continued food, drink and drug poisoning. In order to cure this as well as all other chronic diseases the entire system must undergo a complete regeneration through natural living and treatment. But meanwhile the activity of the kidneys may be increased by the use of mild stimulants such as juniper berries eaten raw or in the form of tea. Kneipp's favourite prescription in such cases was as follows: Take three berries the first day, five the second, seven the third, and so on until the daily dose amounts to twenty-one berries. Then the dose is reduced in the same way at the rate of two berries per day. After the course is completed a rest is taken for a few weeks and then the treatment is repeated if necessary.

5. **Juniper Berry Tea.** This is prepared in the following manner: Upon half a dozen or more macerated juniper berries pour half a cupful of boiling water; let this draw, and sip while warm. A little honey or maple or brown sugar (unrefined) may be added if desired. Two such doses, or in severe cases three, may be taken in twenty-four hours.

6. **Asparagus Tea.** The water in which fresh asparagus has been boiled for from ten to fifteen minutes is also a mild and harmless diuretic. It may be taken in half teacupful doses three or four times a day.

These special treatments for retention of urine should always be accompanied by the general natural treatment, which tends to overcome the constitutional diseases back of the local trouble.

SECTION XX

AIR, LIGHT AND SUN BATHS

What Is the Cause of Poor Skin Action?

Man is naturally an "air animal". He breathes with the pores of the skin as well as the lungs. However, the custom of hiding the body under dense, heavy clothing, thus excluding it from the life-giving influence of air and light, together with the habit of warm bathing, has weakened and enervated the skin of the average individual until it has lost its tonicity and is no longer capable of fulfilling its natural functions. The compact, almost airtight layers of underwear and outer clothing made of cotton, wool, silk and leather prevent the ventilation of the skin and the escape of the morbid excretions of the body. Underwear, if worn at all, should be light and of porous weave, just close enough to absorb the perspiration but not close enough to prevent free escape of the poisonous exhalations of the skin. Thorough ventilation of the skin ensures perfect evaporation of the perspiration, and this not only promotes cleanliness but has a wonderfully cooling effect upon the body in the heat of summer.

1. **The Skin Is an Organ of Absorption.** as well as of excretion; consequently the systemic poisons which are eliminated from the organism, if not removed by proper ventilation and bathing, are reabsorbed into the system just as the poisonous exhalations from the lungs are reinhaled and reabsorbed by people congregating in closed rooms or sleeping in unventilated bedrooms. Who would think of keeping plants or animals continuously covered up, secluded from air and light? We know they would wither and waste away, and die before long. Nevertheless, civilized human beings have for ages hidden their bodies most carefully from sun and air, which are so necessary to their well being. Is it any wonder that the human cuticle has become withered, enervated and atrophied, that it has lost the power to perform its functions freely and efficiently? Undoubtedly, this has much to do with the prevalence of disease.

In the iris of the eye the atrophied condition of the skin is indicated by a heavy, dark rim, called the "scurf rim". It signifies that the skin has become anaemic, the surface circulation sluggish and defective, and that the elimination of morbid matter and systemic poisons through the skin is handicapped and retarded. This, in turn, causes systemic poisoning and favours the development of all kinds of acute and chronic diseases.

2. **The Importance of the Skin as an Organ of Elimination.** Of late physiologists have claimed that the skin is not of great importance as an organ of elimination. Common experience and the diagnosis from the eye teach us differently. The black rim, seen more or less distinctly in the outer margin of the iris in the eyes of the majority of people, had been called the "scurf rim" because it was found that this dark rim appears in the iris after the suppression of "scurfy" and other forms of skin eruptions, and after the external or internal use of lotions, ointments and medicines containing mercury, zinc, iodine, arsenic or other poisons which suppress or destroy the life and activities of the skin. Therefore, when we see in the iris of a person a heavy scurf rim we can tell him at once: "Your cuticle is in a sluggish, atrophied condition, the surface circulation and elimination through the skin are defective and as a result of this there is a strong tendency to systemic poisoning; you take cold easily and suffer from chronic catarrhal conditions." For the same reasons a heavy scurf rim indicates what is ordinarily called a "scrofulous condition", it stands for impoverished and vitiated blood. This certainly shows the great

importance of the skin as an organ of elimination and the necessity of keeping it in the best possible condition. It explains why an atrophied skin has so much to do with the causation of disease and why, in the treatment of both acute and chronic ailments, exposure to air and cold water produce such wonderful results.

The favourite method of diagnosis employed by Father Kneipp, the great Water Cure Apostle, was to examine the skin of his patients. If the "jacket" as he called it, was in fairly good condition he predicted a speedy recovery. If he found the "jacket" shrivelled and dry, weakened and atrophied, he would shake his head and inform the patient that it would take much time and patience to restore him to health. He, as well as other pioneers of the Nature Cure movement, realized that elimination is the keynote in the treatment of acute and chronic diseases.

3. **How to Take an Air Bath.** Everybody should take an air bath daily, for twenty minutes or longer, if possible. It may be advantageously combined with the morning cold rub and exercises as described under Sec. I. Sixteen years ago we constructed the first open-air bath on the roof of our Chicago Sanatorium. I predicted in the Nature Cure Magazine that the time would come when every up-to-date residence would have its air bath as well as its facilities for water bathing. This prediction is already being fulfilled. As a result of Nature Cure propaganda open-air sleeping porches, sun parlours and air baths are rapidly increasing in popularity. All the hospitals built in the neighbourhood of our Chicago Sanitorium have brick and iron enclosures on the roofs, similar to air bath construction. Their patients, however, still take the air and sun while heavily clothed and thus fail to receive the full benefit of air and sunlight.

A regularly constructed air bath is open above (without roof) and surrounded by shutter-like walls constructed of outward and downward sloping slats mortised on the upright posts so as to allow free passage of air and exclude any view of the interior from neighbouring buildings. If surroundings permit, it is better to have the air bath on the ground for reasons explained later. This allows not only nude exposure to the air but also nude contact with the earth which, in itself, is highly beneficial. An air bath on the level ground may be enclosed by shutter work, by solid board walls or by canvas sheets. If possible, spend the hours of rest, and perform such daily tasks as may be feasible, in the air bath. If an open air bath cannot be provided, expose the body to air and light in a room best located for the purpose. In the seclusion of this room remain nude as much as possible. But, after all, the air of a room cannot have the electromagnetic effect of moving currents of open-air breezes, saturated with ozone and sunlight. Many naturists, having experienced the benefits of lying nude in bed, never again wear night clothing even though the bedroom be swept through the night by vigorous breezes. These are the people who have lost the habit of catching cold.

Only those who habitually practise air bathing can appreciate its soothing and tonic effect upon the millions of nerve endings all over the surface of the body. This explains the splendid results obtained by air, sun and cold water bathing in cases of nervousness, neurasthenia, and emotional and mental disorders. Even among the adherents of natural healing methods there are those who think that air and light baths should be taken out of doors in warm weather only, and in winter time only in well heated rooms. This is a mistake. The effect of the air bath upon the organism is subject to the same law of action and reaction which governs the effect of water applications. If the temperature of air or water is the same, or nearly the same, as that of the body no reaction takes place — the conditions within the system remain the same. But if the temperature of air or water is considerably lower than the body temperature there will be a reaction. In order to react against the chilling effect of cold air or water, the nerve centres which control the circulation send the blood to the surface in large quantities, flushing the skin with warm, red, arterial blood. The flow of the blood stream is greatly accelerated and the elimination of morbid matter on the surface of the body is correspondingly increased.

4. **Sun Bathing.** All the good effects of air bathing are intensified by the influence of sunlight. We will see that the effects of sunlight cannot be overestimated when we consider that without it life on this planet would be impossible. Everything that draws the breath of life depends for vital energy upon the life-giving rays of the sun. Beginners, however, must be careful not to expose the body to intense heat and light for too long at a time. This might cause overstimulation with its inevitable reaction, or serious burns. From ten to fifteen minutes may be sufficient to begin with. Dark-skinned people, having more protective pigment, can stand more exposure than can light-skinned people. As the skin bronzes or tans, exposure can be lengthened to twenty or thirty minutes, and gradually to several hours at a time. In the summer time, many of our patients spend all their leisure time in the air bath.

If possible the air bath should contain a spray so that a cold shower can be taken in warm weather while exposed to the air and sun. Allow the body to dry in the sun and air. The alternating influences of air, sunlight and water are as beneficial to the human body as to plant and animal life. Never miss an opportunity to take a nude rain bath. People who are exceedingly sensitive to the effects of sunlight may at least temporarily wear a wrap of white gauze, or seek shelter in shady spots. In bright sunlight it is best to protect the head by a straw hat. Those who are subject to excessive blood pressure to the brain should lay a towel wrung out of cold water over the head. For the treatment of sunburns see Sec. XLII, No. 30.

5. **Earth Magnetism.** While in the air bath, if we lie flat on the earth on the back or stomach we absorb the magnetism of Mother Earth. It is best to lie with the head towards the north in the direction of the magnetic currents of the earth. In order to lie in harmony with the great magnetic earth currents, beds should always be placed with their heads to the north. Sensitives are strongly affected by lying crosswise of the currents; it causes restlessness and disturbed sleep. In many cases of chronic constipation we have observed splendid results from lying on the stomach on the bare ground. The earth magnetism has a tonic effect upon the solar plexus and other nerve ganglia of the sympathetic system. Good effects may be otained while clothed, but nude contact with the earth is better.

6. **Dry Brush Rub.** While taking an air or sun bath rub the body thoroughly with a dry bristle brush, beginning with one not too stiff. The movements should be in one direction only. Sensitive persons prefer the stroking in the direction of the nerves from the spinal cord outwards. This dry rub not only stimulates skin action and circulation, but also removes dead cuticle and impurities from the surface of the body.[1]

SECTION XXI

CORRECT BREATHING

The lungs are to the body what the bellows are to the fires of the forge. The more regularly and vigorously the air is forced through the bellows and through the lungs, the livelier burns the flame in the smithy and the fire of life in the body. Practise deep, regular breathing systematically for

[1]
A great deal of harm to health undoubtedly comes from some of the many cosmetics, scents, deodorants, anti-perspirants, dyes, etc., which are used by all sections of the population. The use of aids to beauty and attractiveness has a very long history and corresponds to a very natural, and indeed laudable, human instinct. However, it would be an improvement if it were more generally realized that health and beauty go together and that real beauty comes from within and cannot be applied on the outside. Skin and hair which are healthy look and feel nice and bodies which are clean within and without smell nice. As Lindlahr points out, the skin acts both as an eliminative and an absorbing organ and therefore nothing should be put upon it or rubbed into it which interferes with its eliminative functions or which, if absorbed, is harmful to the body. As a general rule it may be stated that the putting of chemical preparations of an inorganic kind on the body is harmful but

one week and you will be surprised at the results. You will feel like a different person and your working capacity, both physically and mentally, will be immediately increased. A plentiful supply of fresh air is more necessary than food or drink. We can live without food for weeks, without water for days, but without air only a few minutes.

1. **The Process of Breathing.** With every inhalation, air is sucked in through the windpipe or trachea which terminates in two tubes called bronchi, one leading to the right lung, one to the left. The air is then distributed over the lungs through a network of minute tubes to the air cells, which are separated only by a thin membrane from equally fine and minute blood vessels forming another network of tubes. The oxygen contained in the inhaled air passes freely through these membranes, is absorbed by the blood, carried to the heart and thence through the arteries and their branches to the different organs and tissues of the body, fanning the fires of life into brighter flame all along its course and burning up waste products and poisons that have accumulated during the vital processes of digestion, assimilation and elimination. After the blood has unloaded its supply of oxygen, it takes up the carbonic acid gas which is produced during the oxidation and combustion of waste matter, and carries it to the lungs where the poisonous gases are transferred to the air cells and expelled with the exhaled breath. This return trip of the blood to the lungs is made through another set of blood vessels, the veins, and the blood, dark with the sewage of the system, is now called "venous" blood. In the lungs the venous blood discharges its freight of excrementitious poisons and gases, and by coming into contact with fresh air and a new supply of oxygen, it is again transformed into bright red arterial blood, pregnant with oxygen, the life-sustaining element of the atmosphere. This explains why normal, deep, regular breathing is all-important to sustain life and as a means of cure. By proper breathing, which exercises and develops every part of the lungs, the capacity of the air cells is increased. This, as we have learned, means also an increased supply of life-sustaining and health-promoting oxygen to the tissues and organs of the body.

2. **Bad Effects of Shallow Breathing.** Very few people breathe correctly. Some, especially women with tight skirt bands and corsets pressing upon their vital organs, use only the upper part of their lungs. Others

---

that the use of vegetable and herbal oils and essences is harmless and may up to a point be beneficial. The suppression of perspiration must be wrong. Excessive and offensive perspiration from the body as a whole, or from particular areas, such as the armpits, is a sign that the skin is not healthy or that the circulation to the part is not good or that there is a toxic condition of the body which is not being dealt with satisfactorily by the emunctories as a whole. It may be legitimate to wonder whether some of the trouble that women have with their breasts may not be due to the suppression of perspiration in that part of their bodies.

breathe only with the lower part and with the diaphragm, leaving the upper structures of the lungs inactive and partially collapsed. In those parts of the lungs which are not used slimy secretions accumulate and the tissues become devitalized. Thus a luxuriant soil is prepared for the tubercle bacillus, pneumococcus and other scavenger germs. This habit of shallow breathing, which does not allow the lungs to be thoroughly permeated with fresh air, accounts in a measure for the fact that as much as one third of all deaths result from diseases of the lungs. To one individual perishing from food starvation thousands are dying from oxygen starvation. Lung culture is more important than other branches of learning and training which require more time and a greater outlay of money and effort. In the natural regimen breathing exercises play an important part.

All-important as are the elements of the air in the vital functions of the body, we take in something with breath that is more essential to life than oxygen, that is life itself. That which we call life force, which proceeds from the one central Source of life, intelligence and creative force and permeates all animate things in the sidereal universe, comes and goes, ebbs and flows with the breath. Every living thing inhales and exhales "the breath of life". This life force as it enters the organism is transmuted into electromagnetic energies and other life elements or vitamins.

3. **General Directions.** The effectiveness of breathing exercises and of all other kinds of corrective movements depends upon the mental attitude during the time of practice. Each motion should be accompanied by the conscious effort to make it produce a certain result. Much more can be accomplished with mental concentration, by keeping your mind on what you are doing, than by performing the exercises in an aimless, indifferent way.

Keep in the open air as much as possible, and at all events sleep with windows open. If your occupation is sedentary, take every opportunity of walking out of doors. While walking, breathe regularly and deeply, filling the lungs to the fullest extent and also expelling as much air as possible at each exhalation. This applies to all breathing exercises.[1]

Do not breathe through the mouth. Nature intends that outer air shall reach the lungs by way of the nose, whose membranes are lined with fine hairs in order to "sift" the air, thus preventing foreign particles, dust and dirt, from irritating the mucous linings of the air tract and entering the

[1]
Some writers and doctors of wide experience have thrown doubt on the wisdom of always having the windows wide open at night, especially when the climate is very cold, damp or foggy. They point out that many animals and birds curl up or put their heads under their wings with the obvious purpose of ensuring that the air they breathe when asleep is warm.

delicate structures of the lungs. Also, the air is warmed and moistened before it reaches the lungs by its passage through the nose.

Let the exhalations take about double the time of the inhalations. This will be further explained in connection with rhythmical breathing. Do not hold the breath between inhalations. Though frequently recommended by teachers of certain methods of breath culture, this practice is more harmful than beneficial.

4. **The Proper Standing Position.** Of great importance is the position assumed habitually by the body while standing and walking. Carelessness in this respect is not only unpleasant to the beholder, but its consequences are far reaching in their effects upon health and the well being of the organism. On the other hand, a good carriage of the body aids in the development of muscles and tissues generally, and in the proper functioning of cells and organs in particular. With the weight of the body thrown upon the balls of the feet and the centre of gravity well focused, the abdominal organs will stay in place and there will be no strain upon the ligaments which support them.

In assuming the proper standing position, stand with your back to the wall, touching it with heels, buttocks, shoulders and head. Now bend the head backwards and push the upper body forward and away from the wall, still touching the wall with buttocks and heels. Straighten the head, keeping the chest in the forward position. Now walk away from the wall and endeavour to maintain this position while taking the breathing exercises and practising the various arm movements. Take this position as often as possible during the day, and try to maintain it as you go about the different tasks which must be performed while standing. Gradually this position will become second nature, and you will assume and maintain it gracefully and without effort. When the body is in this position, the viscera are in their normal place. This aids the digestion materially and benefits indirectly the whole functional organism. Persistent practice will correct protruding abdomen and other defects due to faulty position and carriage of the body. Breathing exercises are intended to develop greater lung capacity and to assist in forming the habit of breathing properly at all times. The different movements should be repeated from three to six times, according to endurance and the amount of time available.

5. **Breathing Exercises.** (a) With hands at the sides or on the hips, inhale and exhale slowly and deeply, bringing the entire respiratory apparatus into active play.

(b) (To expand the chest and increase the air capacity of the lungs). Jerk the shoulders forward in several separate movements, inhaling deeper at each forward jerk. Exhale slowly, bringing the shoulders back to the original position. Then reverse the exercise, jerking the shoulders backward in similar manner while inhaling. Alternate the movements, forcing the shoulders first forward, then backward.

(c) Stand erect, arms at sides. Inhale, raising the arms forward and upward until the palms touch above the head, at the same time rising on the toes as high as possible. Exhale, lowering the heels, bringing the hands downward in a wide circle until the palms touch the thighs.

(d) Stand erect, hands on hips. Inhale slowly and deeply, raising the shoulders as high as possible; then, with a jerk, drop them as low as possible while exhaling.

(e) Stand erect, hands at shoulders. Inhale, raising elbows sideways; exhale, bringing elbows down so as to strike the sides vigorously.

(f) Inhale deeply, then exhale slowly. While exhaling clap the chest with the plams of the hands, covering the entire surface.

(These six exercises are essential and sufficient. The following four may be practised by those who are able to perform them and who have time and inclination to do so.)

(g) Stand erect, hands to sides. Inhale slowly and deeply, at the same time bringing the hands, palms up, in front of the body to the height of the shoulders. Exhale, at the same time turning the palms downward and bringing the hands down in an outward circle.

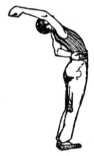

Fig. 7

(h) Stand erect, the right arm raised upward, the left crossed behind the back. Lean far back, then bend forward and touch the floor with the right hand, without bending the knees, as far in front of the body as possible. Raise the body to original posture, reverse position of arms, and repeat the exercise. Inhale while leaning backward and changing position of arms, exhale while bending forward. (Fig. 7.)

(i) Position erect, feet well apart, both arms raised. Lean back, inhaling, then bend forward, exhaling, touching the floor with both hands between the legs as far back as possible.

(j) Horizontal position, supporting the body on palms and toes.

112

Swing the right hand upward and backward, flinging the body to the left side, resting on the left hand and the left foot. Return to original position, repeat the exercise, flinging the body to the right side. Inhale while swinging backward, exhale while returning to position.

6. **Diaphragmatic Breathing.** The diaphragm is a large, flat muscle, resembling the shape of an inverted saucer, which forms the division between the chest cavity and the abdominal cavity. By downward expansion it causes the lungs to expand likewise and to suck in the air. The pressure of air being greater on the outside of the body than within, it rushes in to fill the vacuum created by the descending diaphragm. As the diaphragm relaxes and returns to its original size and position, the air is expelled from the body.

To stimulate the action of the diaphragm, lie flat on floor or mattress, the head unsupported. Relax the muscles all over the body, then inhale deeply with the diaphragm only, raising the wall of the abdomen just below the ribs without elevating either the chest or the lower abdomen. Take about four seconds to inhale, then exhale in twice that length of time, contracting the abdomen below the ribs.

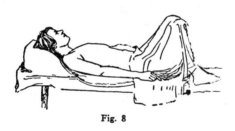

Fig. 8

7. **Internal Massage.** Lie on your back on a bed or couch, knees raised. Relax thoroughly, exhale, and hold the breath after exhalation. While doing so, push the abdomen out and draw it in and up as far as possible each way. Repeat these movements as long as you can hold the breath without straining, then breathe deeply and regularly for several minutes before repeating the massage movements. Next to deep breathing I consider this practice of greater value than any other physical exercise. It imparts to the intestines and other abdominal organs a "washboard" motion which acts as a powerful stimulant to all the organs in the abdominal cavity. Internal massage is especially beneficial in chronic constipation. This exercise may be performed also while standing or walking. It should be practised two to three times daily. (Fig. 8.)

8. **Breathing Exercises to be Taken in Bed.** (a) With hands at side, inhale slowly and deeply, as directed in Exercise No. 5 (a), filling and

113

emptying the lungs as much as possible, but without straining. Practise first lying on the back, then on each side.

(b) (Use one or two pound dumb-bells.) Position recumbent on back, arms extended sideways, dumb-bells in hands. Raise the arms with elbows rigid, cross arms over the chest as far as possible, at the same time expelling the air from the lungs. Extend the arms to the sides, inhaling deeply and raising the chest.

(c) Lie flat on the back, arms at sides. Grasping the dumb-bells, extend the arms backward over the head, inhaling. Leave them in this position for a few seconds, then raise them straight above the chest, and lower them slowly to the original position. Exhale during the second half of this exercise. As a variation, cross the arms in front of the body instead of bringing them to the sides.

9. **Rhythmical Breathing.** We are told in the books of the Ancient Wisdom Religion of India that the life force or prana enters through the nostrils; that in normal rhythmical breathing exhalation and inhalation take place through one nostril at a time—for about one hour through the right nostril and then for a like period through the left nostril. The breath entering through the right nostril creates positive electromagnetic currents, which pass down the right side of the spine, while the breath entering through the left nostril sends negative electromagnetic currents down the left side of the spine. These currents are transmitted by way of the nerve centres or ganglia of the sympathetic nervous system, which is situated alongside the spinal column, to all parts of the body. In the normal, rhythmical breath, exhalation takes about twice the time of inhalation. For instance, if inhalation requires four seconds, exhalation, including a slight natural pause before the new inhalation, requires eight seconds. The balancing of the electromagnetic energies in the system depends to a large extent upon this rhythmical breathing, hence the importance of deep, unobstructed, rhythmic exhalation and inhalation.[1]

In order to establish the natural rhythm of the breath when it has been impaired through catarrhal affections, wrong habits of breathing or other causes, practise water sniffing (Sec. 1, No. 2), and the following exercise, not less than three times a day (preferably in the morning upon rising, at

[1]
The instructions which are given for breathing exercises here and elsewhere would perhaps be more satisfactory and easy to follow if they emphasized the essential difference that there is between inspiration and expiration. The former is something which involves contraction of muscles whereas the latter involves relaxation unless the expiration is very much forced. In fact, to inspire is to do something, whereas to expire is to do nothing. It may be that expiration should take longer than inspiration, but this really means that the muscles should be at rest for longer than they are in activity. Where there is dyspnoea it is as often as not expiratory dyspnoea and is due to an inability to relax and so to empty the lungs. If this can be overcome breathing in can be greatly improved.

noon and at night). This will prove very beneficial in promoting normal breathing and creating the right balance between positive and negative electromagnetic energies in the organism.

10. **The Alternate Breath.** Exhale thoroughly, then close the right nostril and inhale through the left. After a slight pause change the position of the fingers and expel the breath slowly through the right nostril. Now inhale through the right nostril and, reversing the pressure upon the nostrils, exhale through the left. Repeat this exercise from five to ten times, always allowing twice as much time for exhalation as for inhalation. That is, count three or four or six for inhalation and six, eight or twelve, respectively, for exhalation, according to your lung capacity. Let your breath be as deep and long as possible but avoid all strain.

This exercise should always be performed before an open window or, better yet, in the open air, and the body should not be constricted and hampered by tight or heavy clothing. Alternate breathing may be practised standing, sitting or in a recumbent position. The spine should at all times be held straight and free. If taken at night the effect of this exercise will be to induce calm, restful sleep. While practising the alternate breath, fix your attention and concentrate your will power upon what you are trying to accomplish. As you inhale through the right nostril *will* the magnetic currents to flow along the right side of the spine, and as you inhale through the left nostril consciously direct the currents to the left side. There is more virtue in this exercise than one would suspect, considering its simplicity. It has been in practice among the Yogi of India since time immemorial. The wise men of India knew that with the breath they absorbed not only the physical elements of the air but life itself. They taught that this primary force of all forces, from which all energy is derived, ebbs and flows in rhythmical breath through the created universe. Every living thing is alive by virtue of and by partaking of this cosmic breath. The more positive the demand, the greater the supply. Therefore, while breathing deeply and rhythmically in harmony with the universal breath, *will* to open your self more fully to the inflow of the life force from the source of all life in the innermost parts of your being. This intimate connection of the individual soul with the great reservoir of life must exist. Without it life would be impossible.

11. **Warning.** While the alternate breathing exercises are very valuable for overcoming obstructions in the air passages, for establishing the habit of rhythmic breathing and for refining and accelerating the vibratory activities on the physical and spiritual planes of being, they must be practised with caution. These, and other Yogi breathing exercises, are powerful means for developing abnormal psychical conditions. They are therefore especially dangerous to those who are already inclined to be

115

physically, mentally and emotionally negative and sensitive. Such persons must avoid all practices which tend to refine excessively the physical body and to develop prematurely and abnormally the sensory organs of the spiritual body. The most dangerous of these methods are long extended fasting, raw food diet (that is, a diet consisting of fruits, nuts, oils and raw vegetables and excluding the dairy products), Yogi breathing and "sitting in the silence" — that is, sitting in darkness, in seclusion or in company with others, while keeping the mind in a passive receptive condition for extraneous impressions. These practices tend to develop very dangerous phases of abnormal and subjective psychism such as clairvoyance, clairaudience, mediumship and obsession.([1])

SECTION XXII

PHILOSOPHY OF EXERCISE

Next to overeating, lack of exercise in the natural way is one of the leading causes of weakness and ill health. This is true because nature in her wisdom so planned the mechanics and physiology of animal life that activity is essential to maintain normal conditions. In all our preventive and curative work it is of the greatest importance that we study carefully nature's laws and nature's methods and provide conditions as nearly as possible in harmony with them. In this we may derive much help by studying the wonderful correspondences between vegetable, animal and human life based on the unit of life, the primitive single cell.

In the plant kingdom we find that activity or exercise of the unit cell is

---

([1])
The warning which Lindlahr gives here about the dangers of Yogi breathing and other Yogi practices would seem to be somewhat exaggerated. It is hard to see how any great harm could result from taking up Hatha Yoga for the purpose of attaining a condition of physical well being. However, more advanced forms of Yoga should undoubtedly not be undertaken except under the guidance of an honest and competent teacher and to attempt to do so may lead to serious physical and psychical disorders. This is discussed in the Introduction to Indra Devi's book "Forever Young, Forever Healthy". Also it would seem doubtful whether Lindlahr is right in condemning, as he seems to do, all forms of clairvoyance, clairaudience and mediumship. It would seem that there are good and bad forms of these things. It is certainly possible, as Lindlahr here says, to develop a form of clairvoyance or clairaudience which leads to connection with and dominance by spiritual influences on a very low plane. On the other hand there are an increasing number of people who do or can develop forms of extra-sensory perception which are good and useful. Moreover, all great religions and civilizations have developed techniques of prayer and meditation designed to make contact with high spiritual planes and powers.

provided for by the wind, rain, and by changes in temperature and light. In the animal kingdom exercise is called forth by the search for food, by play and by aggressive and defensive warfare. In the human kingdom exists the same necessity for activity in search for food, provision for shelter, in play, and in defence against nature's destructive forces and against animal and human enemies. But man, loving leisure better than exertion and being a free moral agent, has followed the lines of least resistance. He enslaved the horse to draw his vehicles; invented railroad carriages, automobiles, bicycles and all kinds of labour-saving machinery in order to gain speed and to avoid the necessity for physical exertion. The unnatural conditions of civilized society have overburdened some with hard physical labour and condemned others to indoor, sedentary occupations which compel almost complete physical inactivity. Systematic, corrective exercises are needed to counterbalance both extremes.

Most persons who have to work hard physically are under the impression that they need not take special exercise. This, however, is a mistake. In nearly all kinds of physical labour only parts of the body are called into action, certain sets of muscles are exercised while others remain inactive. This favours unequal development, which is injurious to the organism as a whole. It is most necessary that the ill effects of such one-sided activity be counteracted by exercise and movements that bring into active play all the different parts of the body, especially those that are neglected during the hours of work. Hard gymnastic exercises such as weight lifting, boxing, wrestling and athletic feats which require great physical exertion are not conductive to normal development and longevity. On the contrary, steady hard physical labour and severe, long continued gymnastic and athletic training overstimulate and overdevelop the muscular structures of the body at the expense of the vital organs and of the brain and nervous system. This tends to coarsen the body. The animal nature in time reveals itself in outward appearance in the coarsening of the features, in the disproportionate and distorted physique, and in stunted intellectual and aesthetic development. For these reasons Natural Therapeutic philosophy does not favour strenuous physical and physiological exercise, but advises the lighter forms of physiological combined with psychological exercise.

117

SECTION XXIII

PHYSIOLOGY OF EXERCISE

Aside from breathing gymnastics, general exercises should be taken every day. In case of illness or deformity special corrective and curative exercises should be taken. Physical exercise has effects upon the system similar to hydrotherapy, massage and neurotherapy. It stirs up the morbid accumulations in the tissues, stimulates the arterial and venous circulation, expands the lungs to their fullest capacity, thereby increasing the intake of oxygen, and most effectively promotes the elimination of waste and morbid materials through the skin, kidneys, bowels and the respiratory tract. Furthermore, well adapted, systematic physical exercises tend to relax and soften contracted and hardened muscles and ligaments and other connective tissues and to tone up those tissues which are weakened and abnormally relaxed. Such exercises should always be prescribed during and after the correction of lesions of the spinal column and of other parts of the framework of the body. Regular physical exercise means increased blood supply, improved nutrition and better drainage for all the vital organs of the body. By means of systematic exercise, combined with deep breathing, the liberation and distribution of electromagnetic energy in the system is also greatly promoted.

Increased physical activity means increased oxidation of fuel and waste materials which in turn necessitates a greater intake of oxygen and compels deeper and more rhythmic breathing. This means not only a fuller intake of the elements of the air, but also a greater inflow of the life force itself. This primary force of all forces comes and goes, ebbs and flows in all living beings with inspiration and expiration. The Hindu wise men call life the "breath of Brahm". Some use the expression "breath is life". To this I cannot subscribe. I would say breathing is the mechanical and physiological vehicle through which the life elements enter living forms. From this it follows that the deeper and more regular and more rhythmical the breathing, the greater the inflow of the life force into the living organism. As it enters the body through the sympathetic nervous system it is transmuted on the physical plane into electromagnetic energy; on the vegetable plane into vitochemical energy; on the animal plane into mental and emotional energy; and on the human plane into the higher psychical activities. Each plane in addition to its higher properties retains the properties of the lower life elements. These life elements of natural philosophy are identical with the "newly discovered" vitamins of orthodox medical science.

Systematic physical exercise is an absolute necessity for brain workers

118

and those following sedentary occupations. They not only need breathing gymnastics and corrective movements mornings and evenings, but should take regular daily walks no matter what the condition of the weather. Unless they do this faithfully their circulation will become sluggish and the organs of elimination inactive. The cells and tissues of the body will gradually become clogged with morbid encumbrances and this will inevitably lead to physical and mental deterioration.

General Rules

(a) Weak persons and those suffering from malignant diseases such as cancer, tuberculosis, heart trouble, asthma, or from displacements and ruptures, or who are liable to apoplectic seizures, etc., should not take these or any other vigorous exercises except under the supervision of a competent physician.

(b) At least twice a day all parts of the respiratory apparatus should be thoroughly exercised (Sec. XXI). Deep breathing should accompany every corrective movement, whether it be a special breathing exercise or not.

(c) Begin the exercises each day with light movements and change gradually to more vigorous ones, then reverse the process, ending with light, relaxing movements.

(d) When beginning to take systematic exercise do not make the separate movements too vigorous or continue them too long. If any of them cause pain or considerable strain omit them until the body becomes stronger and more flexible. The muscular soreness often resulting from exercise at the beginning is, as a rule, of little consequence and soon disappears. The various movements should be practised in spite of it, because it is the only way to relieve and overcome this condition.

(e) Stop when you begin to feel tired. Never overdo. You should feel refreshed and relaxed after exercise, not tired and shaky.

(f) Do not take vigorous exercise of any kind within an hour and a half after eating, or immediately before meals. It is a good plan to rest and relax thoroughly for about fifteen minutes before sitting down to the table.

(g) Whenever practicable exercise out of doors. If indoors, perform the movements near an open window or where there is a current of fresh air.

(h) Exercise undressed, if possible, or in a regular gymnasium suit which gives free play to all the muscles. If dressed, loosen all tight clothing. If shoes are worn, they should be without heels and wide enough to allow the toes to spread naturally when the weight is upon them.

(i) Always relax physically and mentally before taking exercise.

(j) Apparatus is not necessary to produce results. However, dumb-bells, wands or Indian clubs may be used, but they should not be too heavy. One pound dumb-bells are sufficiently heavy in most cases. The exercises here described are intended for muscular control, flexibility, improvement of the circulation and increased activity of the vital functions rather than for mere animal strength. In the following paragraphs we offer a selection of corrective movements graduated from the more simple to those requiring considerable agility and effort. In practising the exercises, it is best to alternate them, that is, to select, say, six or seven movements suited to individual conditions with a view to securing all-round general development and special practice for those parts and organs of the body which need extra attention. The time at your disposal will also have to be considered. Practise these exercises daily for a week. For the following week select six different exercises, then six more for the third week and so on, supplementing the list here given as may be required by your particular needs. Then start all over again in a similar way. This is better than to do the same stunts every day. It promotes all-around development of the body and keeps the interest from flagging.

Corrective Gymnastics

1. Raise the arms forward (at the same time beginning to inhale), upward above the head, and backward as far as possible, bending back the head and inhaling deeply. Now exhale slowly, at the same time lowering the arms and bending the body downward until the fingers touch the toes. Keep the knees straight. Inhale again, raising the arms upward and backward as before. Repeat from six to ten times. This exercises the muscles between the ribs and the abdominal region muscles in the back.

2. Inhale slowly and deeply with arms at side. Now exhale and at the same time bend to the left as far as possible, at the same time raising the

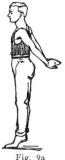

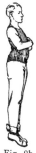
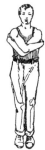

Fig. 9a   Fig. 9b   Fig. 9c

right arm straight above the head and keeping the left arm close to the side of the body. Assume the original position with a quick movement, at the same time inhaling. Exhale as before, this time bending to the right and raising the left arm. Repeat a number of times. This exercise makes the chest flexible and is excellent for the digestive organs.

3. This chest-stretching exercise must be performed vigorously, the movements following one another in rapid succession. Stand erect. Throw the arms backward so that the palms touch (striving to bring them higher with each repetition), at the same time rising on the toes and inhaling. Without pausing, throw the arms forward, the right arm uppermost, striking the back with both hands on opposite sides, at the same time exhaling and lowering the toes. Throw the arms back immediately, touching palms, rising on toes and inhaling as before, then bring them forward and across the chest again, left arm uppermost. Repeat from ten to twenty times. This is an excellent massage and a vibratory movement for the lungs. (Figs. 9a, b, c, p. 120.)

4. Exercises for filling out scrawny necks and hollow chests:

(a) Stand erect. Without raising or lowering the chin and without bending the neck, push the head forward as far as possible, then relax. Repeat a number of times. Push the head straight back in similar manner, making an effort to push it farther back each time. Do not bend the neck. Repeat.

(b) Stand erect. Bend the head toward the right shoulder as far as possible, then relax. Do not rotate the head. Then bend the head to the left shoulder in a similar manner. Then continue, alternating the two movements.

(c) Stand erect. Bend the head forward as far as possible, making an effort to bring it down farther each time. Relax. Then bend the head backward as far as possible. Repeat, alternating the two movements.

5. For exercising the muscles of the chest and upper arm: Stand erect, elbows to sides, hands closed on chest, thumbs inward. Thrust out the arms vigorously and quickly, first straight ahead, then to the sides, then straight up, then straight downward, then backward. Repeat each movement a number of times, then alternate them, each time bringing back the arms and hands to the original position quickly and forcefully. As a variation, raise the elbows sideways to shoulder height with fists on shoulders, then strike vigorously as before, opening the palms and stretching the fingers with each thrust.

6. Stand erect, hands on hips. Keeping the legs straight, rotate the trunk upon the hips, bending first forward, then to the right, then backward, then to the left. Repeat a number of times, then rotate in the opposite direction. Especially valuable to stir up a sluggish liver.

7. Lie flat on your back on a bed or, better still, a mat on the floor, hands under head. Without bending knees, raise the right leg as high as possible and lower it slowly. Repeat a number of times, then raise the other leg, then alternate. As the abdomen becomes stronger, raise both legs at once, keeping knees straight. It is important that the legs be lowered slowly. This is for exercising the abdominal muscles and strengthening the pelvic organs. With the following exercise it is especially valuable for remedying female troubles.

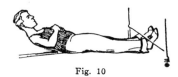

Fig. 10

8. Lie flat on back, arms folded on chest. Place the feet under a chair or bed to keep them in position. Raise the body to a sitting posture, keeping knees, back and neck straight. Lower the body slowly to its original position. Repeat from five to ten times according to strength (Fig. 10).

Supplementary Exercises

9. Stride-stand position (feet about one half yard apart). Raise the arms sideways until even with the shoulders, then, without bending the back, rotate the trunk upon the hips, first to the right, then to the left. As a variation, rotate from the waist only, keeping the hips motionless. An excellent massage for the internal organs.

10. See-saw motion: Stride-stand position, arms raised sideways. Bend to the right until the hand touches the floor, left arm raised high. Resume original position. Repeat several times, then bend to the left side, then alternate.

11. Chopping exercise: Stride-stand position. Clasp the hands above the left shoulder. Swing the arms downward and between the legs, bending well forward. Return to position and repeat a number of times, then repeat with hands on right shoulder, then alternate.

12. Cradle rock: Clasp hands over head, elbows straight. Bend the trunk to the right and left side alternately and without pausing, a number of times.

13. Stand erect, feet together. Jump to the stride-stand position, at the same time raising arms sideways to shoulders; jump back to original position and lower arms. Repeat from ten to twenty times.

14. Lie flat on back, arms at side, legs straight. Raise both legs till

they are at right angles with the body.　From this position sway legs to the right and left side alternately.

15. Lie flat on back, arms extended over head.　Swing arms and legs upward simultaneously, touching the toes with the hands in mid air, balancing the body on the hip bones and lower part of spine.　Return to original position and repeat.　This is a difficult and strenuous exercise, and should not be attempted at first.

16. Lie flat on the stomach, hands under shoulders, palms downward, fingers turned inward, about six inches apart.　This will give free play to the muscles of the chest.　Raise the upper half of the body on the hands and arms as high as possible, keeping the body straight.　Return to position and repeat until slightly fatigued.　(Fig. 11.)

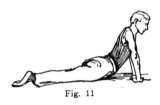

Fig. 11

17. Same position as before.　Raise the entire body on hands and toes, keeping arms and legs straight.　Return to relaxed position and repeat the exercise.　As a variation, sway forward and backward while in the raised position.

18. Lie flat on stomach, arms extended in front.　Fling the arms upwards and raise the upper part of the body as high as possible, keeping the legs straight.　Return to position and repeat, but avoid excessive strain.

19. Same position as before, but hands on hips or clasped in back. Raise upper part of the body without assistance from hands or arms.

20 Rocking chair motion.　Sit on a mat or bed, legs straight, arms at side.　Recline so that the upper part of the body almost touches the mat, at the same time swinging the legs upward.　Return to original position and repeat without any pause between the movements, rocking back and forth until slightly tired.　As you get stronger, clasp the hands behind the head.　As a variation, rock with the knees bent, hands clasped below them.

Special Exercises for Reducing Flesh and Strengthening the Abdominal Organs

21. Lie flat on stomach, heels and toes together, hands stretched out in front.　Fling head and arms upward, at the same time raising the legs, knees straight.　Avoid straining.

123

22. Same position, hands clasped on back, feet together. Roll from side to side.

23. Lie flat on back, seize a bar (bed rail or rung of chair) just behind the head. Keeping the feet close together, raise the legs as high as possible, then swing them from side to side. As a variation, swing legs in a circle without flexing the knees.

24. Same position. Raise and lower the legs without letting them touch the floor, keeping the knees straight.

25. Lie flat on the back, fold the hands loosely across the stomach. Raise and lower the upper body without quite touching the floor.

26. Stand erect, heels together, arms raised above the head. Bend forward and downward, endeavouring to place the palms of the hands on the floor in front of the body without flexing the knees. Return slowly to original position and repeat.

27. Stand erect, hands on hips. Keeping the body motionless from the hips downward, sway the upper part of the body from side to side and forward and backward, and in a circle to right and left.

28. Stand erect, raise the arms above the head. Rotate the trunk upon the hips with extended arms, bending as far as possible in each direction, but avoiding undue strain. These are strenuous movements and should not be carried to excess or performed very long at a time.(¹)

Physical Exercises for Invalids

29. Persons who are very weak and unable to be on their feet for any length of time need not, for this reason, forgo the benefits to be derived from systematic physical exercise. A low chair, with a straight or very slightly curved back and no arms, or a rocking chair of similar construction with a wedge placed under the rockers in such a manner as to keep the chair steady at a suitable angle, is well adapted to the practice of a number of corrective movements, such as rotating of hips and waist, forward and sideways bending of the trunk, the various arm and neck exercises, bending and twisting of feet and toes, and the internal massage (Sec. XXI, No. 7).

(¹)
There is a remarkable classic, "The Culture of the Abdomen", by F. A. Hornibrook (William Heinemann) which is now out of print but which rightly had an enormous vogue earlier in the century. This book sets forth a simple but very effective exercise routine for the cure of obesity and constipation and the improvement of posture. It is profusely illustrated and carries conviction.

SECTION XXIV

PSYCHOLOGICAL EXERCISE

You may ever so often go through the ordinary forms of physical gymnastic exercises in a listless, inattentive way without deriving much benefit aside from a certain amount of development of the muscular structures. In order to derive from exercise genuine curative effects, mind and will must govern and vitalize the purely physical activity. While it is true that the vital activities of the living organism continue independently of the individual consciousness, being under the control of the universal intelligence, we can learn to reinforce and to stimulate, or if necessary to relax and soothe the vital activities by the exercise of our own intelligence and power of will. This is proved by the following experiments: Let the physical culture class perform certain feats in weight lifting, instruct them to use all the physical energy at their disposal, and carefully record the results as to the amount of weight lifted, length of time required, etc. Then give to the class some brief explanation of the power of mind over matter and over the physical constituents of the body, and ask them to exert the power of their will to the uttermost while repeating the same feats. It will be found that the lifting power of the members of the class, thus reinforced by intellectual effort and the power of the will, can be increased from one third to one half.

I have seen a weak little woman under the control of a hypnotist display sufficient physical energy to overcome the concentrated efforts of four strong men to lift her from the floor or to move her from her place. I have seen her lift weights which could not be raised by two or three strong men. On another occasion I saw a weak boy carry the hypnotist, a man weighing over a hundred and seventy pounds, on his outstretched, unsupported arm. The hypnotist in these cases was not reinforcing his subjects by his own muscular strength. Their greatly increased physical strength and stamina were entirely due to the power of his will, acting on their subconscious minds through hypnotic control. I have explained the nature of this phenomenon more fully in Chap. XXX of "The Philosophy of Natural Therapeutics". I do not mean by this to extol the practice of hypnotism, which is always destructive in its effect upon the mind and soul of the subject as well as of the hypnotist, but these phenomena give us a marvellous demonstration of the power of concentrated will over matter and over the physical organism.

The cells and organs making up the great commonwealth of the human body are or should be under the complete control of mind and will. The cells, tissues and organs of the body are or should be physiologically and psychologically negative to the positive mind. In most people the normal polarity is reversed. Their minds and souls are negative and subjective to the constituents of the physical body. The slightest pain or discomfort fills their minds with fear and anxiety. There is no better method to establish normal polarity — the dominion of the conscious mind over the cells, tissues and organs of the body — than systematic psychological exercise. Some exercise does not depend so much upon physical exertion as upon the action of the mind and will upon the nerves and nerve centres which control physical activity. For instance, if the shutting and opening of the hands is intensified by mental effort and by the conscious exertion of the will, it will be of more benefit to the vitalizing of the muscular structures of the arm as well as to the energizing of the brain and nerve centres concerned in the transaction, than the lifting of heavy weights which would unduly exercise the fleshy structures at the expense of the brain and nerve centres.

Psychological exercise becomes still more valuable for the strengthening of mental control over physical activity when the tensing of one part is accompanied by simultaneous relaxation of the companion part — for instance, when the tensing and bending of one arm is accompanied by simultaneous relaxation and unbending of the other arm. The same principle may be applied to all other companion parts of the body in so far as this is possible. The conscious tensing and relaxing exercises must be accompanied always by deep, rhythmic breathing.

From the foregoing it becomes apparent that psychological exercise is one of the most important methods in the treatment of physical disease; for anything and everything which helps to normalize and energize the functions of the body removes the underlying causes of disease.

Effects of Psychological Exercises on Mental and Psychical Ailments

In the treatment of mental and psychical disorders, psychological exercise is of special importance and of wonderful efficacy in bringing about improvement and cure where in the nature of the case that is at all possible. In all mental and psychical derangements one of the primary manifestations is a weakening of reason, will and self control and the gradual loss of control of the mind and will over the physical functions of the body. For the reasons before explained it becomes evident that there can be no better way to strengthen will power and self-control, to re-establish coordination of mental and physical functions and thereby to strengthen the control of mind and will over the body and indirectly in other directions, than by systematic psychological exercises. It is, therefore, one of the most important features in our institution in the treatment of mental, emotional and psychic diseases.

Natural Exercise

Regular outdoor work sufficient to produce good perspiration, where one is in the closest touch with nature, is the best of all exercise for human beings. The work itself should be constructive to the extent that it provides some of the necessities of human life and calls forth the best instincts of human nature. There is none better than the tilling of the soil for the production of vegetables, fruits and flowers.

Elimination through perspiration produced by vigorous outdoor activity — bareheaded and barefooted — is best of all. Numerous experiments have demonstrated that perspiration resulting from actual work or play is far more effective in the elimination of morbid matter from the human body than perspiration induced by steam baths, hot air, electric light baths or other artificial contrivances. It is also true that actual outdoor exercise in the shape of work or play produces much better results than exercise taken with special apparatus in heated buildings.

Next to the tilling of the soil, outdoor play is one of the best forms of exercise — such games as lawn tennis, golf, volleyball, football or baseball bring into activity the whole muscular system, provide the best possible exercise of the lungs, the heart and the vital organs, and at the same time call forth intense brain activity and concentration of mind by the competition and rivalry.

Next to outdoor sport, the best natural form of exercise is walking. To attain the best results walks should be taken not alone but in company with some congenial companion. Select some objective point and make the walk vigorous and rapid, the arms swinging free from the shoulders, the breathing deep and vigorous, the carriage of the body erect. Now and then take a "chest lift". This is done while walking. Hold the entire body erect, draw in a breath; after a few seconds, without exhaling, draw in another and, after a further interval of a few seconds, still another. After the third inhalation vigorously expel all the air. The object of this is to inflate the chest to its fullest capacity. Four or five miles are not too much for a good vigorous walk, although one or two miles a day may be all the average city dweller can afford. To get the best results from any form of exercise the clothing should be removed immediately afterward and a cold rub or cold sponge bath taken, followed by a brisk rub with a dry towel. This in turn should be followed by a few minutes' rest or thorough relaxation in order to allow the system to resume its normal functions.

Since a large proportion of people who live in cities find it absolutely impossible in their regular daily life to take natural exercise in the shape of work, play or walking, they must have some substitute in the way of indoor exercise. Many people believe that the chief object of exercise is to develop large muscles and unusual strength, and for that purpose all kinds of special apparatus, weights and various other contrivances have been devised and sold at fancy prices. Apparatus is entirely unnecessary for good physical development and for maintaining normal health. The leading authorities on physical culture agree that best results may be obtained by the simple exercises, resisting, tensing and relaxing, without the use of weights or special apparatus.

Exercise in order to produce best results must be regular. Set aside a certain time each day for this purpose and adhere to it. The body becomes accustomed to duties of this kind, performed at regular times each day. The entire reserve force of the organism is brought into play at these times and great benefit is derived not only from the physical effects but also from the concentration of mind and will on the work in hand, and this will gradually extend to all other forms of physical and mental occupations.

The following simple movements cover the whole range of psychological exercise. They may be modified or added to according to individual needs. The number of times each shall be done also depends upon individual conditions and requirements. Never hold the breath while exercising. At first continue the exercises until slight fatigue is felt. On an average fifteen to twenty times will be enough for each movement. As a final warning, remember that tensing in the sense used in these directions does not mean straining. Tensing to the point of straining and exhaustion would be decidedly harmful.

Psychological Exercises

1. Stand erect, hands on chest, extend arms forward with a jerk, horizontally from the shoulders, tensing all muscles at the end of the movement. This should be done at the rate of about one movement per second.

2. Same as No. 1, except that the arms are extended downwards at the sides full length.

3. Strike out from the shoulder alternately with each arm, aiming at some imaginary point in front of you.

4. Clinch the fist tightly and strike a vigorous blow from the left hip towards the right ear and across the shoulders. Alternate with the right. As before, end the movement by tensing all muscles.

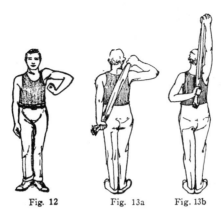

Fig. 12   Fig. 13a   Fig. 13b

5. Stand erect, bring up the knees alternately as high as possible, stopping the movement by tensing all muscles.

6. Stand erect, make a vigorous kick toward the front, first with the left and then with the right foot. Bring the leg to a sudden stop by tensing all the muscles. Extend the toes as far forward as possible when making the kick. The value of this exercise depends on the energy put into it. Do the same by kicking toward the rear.

7. (Fig. 12.) Stand erect. Clinch the right fist, contract the arm, and bring the hand up under the right shoulder, raising the shoulder in the meantime as far as possible, and tensing all the muscles at the end of the stroke. Do this alternately with the left hand. While tensing one arm relax the other.

8. (Figs. 13a, b.) Take an ordinary bath towel, grasp one end in the right hand, over the right shoulder, pass the left hand around below the waist and grasp the other end. Now raise the right arm to an extended position, resisting with the left arm. Return to the original position, maintaining the resistance all the time. Change to the left arm over the shoulder and the right arm down to the hips and repeat.

9. (Fig. 14.) Grasp one end of a Turkish towel with the right hand raised to the shoulder, and the other end with the left hand raised to the shoulder, the towel passing behind the neck. Extend the right arm full length, resisting with the left arm. Return to the first position, maintaining the resistance all the time. Repeat the exercise with the towel passing in front of the neck.

10. Stand erect, with both arms extended downwards; tense the muscles of the upper forearm, hand extended, and raise the right hand to the shoulder, resisting the biceps muscles in the upper arm by the triceps

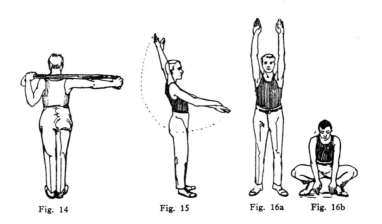

Fig. 14   Fig. 15   Fig. 16a   Fig. 16b

muscles. Return to the original position, still tensing the muscles, at the same time raising the left arm to the shoulder. Repeat.

11. Extend the arms out to the sides in horizontal position, tense all muscles of the arms and shoulders, and bring the arms down close to the body. Repeat.

12. (Fig. 15.) Raise the arms high above the shoulders and a little backward, tense all the muscles, and circle the arms outward and down in front of the body, crossing the hands in front of the abdomen.

13. (Figs. 16a, b.) Raise the hands straight above the head, inhaling a full breath; gradually assume a squatting position as close to the floor as you can get, with the arms down between the knees, the head bent over, and the diaphragm muscles contracted. This is for the purpose of expelling all the air from the lungs.

14. Stand erect, with arms high over the shoulders. Bend over and touch the floor in front of the feet with the hands, the feet remaining flat on the floor, the knees stiff. On returning to upright position tense the muscles in the small of the back.

15. (Fig. 17.) Stand erect, raise the right arm fully extended, swing it up over the head, bend the body as far as possible straight to the left, keeping both feet solid upon the floor; then swing the body as far as possible to the right, raising the left arm and lowering the right. Keep both feet solidly on the floor. Tense the muscles of the arms while doing this exercise.

16. (Fig. 18.) Stand erect, place the hands on the hips, the feet firmly on the floor. Twist the body slowly to the right and then slowly to the left. Do not move the feet. Tense the muscles of the back and abdomen at the extreme end of each movement, and turn the head as far as possible in the direction of each movement.

130

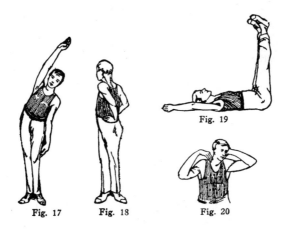

Fig. 19

Fig. 17   Fig. 18   Fig. 20

17. Lie flat upon the floor or upon a bed, arms extended above the head. Raise the arms and the head the shoulders as far as possible from the floor, contracting or tensing the muscles of the abdomen. Relax, and lie again upon the floor, drawing the hips up towards the shoulders, contracting or tensing the muscles of the back.

18. (Fig. 19.) Lie flat upon the floor, arms extended above head. Now raise both feet up over the chest, tensing and contracting the muscles of the abdomen. This exercise may be made more strenuous by tensing the muscles of the legs and raising them up and down from five to ten times without touching the floor. Also extend the arms above the head and grasp an iron bedstead or any other apparatus available, with the hands; then raise the legs from the floor and gradually the hips until the legs pass over and beyond the head. You may also swing the legs from one side to another or in circle.

19. Stand erect. Have the head well poised; bend it as far forward as possible till the chin touches the chest, and then as far backward as possible, without moving the body. Second, have the head well poised, and then turn the head over to the right as far as possible.

20. (Fig. 20.) Have the head well poised and turn it to the right and left alternately without moving the body. While doing this exercise tense the muscles of the back, and if desired, you may resist the neck movements by either hand.

21. Stand erect, heels close together; raise the body on the toes as high as possible. Resume normal position, the heels remaining on the floor. Repeat this with the feet ten inches apart. Repeat again with the feet eighteen inches apart.

22. For cold feet sit upon a box or bench or chair high enough so that

131

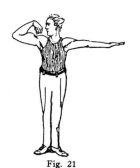 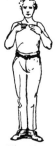 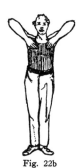

Fig. 21   Fig. 22a   Fig. 22b

the feet swing clear of the floor; work the ankle joints vigorously, raising the ball of the foot as far as possible toward the knee, and then lowering it as far as possible. Do this for about one minute to begin with, and gradually increase to from two to five minutes. This will start the circulation of the blood in the feet.

23. (Fig. 21.) Raise arms horizontally at sides, palms up. Contract right arm, bringing fist towards head and turning the face towards it simultaneously, resisting biceps muscle with triceps muscle, left arm extended outward relaxed — then reverse.

24. (Figs. 22a, b.) Hands on chest. Raise elbows up as high as possible and down again. Inhale while raising, exhale while lowering. Then reverse.

SECTION XXV

NATURAL TREATMENT FOR THE EYES

The health of the eyes, as well as that of all other parts of the body, depends upon perfect nutrition, drainage and nerve supply. Diseases of the eyes, unless caused by external injury, excessive strain under inadequate light or exposure to brilliant light, are due to constitutional conditions. The sensory organs do not weaken and become diseased unless there is something wrong with the three primary life requirements — nutrition, drainage and nerve supply. Most of the work of the eye specialists, as long as they do not treat constitutional causes, is, therefore, not curative but symptomatic and suppressive. The delicate mechanism of the eye becomes easily obstructed with pathogenic encumbrances which cause interference with the circulation of blood, lymph and nerve currents. Cataract is nothing but an infiltration of the lense with pathogenic materials. The same uric acid and crystalloid earthy substances which form deposits in the rheumatic joints also accumulate in the lenses of the eyes and cause them to become milky and impervious to light. All the various forms of inflammation of the eye, if not caused by injury from without, are due to pathogenic obstruction, like all other forms of inflammation in the body.

The natural treatment of the eyes, therefore, aims to remove pathogenic encumbrances and to adjust the mechanical lesions or abnormalities in such a way as to establish perfect nutrition, drainage and nerve supply. This accomplished, ailments of the eyes become a thing of the past and good sight may be maintained to the end of life. From the foregoing it follows that the treatment of the eyes must begin in the first place with the natural treatment of the body as a whole. This is accomplished by faithful adherence to the regimen for wholesome living outlined in Sec. 1. This, with neurotherapy, has in many instances sufficed to cure serious chronic ailments of the eyes. Many people have come to us for the treatment of chronic constitutional diseases, not expecting their weakened eyes to be especially benefited, believing this to be impossible. They were most pleasantly surprised when they found that together with constitutional improvement came also much better eyesight and keener hearing.

But hand in hand with constitutional regeneration should also go special treatment of the eyes themselves. This consists in an adaptation of several important natural methods of treatment; namely, hydrotherapy, eye gymnastics and massage. In many cases it may be necessary to supplement this combination by neurotherapy in order to correct mechanical lesions and abnormalities in the spinal column and nerve tissues which may interfere with the blood and nerve supply of the eyes and with adequate drainage.

1. Water Treatment. For the eye bath the temperature of the water should be as cold as the sensitive eyeball can stand, but not cold enough to cause serious discomfort. A few grains of salt may be added to make the water slightly saline.

(a) Submerge forehead and eyes in a basin of water, open and close the lids under water from six to eight times. Repeat a few times.

(b) Fill an eye-cup with water, bend the head forward and press the cup securely against the eye; then bend backward and open and shut the lid a number of times.

(c) Bend over a stream of water running from a tap or over a large dish containing water of natural temperature; then scoop up the water in the hollow of the hands and throw it into the open eyes, at the same time moving the eyeballs sideways in circular or up and down motion. This is done in order to permit the water to reach all parts of the eyeball equally.

The cold bathing is continued until the eyes cease smarting and perfect reaction is established. This may require about a minute.

2. **Massage and Vibratory Treatment.** We have learned in other parts of these volumes that massage has very much the same effect upon the circulation of the blood, lymph and nerve currents as hydropathic treatment. It stirs up the pathogenic deposits in the tissues and actually squeezes them into the lymphatic and venous circulation, thus allowing a free inflow of the red arterial blood with its freight of life-sustaining oxygen and other elements of nutrition. Like the cold water, it stimulates the flow of the sluggish, pathogenic-laden lymph and venous blood towards the heart and organs of elimination. Another very important effect of massage of the eyes lies in the fact that it makes the eyeball more elastic and resilient, thereby correcting abnormal depressions and inequalities of the surface; in other words, it rounds the eyeball more perfectly. This is a simple and natural way of curing astigmatism, which the oculist tries to overcome by specially ground lenses. It is easily to be seen which of these methods is the more natural and rational. The one endeavours to overcome a symptom; the other removes the cause and actually corrects the abnormal condition. Both massage and hydropathic treatment, aside from their mechanical effects upon the circulation, nutrition and drainage, also arouse and stimulate the latent electromagnetic energy. This, together with a more liberal supply of alkaline mineral elements in food and drink, raises the positivity of the organism, which means greater vitality and recuperative power. The best massage movements adapted for the eye treatment are the following:

3. **Massage Movements.** (a) *Kneading.* In order to execute this movement, press the eyeballs out of their sockets with the tip of one or two fingers of each hand. Continue this until the eyeballs have received a thorough kneading, as far back in the sockets as possible. You need not be afraid of injuring the eyes by this treatment unless you exert undue or excessive force.

(b) *Vibrating.* Vibrate the eyeball all over its surface as far as you can reach it, first with one, then with two and lastly with three fingers — the thumb, forefinger and middle finger brought to a point. The movement is executed by a quick vibratory motion of the hand in the wrist joint. It may require some practice before perfect vibratory motion is attained, but when once acquired it is very beneficial for the purposes described in this book. After thoroughly vibrating the eyeball for about a minute, finish with the stroking movements.([1])

(c) *Stroking.* This movement is executed by stroking the eyeball, first gently, then gradually more and more strongly, with one and later two finger tips. The stroking proceeds over the upper and lower lids from the inner corners of the eyes outward; then reverse and stroke from the outer corner of the eye in a half circular motion to the other corner. These movements also are repeated from a dozen to two dozen times, according to the endurance and time available.

The stroking is applied first gently and with gradually increasing pressure until the eyeball has become seemingly insensible. As before stated, none of these treatments, if executed with a little care and common sense, can possibly inflict any injury. Although the mechanism of the eye is very complicated and highly sensitive, it is at the same time very tough and resilient. Cures of serious eye troubles which are little short of miraculous have been effected by this simple treatment. If faithfully applied at least twice a day, and, if possible, in conjunction with the general regimen for natural living and with neurotherapy, it will do away in a great many cases with the necessity for the wearing or glasses, and will preserve excellent eyesight under strenuous usage, even to extreme old age.

4. **Eye Gymnastics.** After the eyes have recovered sufficiently from the cold bathing, practise eye gymnastics. Stand erect, or if too weak, assume a comfortable position in a chair, then move the eyes upward and downward, as far as the mobility of the eyeballs will permit, along an imaginary vertical line on the wall opposite you. Repeat this from twelve to twenty-four times. Then in like manner move the eyeballs as far as you can force them from right to left on an imaginary horizontal line in front of you on a level with your eyes. Move the eyeballs in similar manner diagonally from the highest point on the right to the lowest point on the left, and then reverse. Finally, roll the eyeballs in circular motion from right to left and then from left to right.

The special value of these eye exercises lies in the fact that the movements of the eyeball are regulated by four sets of muscle which pull the eyeball upward, downward, to the right and to the left. The ordinary use of the eyes in certain occupations such as reading, playing the piano, etc.,

[1]
Vibration, massage and exercise is good for all tisues in which lymph vessels run. The valves in lymph vessels consist of two tiny flaps which come together. Hence any squeezing of the lymph vessels through exercise or vibration forces the lymph through the valves which then close so that there is no return. In other words it produces a flow of lymph and relief of lymph back pressure on the cells which it drains. New nutriment can then ooze into the cells, bringing them new life and comfort.

may exercise the eye muscles unequally and thus overwork and strain some of them while others are weakened through lack of exercise.   In time this is bound to result in unequal development of these muscles and in one-sided strain.   This in turn results in unequal focusing of the eyes, which seriously interferes with normal vision.   This is usually corrected by fitting lenses specially adapted for this purpose, but it is obvious that the better adjustment consists in equalizing the strength of the four muscles which control the movements of the eyeball.

SECTION XXVI

CONSTIPATION

Constipation is characterized by sluggish action of the bowels.   For some reason the evacuation of waste matter from the colon has become difficult.   Normally a person should have a copious movement of the bowels once in twenty-four hours — twice is better.   Constipation has become so common among people of civilized countries that this has been called "the age of constipation".   At least three-fourths of the chronic patients that come to us for treatment suffer from chronic constipation in its worst forms.   Many of them tell us that they have not had a natural movement of the bowels for many years.   This alone is sufficient to show that the ordinary methods of living and treating human ailments are faulty and inadequate.   While itself a form of disease, constipation becomes in turn one of the primary causes of other constitutional diseases.   Inactivity of the eliminating organs, the skin, the kidneys and the bowels, causes retention of waste and morbid matter which results in systemic poisoning or autointoxication.   Any system of treatment which cannot restore the normal activity of the organs of depuration cannot accomplish anything else.

The medical treatment of constipation, consisting largely in the administration of laxatives and cathartics, gives only temporary relief and tends to benumb and paralyse the intestines more completely.   This has been explained in Vol. 1, Chap. VII.   All laxatives and purgatives are poisonous to the system or they would not produce their peculiar drastic effects. They do not act upon the system, but the system acts upon the drugs. Being poisons, the organism tries to expel these enemies to health and life by copious excretions from the liver and the walls of the intestines.   This eventually produces an evacuation of the contents of the bowels, but every time such violent artificial stimulation is resorted to, the liver and the membranous linings of the intestinal tract, and the nerves which supply them, become more benumbed and inactive. This progressive atrophy is revealed in the iris by the darkening of liver and digestive areas, located directly around the pupil. As constipation becomes more stubborn, this region becomes darker, with brown discolourations, turning gradually black in places. In cases of serious atrophy of the membranes, the intestinal area presents a uniform black appearance. We find this frequently in people who have habitually used calomel or have taken other mercurial treatment. Quinine and the derivatives of opium also have a very paralysing effect upon the digestive tract. The acute catarrhal conditions characterized by frequent purging are indicated in the iris by white signs in the intestinal area.

Other causes of constipation are: (1) congestion of the liver, causing insufficient or abnormal secretion of bile; (2) interference with the blood supply of the intestines, causing insufficient secretion of mucus, thus reducing lubrication and causing excessive dryness of faecal matter; (3) interference with the motor nerve supply to the muscular walls of the intestines (partial paralysis), thus reducing their peristaltic action, which in turn causes stagnation and fermentation of faecal matter; (4) spasm of the sphincter muscles of the rectum, inhibiting the act of evacuation; (5) mechanical pressure upon the intestines by new growths, tumours or adhesions.

Chronic constipation is usually preceded by periods of diarrhoea. Hyperactivity, due to excessive stimulation, is always followed by corresponding weakness and gradual atrophy. The ordinary high protein and starchy diet produces, as we have learned, excessive amounts of poisonous acids, ptomaines, alkaloids, xanthines (collectively called pathogen). These morbid materials are powerful stimulants. Their effects are frequently mistaken for increased vigour, as in the case of meat and coffee poisons. They overirritate and overstimulate the liver and the membranes of the intestines, causing an excessive flow of secretions and increased peristaltic action of the bowels. This results at times, when the digestive organs become clogged with pathogenic matter, in periodic diarrhoea. This is the rule during infancy and youth. Gradually, however, continual irritation and overstimulation, with the attendant purging, changes, in accordance with the laws of action and reaction, into the opposite condition of chronic constipation which is aggravated and made more stubborn by the use of laxatives and cathartics.

Constant clogging of the liver with the morbid by-products of a high protein and starchy diet leaves that organ in a congested and inactive condition.   This interferes with the secretion of bile, which in turn causes dryness of the contents of the bowels and deprives them of the lubricants necessary for the easy evacuation of the faeces.   Continual overirritation and overstimulation resulting from pathogenic poisoning also benumbs and paralyses the motor nerves which supply the muscular walls of the intestines, resulting in partial paralysis and diminished peristaltic action. This is aggravated by the continual intake of food materials deficient in cellulose and woody fibre, such as white flour products and polished rice. The hulls of cereals, which act as natural stimulants to the peristaltic action of the bowels, are removed in the modern "refining" milling process.   The particles of hull in whole grain meals serve to keep the starchy parts of the creals from coagulating into lumpy masses and thus facilitate the penetration of the digestive juices into the starchy mass.   It is for this reason that the followers of Nature Cure have always advocated the use of whole grain foods and the liberal consumption of fruits and vegetables whose fibrous waste serves as scouring material for the intestinal tract and as a natural stimulant for peristaltic action.

Spasm of the sphincter muscles of the anus, or spasm of the rectum, is usually caused by long continued overirritation with systemic poison or by the paralysing effect of drug poisons.   Many such cases I have traced back to suppression of gonorrhoea or haemorrhoids.   Such chronic paralysis and inhibition must be overcome through general constitutional treatment, cold tonic sitz baths and tonic manipulative treatment.

Mechanical pressure upon and resulting obstruction of the intestines caused by tumours, new growths or adhesions must be removed through absorption of the abnormal growths and adhesions by natural living and treatment, with strict vegetarian diet and occasional fasting periods.   Hydrotherapy and manipulative treatment are necessary to achieve satisfactory results.   Such deep-seated chronic conditions, therefore, require systematic institutional treatment.

Mental and emotional conditions exert a powerful influence upon the alimentary tract.   Certain emotions have a benumbing, others a stimulating effect upon the secretions and peristaltic action of the bowels.   A few days ago I read about certain experiments made with living animals.   X-ray pictures were taken of a healthy cat whose peristaltic movements were normally active.   The animal was suddenly confronted with an angry dog barking at her fiercely.   Instantly, as the hair on her body and her tail went up as the result of sudden fright and anger, the peristaltic action of the stomach and bowels ceased entirely and did not revive until the animal had thoroughly recovered from its emotional excitement.   It has also been proved by experiments on living animals that sudden emotional excitement stops the secretion of the gastric and pancreatic juices.   The nature and treatment of nervous, mental and emotional disorders is fully discussed in Sec. XXIX and XXX.

The most remarkable case of constipation which has come under my observation was that of a woman suffering from a severe attack of appendicitis and general peritonitis. She had been under Christian Science treatment for six days, her condition in the meantime becoming more aggravated until she was in a dying condition. Cold water compresses and manipulative treatment relieved her intense suffering almost instantly. We tried to empty the colon by repeated flushings, but without success. The bowels did not move for twenty-eight days, then they moved naturally without artificial aid. From that time on the patient made a rapid and perfect recovery. During the four weeks she had received no food whatsoever. The usual hydropathic and manipulative treatment controlled the fever and gradually revived the peristaltic action of the paralysed intestines. Eating at any time during the period of constipation would have meant sure death.

As before stated, habitual constipation means not only deficient elimination but also reabsorption of toxins from the putrefying materials in the intestinal canal, especially in the descending colon and rectum. Appendicitis is practically always preceded by an inactive, atrophic condition of the intestines, which favours the accumulation of faecal matter in the caecum and ascending colon, which in turn leads to inflammation of the caecum and appendix. The causes and treatment of appendicitis have been fully described in Vol. 1, Chapt. XIII.

In the urine of people suffering from chronic constipation we usually find considerable amounts of indican, a poisonous ptomaine which forms in putrefactive processes in the intestines. This is absorbed into the general circulation and partially eliminated through the kidneys. In like manner many other alkaloids of putrefaction are absorbed from the stagnant, putrefying materials in the sluggish intestines, causing headache, nervousness, muscular fatigue, sluggish mentality and many other ailments. Arteriosclerosis, Bright's disease, diabetes and premature old age are caused or aggravated by continual absorption of intestinal toxins. Post-mortem examinations often show the lining membranes of the colon, caecum, and certain parts of the small intestine covered with adhesive, putty-like faecal materials. Such a clogged condition of the intestinal membranes interferes with assimilation as well as with elimination. This leaves the blood in an impoverished condition and overcharged with systemic poisons, causing on the one hand, nerve starvation, and on the other hand, nerve poisoning. This condition of the intestines is revealed in the iris by a darkening and brown discolouration of the digestive area and by the lymphatic rosary. Frequently when I tell patients that their intestinal tract is in a clogged and atrophic condition, they seem surprised, saying there is nothing the matter with their bowels because they move regularly. This, however, is not evidence that the bowels are in a normal condition or that the person is free from intestinal autointoxication. As before explained, the intestines, particularly the colon down as far as the sigmoid flexure, may be encrusted with adhesive faecal matter, leaving a clear way in the centre for the passage of recently formed waste products. In such cases it is necessary to resort to measures which are somewhat drastic to cleanse the colon quickly and thoroughly.

Treatment

1. It must be understood that the first requisite in the treatment of any disorder, and especially of constipation, is a change of diet. The diet for a person suffering from constipation must be of such a nature as to preclude the possibility of the formation of toxins and at the same time to assist in the removal of morbid accumulations from the alimentary tract. Finally, the diet must contain the positive mineral elements necessary to neutralize the negative pathogenic substances in the circulation and in the tissues of the body. Meat, coffee, fermented cheese, fried foods, white bread, pastry and all other white flour products must be strictly avoided, as also the habitual use of condiments, spices and white sugar. A raw food diet, rich in fruit and vegetables, low in proteins, starches and fats, is the best adapted quickly to bring about the desired results. All kinds of fruit, fruit juices and leafy, juicy vegetables are of the utmost value, but a mixture of many at one meal is not advisable. Salads, consisting of lettuce or other leafy vegetables and raw carrots, turnips, parsnips, celery, young onions and radishes, with a dressing of lemon juice and olive oil, should form the basis of the diet. Bran biscuit, health bread, steamed wheat, dates, figs, raisins, grapes, acid and subacid fruits and berries will furnish sufficient nourishment and will serve to stimulate the peristaltic action of the bowels.

2. **A Sample Diet.** *Breakfast*, any kind of acid or subacid fruit or berries. *Luncheon*, raw vegetable salads with dressing of lemon juice and olive oil; dates, raisins and a small amount of either whole wheat bread, bran biscuit, shredded wheat or whole steamed wheat. *Dinner*, raw vegetable relishes and salad of green, leafy vegetables with raw grated carrots or turnips; cooked leafy vegetables such as spinach, cabbage, or Swiss chard; one potato, or in place of it a slice of whole grain bread; some sweet, alkaline fruit for dessert; buttermilk or yogurt. Fruit juices, either pure or dilute, may be taken between meals. This diet should be followed for two or three weeks.

3. **A Natural Laxative.** The treatment of constipation may begin by

taking a mixture of bran, agar-agar and flaxseed to be used two or three nights in succession in the following proportions: mix two tablespoonfuls of bran, one tablespoonful of agar-agar and one of flaxseed. This must be eaten dry before retiring.

In order to soften and to remove old, hard faecal encrustations from the colon a few colon flushings may be taken at the beginning of the treatment. Descriptions of colon flushing and of the necessary apparatus, posture, etc., are given in Sec. XVIII, No. 7. While it is permissible to resort to a few thorough colon flushings at the beginning of the treatment, I am strongly opposed to the habitual use of enemas. This is bound to result in greater weakness and atrophy of the intestines. Filling the lower part of the intestinal tract habitually with large amounts of warm water not only dilates the already weakened intestinal wall but takes away the natural impetus to secretion. In other words, the more you flush, the more lazy the bowels become. I have met many victims of this weakening practice who assured me that the longer they used the "rubber doctor" the more relaxed and weakened the intestines became and the more they suffered from indigestion, fermentation, gas formation and the effects of systemic poisoning. Therefore we resort to colon flushing only as a "crutch" in the beginning of treatment until the intestines become alive and active under natural diet and treatment. We advise patients to resort to flushing only when it becomes absolutely necessary. In that way they learn to take enemas at increasingly long intervals, forcing nature to do the work in the natural way. Natural evacuation will be hastened and facilitated by going to the stool at certain stated times.

4. **Hydrotherapy for Constipation.** A cold sitz bath should be taken every evening (with the usual restriction for women). It has a splendid cooling and relaxing effect upon the abdominal organs (Sec. XIII, No. 13). The abdominal bandage has an effect similar to that of the sitz bath. It is cooling and relaxing, thus relieving the overheated condition of the intestines.

5. **Exercises.** The best exercises for overcoming constipation are those which bring the abdominal muscles into play (Sec. XXI, No. 16, and Sec. XXIII, Nos. 6, 7, 8, 9, 14, 23). Aside from these special exercises brisk walks in the fresh air have a splendid tonic effect upon the muscular apparatus of the digestive tract.

6. **Massage.** In stubborn chronic cases abdominal massage is absolutely necessary to attain speedy and satisfactory results (Sec. XVIII, No. 1).

7. **Neurotherapy.** If lesions are present in that region of the spine which gives rise to nerves which supply the intestines, no permanent results can be expected until these lesions are corrected.

141

8. **Orificial Dilatation.** This is one of the most effective methods for the treatment of chronic constipation. It is fully described under Sec. XXVIII.

SECTION XXVII

HEADACHE

Headache is usually but a symptom of disease somewhere in the body, though it may be due to irritation by systemic or drug poisons. Diseased conditions and irritation anywhere in the system are telegraphed to headquarters in the brain and there manifest in the form of various symptoms, the most frequent of which is headache. Sometimes it is caused by defects in vision, or eye strain, and may be alleviated by properly fitted glasses. This, however, cannot take the place of removing constitutional causes. Frequently the wearing of "eye crutches" prevents the locating and removal of the underlying causes and thus condemns the individual to the lifelong use of glasses, to constantly weakening eyesight and to chronic constitutional disease. One of the most common causes of headache, as well as of eye trouble, is uric acid or pathogen poisoning. This has been fully described in Vol. 1, Chap. XXIX. A typical uric acid headache is migraine or one-sided headache, particularly annoying in the morning when the blood is loaded with pathogenic materials.

1. **Bilious or Sick Headaches.** Another common type is the so-called bilious headache. While usually attributed to an inactive liver, it may be caused in various ways. Pathogenic clogging of the liver will interfere with the elimination of bile products; these will remain in the circulation and cause general symptoms of biliousness, jaundice, nausea, vomiting and headache. Pathogenic obstruction may be due to overeating, to the excessive intake of starchy, protein and fatty food, and to a deficiency of fruits and vegetables in the diet; or the discharge of the bile may be obstructed by sticky, colloid accumulations in the gall bladder and bile duct. In other cases the bile duct is contracted and obstructed through inflammation of the duodenum. Anything which interferes with bile formation in the liver or its discharge from the gall bladder or bile duct not only causes surging back of the bile into the general circulation but also a deficiency of it in the intestinal tract, which in turn gives rise to acidity of the intestinal contents, indigestion, constipation, fermentation and gas

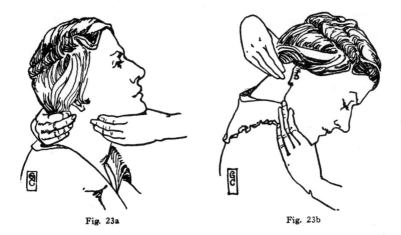

Fig. 23a   Fig. 23b

formation. This intestinal toxaemia is reflected to the brain in the form
of congestion and headache, and favours the formation of emboli (ob-
structive plugs) and the development of apoplectic strokes. Anything
which tends to cause constipation and thereby intestinal toxaemia or
autointoxication will also help to produce acute or chronic headaches.

The headaches so far described are of the congestive type, characterized
by excessive blood pressure to the brain. Anything which tends to raise
the blood pressure will therefore create or aggravate these ailments. A
common cause is pathogenic obstruction of the capillary circulation,
which results in active congestion in the internal organs and the brain; or
pathogenic obstruction in the lymphatic or venous drainage which interferes with the flow of the blood from the brain and thus causes passive
congestion. The foregoing remarks explain the effectiveness of a simple
manipulative treatment which any layman can apply. The subject assumes a sitting position. The operator stands on either side, applies the
thumb and the first and second fingers of one hand firmly to the base of
the skull, while with the other hand under the jaw he lifts the head and
stretches the neck gently but firmly upward and backward. The stretching should continue from thirty to sixty seconds. This movement kinks
the arteries and straightens and drains the veins, thus relieving the congestion in the brain. After slowly releasing the pressure, the operator firmly
strokes the neck downward along the course of the main arteries and
veins, on both sides. The stretching should be followed by magnetic
treatment. The operator takes the head of the patient between his hands
and with this thumbs stretches the skin of the forehead outward, half a
dozen times, and then makes the regular magnetic strokes from the forehead downward and outward along the neck and arms. The various

143

forms of magnetic treatment are fully described in Vol. 1, Chap. XXXIV. The operator, while giving the manipulative and magnetic treatment, must combine with these the right mental and psychical attitude as described in the chapter just referred to. If one of these combination treatments does not bring the desired result, it may be repeated. If the attention of the subject can be temporarily distracted from his ailment, so much the better. After an interval of five or ten minutes his headache will usually have disappeared. (Fig. 23a.)

2. **Anaemic Headache.** This type of headache is caused either by great impoverishment in the quality of the blood or a deficiency of it in the brain. This condition frequently obtains in cases of anaemia, leukaemia, pernicious anaemia, or where the flow of blood to the brain is interfered with by a tumour, aneurysm or other mechanical obstruction. While the congestive headache has violent, throbbing, paroxysmal pains, the anaemic headache is accompanied by extreme dullness and lassitude. The former is characterized by heat and redness of the face, the latter by coldness, clamminess and pallor. The manipulative treatment for the anaemic headache is similar to the other. The hands are applied to the nape of the neck and under the jaw in the same manner, but instead of stretching the neck upward and backward, it is stretched upward and forward. This movement kinks the veins and straightens the arteries, thus allowing a greater flow of blood to the brain. The magnetic, mental and psychic treatments are the same in either case. (Fig. 23b.)

In all types of headache the dietetic treatment must build up the blood on a natural basis and eliminate pathogenic encumbrances. The various regimens for this purpose have been given under Secs. 1 and X. In headaches of the congestive type, fasting is of particular value. If the trouble is caused by indigestion, biliousness and foetid condition of the stomach, copious draughts of water as warm as it can be swallowed sometimes give quick relief. If the "warm water flushing" causes vomiting, so much the better.

3. **Nervous Headaches.** These may be caused by sudden fear, shock, excessive worry or anxiety. The preventive and curative treatment is given under "Nervous, Mental and Emotional Disorders". But even for nervous headaches constitutional treatment is essential. Persons in perfect physical condition are not likely to suffer from nervous, mental or emotional disorders of any kind.

4. **Mechanical Lesions.** In many instances headaches are caused by the impingement of luxated bones or strained muscles or ligaments on blood vessels or nerves supplying the brain or eyes. Luxation of the atlas, the topmost bone of the spinal column which carries the skull, frequently gives rise to this sort of headache. Luxations of one or more of the

cervical vertebrae may have a similar effect. Such mechanical lesions must be corrected by manipulative (neurotherapy) treatment.

5. **Drug Poisons.** The most obstinate and severe types of chronic headaches are caused by drug poisoning. Nature has made ample provision for the elimination of systemic waste, but she never intended that the many forms of powerful poisons given under the guise of medicines, tonics and stimulants should enter the human body. Therefore the organs of depuration have not been constructed for the elimination of these poisons. They accumulate in the system in certain parts and organs for which they exhibit special affinity, and there become the source of constant irritation, frequently of actual destruction. Through diagnosis from the iris we have traced hundreds of cases of stubborn chronic headache to the action of powerful drug poisons in the brain itself or in other organs. Many such cases have been described and illustrated in "Iridiagnosis", another volume of this series. The only way to overcome such headaches is to remove the poisonous irritants and stop their destructive effects by thorough systematic natural treatment as outlined under the sections dealing with chronic diseases.

SECTION XXVIII

ORIFICIAL TREATMENT

The following principles underlie the various methods of orificial treatment.

(a) All the involuntary functions of the body such as circulation, respiration, digestion, secretion, elimination, etc., are under the control of the sympathetic nervous system.

(b) Each of the pelvic outlets of the body is guarded by two sphincter or circular muscle bands. The lower (external) sphincter is under the control of the will and is supplied by the cerebro-spinal nervous system. The upper (internal) sphincter is not under the control of the will and receives its nerve supply from the sympathetic nervous system. In this way the most important connection is established between these two nervous systems.

(c) Overtension of these sphincter muscles produce impingement of the sympathetic nerve endings, thus lowering the vitality by exhausting the sympathetic nerve force, on the same principle that electric energy is wasted by pressure on the button which rings the bell. In time such spastic contraction results in hypertrophy and atrophy.

(d) By dilating the abnormally tensed outlets, this irritation of the sympathetic nervous system is relieved. Thereby nervous energy is economized, undue tension removed and functional activity of all the internal organs enhanced.

(e) Dilatation of the sphincters of the orifices relaxes the vasomotor nervous system, which is under the control of the sympathetic, and thereby causes a widening and well marked flushing of the capillaries over the entire body, thus aiding metabolism, oxidation and elimination of tissue waste and promoting the repair of diseased or injured tissues.

Orificial surgery, as the name implies, in order to relax contraction of the sphincter muscles relies to a large extent upon surgical treatment. This, however, is not natural treatment. We avoid wherever possible any and all mutilations of tissues and organs because these are always followed by more or less harmful after-effects. Surgical treatment usually means serious injury to nerves, blood vessels, muscles, ligaments, and the formation of scar tissue or adhesions which, in turn, may cause impingement and interference with normal functions. From our point of view such surgical mutilations are not only harmful but in most cases absolutely superfluous, because in natural methods of treatment we possess the means for relaxing abnormal contraction of tissues in any part of the body. I shall describe the most common lesions of this character and their natural treatment.

1. **Phimosis.** Frequently the foreskin or prepuce of the penis of a male child or of an adult is so tightly contracted around the head or glans of the organ that it cannot be retracted. Sometimes the opening of the foreskin is constricted to the size of a pinhead, causing interference with the free discharge of the urine. Smegma, a sebaceous secretion of the glans of the penis, may accumulate under the tightly adherent foreskin and cause irritation, which frequently results in serious affection of the nervous system. The intolerable itching caused by such irritation not infrequently leads to masturbation.

The remedy of the orificial surgeon, as well as of the medical profession in general, consists of circumcision, that is, complete surgical removal of the foreskin. I have never been able to conceive of a valid reason for this barbarous practice, which always means mutilation of one of the most highly sensitive nerve centres of the body. It is a fact well known to Nature Cure physicians that cooling applications in the forms of sitz bath or friction bath have a cooling and relaxing effect upon all the abdominal organs, indicating that there must be intimate nerve connection through the sympathetic and cerebro-spinal nerves between the internal organs

146

and the glans penis and prepuce. Mutilation of the sexual organs seems inexcusable when there are natural ways of attaining the desired results. In the majority of cases all that is necessary is to lave the head of the penis with cold water for a few minutes in order to produce partial anaesthesia, and then to exert gentle traction on the foreskin. This treatment usually succeeds in from two to ten days in loosening and drawing back the foreskin. If, however, the constriction be so severe that traction does not succeed in overcoming it, or if the prepuce is adherent to the glans penis, a probe may be employed to loosen it or a small penile syringe may be inserted within the orifice of the foreskin so that water may be forced into the cavity between the glans and foreskin. Drawing the prepuce over the end of the syringe, an injection is made of warm water mixed with a little Castile soap. This should be followed by two or three injections of clear warm water. This procedure not only removes foetid accumulations but also separates and dilates the adherent foreskin without irritation or injury to the parts. It expands the prepuce with an all-round even pressure. This treatment should be followed by gentle backward traction. Among several hundred cases thus treated I have only found two which demanded surgical treatment, because the prepuce had grown so fast to the glans penis that it could not be removed by the natural treatment.

2. **Paraphimosis.** Paraphimosis results when the contracted prepuce yields to traction or slips back of its own accord, causing strangulation of the neck of the penis behind the corona. This results in compression of the urethra, retention of urine, and in shutting off the circulation in the extremity of the organ. The gland becomes congested and inflamed, and the foreskin is swollen with serous exudates. In order to prevent ulceration and sloughing of the parts, the foreskin must be brought forward over the glans penis. I have always succeeded in accomplishing this by cooling water applications and absorbent packs followed by gentle dilatation and forward pulling of the constricted prepuce. In no case was it necessary to resort to surgical treatment.

3. **Hooded Clitoris.** The clitoris of the female corresponds anatomically and sexually to the penis of the male. It is a small erectile organ concealed beneath the labia minora, just in front of the urethra. The free extremity of the organ (glans clitoridis) is a small round tubercle of spongy erectile tissue, and highly sensitive. This protuberance is not infrequently covered by a membrane under which secretions may accumulate as under the adherent male prepuce, resulting in nervous irritation. Many serious nervous ailments have been traced to this cause. The natural treatment here, also, consists in cooling applications and gentle backward traction or in loosening the skin with a probe. As a rule the difficulty is overcome more easily than in phimosis. In rare instances where the covering mem-

brane is so tough and tightly adherent that it will not yield to the natural treatment, a small V-shaped incision may have to be made in order to free the organ.

4. **Dilatation of the Lower Orifices of the Body.** The sex organs, as well as the entire system, receive their influx of life force through the sympathetic. The tonicity of the sexual organs therefore depends upon the integrity of the part of the sympathetic which supplies the pelvic organs. Since the secretions of the ductless glands of the sex organs exert a profound influence on the organism in general, it will be seen how important it is that the sympathetic nerve supply to these organs be not interfered with in any way. Such interference results when the genito-urinary organs are either in an overirritated or atrophic condition. Irritation of the urethra or prostate gland by acute or subacute inflammatory processes causes sexual hyperactivity and a great waste of nervous energy, and through the ramifications of the sympathetic, it produces by reflex action nervous irritation in neighbouring or even the most distant parts of the body.

Excessive irritation of the genital organs or the rectum, communicated to the vasomotor centres, may cause constriction of the blood vessels and thereby congestion, pathogenic obstruction and inflammation in nearby or distant parts of the body predisposed to these conditions. On the other hand, sexual weakness or atony diminishes the secretions of the sex glands, benumbs the nervous activities and retards heart action and circulation. Aside from excessive drainage of the sex fluids nothing else produces these debilitating effects upon the system like permanent contraction and hypertrophy of the rectal sphincters and of the tissues of the penis and the prostate gland. Such contraction may be the result of long continued irritation and hyperactivity due to excessive indulgence or self abuse, or it may be caused by gonorrhoeal inflammation, irritating drug poisons, or by long continued constipation with its deadening effects upon the sphincter ani.

The expenditure of nerve force is reduced to a minimum through complete rest and relaxation and its expenditure through voluntary activities ceases entirely during sleep, sound sleep, as is indicated by the disappearance of the aura. Anything which causes abnormal irritation, while awake or asleep, involves unnecessary expenditure.

At this point it may be well to enumerate the various causes of nerve waste described in this chapter and in connection with other subjects:

(a) Acute and subacute inflammatory processes affecting any part of the sympathetic or cerebro-spinal system.

(b) Roughened surfaces of internal membranes, especially at the orifices, fissures, papillae, piles, incipient tumours and other adventitious

148

tissues (new growths) in the rectum, genito-urinary organs or in any other part of the body.

(c) Nerve irritation caused by impingement or pressure on nerve matter as the result of structural and mechanical abnormalities and defects in the body.

(d) Nerve irritation due to discordant and destructive mental and emotional activities such as impatience, irritability, fear, worry, anxiety, anger, rage, fury, jealousy, self pity, as described in Sec. XXIX.

Nervous irritation from any of these causes if continued for a long enough time will result in atony, hypertrophy and atrophy of connective tissue and nerve matter, which in turn results in obstruction to the inflow of vital energy and its distribution through the organism. Acute and subacute irritations are indicated in the iris by white nerve rings; atony and atrophy by black nerve rings, as explained in our iridiagnosis volume.

5. **How to Stop the Leaks.** Aside from the ordinary natural methods of living and of treatment there is nothing more effective for the relaxation and invigoration of the lower intestinal tube and of the sex organs than dilatation of the rectal sphincters, male urethra, and of the sphincter muscles of the vulvae, vagina and uterus. Alternating compression and relaxation of the sphincters of these orifices has a wonderful relaxing and tonic effect upon the organs themselves and upon the entire organism. It relieves abnormal tension and thereby allows a more copious inflow of vital energy through the sympathetic and prevents its waste through continual irritation while waking and sleeping. This restores the normal tonicity of the rectum and of the sex organs, which in turn ensures normal evacuation of faeces and urine, increased secretion of the ductless glands, and greater activity of all the vital functions of the organism, physical as well as mental and psychical. Manual or mechanical dilatation of the lower orifices of the body is more invigorating than any medical tonic or stimulant, without producing deleterious after-effects. It is a splendid means of reviving persons suffering from fainting fits, anaesthesia, epileptic seizures, from opium or other poisoning, and from asphyxiation or drowning. Rectal dilatation is a splendid aid to promote recuperation from serious acute diseases, and to start the normal breath of the new born infant.

A writer on orificial surgery discusses diseases of the lower intestinal canal as follows: "Diseases of the lower portion of the intestinal canal are exceedingly common. There is probably no one organ or locality of the human body so subject to a variety and complexity of diseased conditions as this. Experience and observation for many years have convinced us of the fact that rectal diseases are the foundation and cause of very many other grave forms of chronic disease which it is impossible to cure so long

149

as the rectal lesion holds. Very many serious uterine affections that baffle the skill of the practitioner are thus obstinate because he has failed to discover or cure the rectal complications. We have no doubt but that many cases of mental aberration are caused by lesions of the intestinal canal and especially of the rectum."

6. **Contraction of the Sphincters of the Rectum and its Causes.** This condition interferes seriously with the evacuation of the faeces; it frequently results in stubborn constipation, reabsorption of toxic materials from the lower sections of the intestinal canal and in all the evils of autointoxication. In many cases overtension of the sphincter muscles is due to reflex irritation associated with disturbances of the rectum, uterus, urethra, prostate, bladder, etc., caused by acute or chronic inflammation, tumours, haemorrhoids, fissures, rectal pockets which retain faecal matter, etc. In discussing the effects of rectal pockets and papillae, Dr. Pratt states that they "induce sexual over activity, disturb colonic peristalsis and lower vitality by inducing chronic over tension of the internal sphincter and shallow respiration, inviting stomach, heart, lung and head troubles, as well as interfering with capillary circulation throughout the body". Granting that artificial dilatation will beneficially influence these conditions by relieving nervous irritation, the fact remains that the rightening of sphincters is a symptom, not a primary cause of the condition, and these primary manifestations of disease must be removed by natural methods of treatment.

7. **Technique of Rectal Dilatation.** Alternating compression and dilatation of the sphincter and of the ganglion impar situated on the internal convexity of the coccyx, and of the sympathetic nerves which radiate from it to the lower part of the rectum and the pelvic organs, is best produced by manual treatment. The operator inserts the forefinger as deeply as possible and exerts firm pressure necessary to obtain the best results can be regulated much better by manual treatment than by a mechanical instrument. It offers the only means of forcing back into normal position the bent coccyx which frequently causes pressure on the rectum and the ganglion impar, or tension of muscles and ligaments attached to the coccyx, which may result in spastic contraction of the rectum and the most stubborn constipation. A rubber glove is worn while giving the treatment.

8. **Mechanical Dilatation.** Several types of rectal dilators are on the market for the use of the laity. The results of such home treatment are not always satisfactory because rectal dilatation requires the skill of a physician who can judge the degree of dilatation necessary in each case, the length of each treatment and the frequency with which it should be repeated. It is essential that the internal sphincter should be dilated without exerting undue force on the external sphincter. When this has

150

been accomplished the speculum is withdrawn without closing it so as to dilate the external sphincter from within outward, thereby imitating nature's way of evacuating faeces which produces natural dilatation of the sphincter ani with its tonic effects upon the system.

9. **How to Use Rectal Dilators.** Dilators made of hard rubber, wood or glass may be procured in any drug store. They come in sets of four. One should begin with the largest size consistent with comfort. The dilator should be lubricated with clean olive oil, vegetable oil or pure Castile soap. The size of the dilator to be employed depends upon the size and relaxability of the sphincters; the length of time it is allowed to remain should be determined by the individual condition and the amount of reaction to be desired. Respiration and capillary circulation are more profoundly stimulated by rectal dilatation than by the treatment of the genito-urinary orifices. The instrument is gently passed well into the rectum, as far as the flange or rim will admit it. The flange prevents the dilator from slipping in too far. The best position for the patient to assume is lying on the side with the knees drawn up. Hold the dilator in place for a few moments, until the inner sphincter closes tightly around it. Then it will be retained. It may remain in position from ten minutes to half an hour, or as long as one or two hours. The dilator may be inserted either on retiring at night or on waking in the morning, or at any other convenient time during the day. In case of obstinate constipation it should be inserted after waking in the morning and retained about half an hour or more. This usually induces a natural bowel movement. If used at night it will promote natural, refreshing sleep. The patient should go to sleep if possible and not lie awake to time himself, as no harm can result if the dilator is retained all night. Dilatation may be repeated daily, every second day or a few times a week, according to individual needs.

Since it has taken years of wrong living, neglect and abuse by drugs, to create the chronic conditions, results cannot be expected within a few days or weeks. While some stubborn cases show improvement at once, others require time and patience. As before stated, in order to attain quickest and best results the mechanical treatment must always go hand in hand with the general natural regimen and neurotherapy. By improving nerve and blood supply and by establishing better drainage, rectal dilatation will not only help to overcome stubborn constipation but also promote the absorption of piles, fissures, rectal pockets, papillae and other abnormalities. More efficacious and safer than the ordinary rectal plug are instruments especially designed for this purpose, in the hands of the trained physician or nurse. Best adapted are the rectal speculum or instruments of similar construction.

10. **Dilatation of the Sphincters and Tubes of the Genital Organs.** One

of the common causes of sexual weakness or complete impotence, as already explained, lies in contraction, hypertrophy and atrophy of the sphincters of the rectum. These conditions curtail the inflow of vital energy into the sexual organs and obstruct the blood supply to the erectile tissues of the penis or the clitoris. Similar effects upon the sex functions result from contractions and structures of the tissues of the penis and prostate glands. Aside from rectal dilatation, the passing of graded steel sounds, either cold or at blood heat temperature, is the best remedy for correcting the abnormalities just described. Sounds, as well as rectal plugs, have both local and general effects upon the circulation and the nervous conditions of the system. In cases of excessive irritability and abnormal sexual excitation leading to involuntary emissions and masturbation, the mere introduction and removal of a warm sound will immediately reduce the hyperaesthesia and restore the sympathetic to its normal tone. Where excessive irritability has become chronic the treatment must be repeated daily or a few times a week until the desired results are obtained. In states of sexual weakness or impotence, which may result in a sluggish, indolent condition of the entire organism and in physical and mental debility, it may be best to leave a warm sound in position for from a few minutes to one or two hours, and to follow this with the introduction of a cold sound which should be left in position no longer than a few minutes. This treatment may be repeated once, twice or, in stubborn cases, three times a week, until normal tonicity of the sex organs and of the system in general has been restored or at least greatly improved.

No routine rules for the use of sounds can be prescribed; this treatment must be adapted to individual conditions. The treatment is very beneficial for the cure of gleet and strictures. It is equally as serviceable in spastic contractions of the urethra and prostate as in relaxed and flabby conditions of these organs. In order to ensure good results from the passing of steel sounds for any purpose whatsoever they should be made to pass as far as the interior of the bladder. Their good effects locally and constitutionally depend on their action upon the prostatic inch of the urethra.

11. **Dilatation of the Sphincters of the Female Organs.** Dilatation applied to these parts is beneficial to relieve irritation as well as abnormal relaxation and atony. In other words, it is effective for the cure of spastic contraction as well as for atony, atrophy and paralysis. The former conditions of the vulvae, vagina and uterus occur most frequently in unmarried women and in those of the married who have never borne children. Abnormal relaxation of the parts is frequently the result of sclerosis of the spinal cord, of tubercular processes and of excessive strain in delivery.

The various parts of the female sexual apparatus are so closely related and associated in construction and function that tension or relaxation in one part effects the other parts as well. Undue tension of the vagina may be overcome by careful dilatation with the rectal bivalve, but care must be taken not to injure the vaginal walls, as this might have a tendency to aggravate rather than to relieve the abnormal irritation and contraction of the parts. Dilatation of the uterus is accomplished in similar manner as that of the male urethra by the insertion of graded steel sounds; first smaller, then larger sizes are employed until resistance increases sufficiently to procure the necessary dilatation of the sphincters of the external and internal mouth of the uterus. Dilatation of the sphincters of the atonic female organs not only raises their tonicity but through increasing the supply of vital energy, stimulating the capillary circulation and procuring better drainage, greatly facilitates the absorption of roughened membranes, papillae, fissures, scars and incipient tumours; however, the treatment must be executed only by physicians well trained and experienced in the use of the instruments. The latter must always be well sterilized and dipped in clean olive oil before insertion.

12. **Dilatation by Neurotherapy Treatment.** All the beneficial effects resulting from mechanical dilatation of the lower orifices of the body can be obtained also, more or less completely, by neurotherapy and hydrotherapy treatment. To procure the best results all three methods should be applied in proper combination.

13. **Coccygeal Lesions.** (a) *Anatomy of the Parts.* The coccyx or end of the spine consists of four small bony segments which are fused into a single curved bone about one inch in length. At the junction between the coccyx and the sacrum, spinal nerves emerge which supply the external sphincter muscle which guards the lower opening of the bowel.

(b) *Occurrence of Lesions.* Notwithstanding the fact that injuries of the coccyx frequently give rise to obscure neurotic disorders, the literature on this subject is deplorably meagre. Evidently the reason why so few cases are reported in professional journals and text books is because sufferers from an annoyance "at the end of the spine" will, from motives of delicacy, adopt semi-invalid ways rather than seek professional aid. Coccygeal lesions occur most frequently in women, and play an important part in the large number of diseases peculiar to the female genital apparatus.

14. **Causes of Lesions.** (a) Falls or blows on the base of the spine are mishaps which the majority of us have experienced at some time during our lives. (b) Jars to this region occur while riding on horseback. (c) Faulty posture while sitting, if continued for any considerable period of time, frequently gives rise to coccygeal lesions. (d) Childbirth. Injuries are

153

frequently sustained to the coccyx at childbirth, owing to pressure of the child's head during its passage through the outlet of the pelvis. Normally the pelvis yields to the head of the child so as to increase the diameter of the pelvic outlet, but in cases where the pelvis is too small or where the head of the child is abnormally large, or in cases where women give birth to their first child at an age when the coccyx is partially or completely ossified to the end of the sacrum, the coccyx is very susceptible to injury. The exact manner in which these lesions as well as all other spinal lesions are produced is described in Vol. 1, Chap. XXXII.

15. **Effects of Coccygeal Lesions.** An abnormally anterior position of the coccyx encroaches upon the posterior wall of the rectum, thus mechanically giving rise to rectal constipation with its train of complex after-effects. Impingement of the coccygeal nerves produces overtension of both internal and external sphincters of the anus and thereby wastes nerve energy as previously described. In persons with rheumatic or gouty tendencies an inflammatory condition called coccydynia frequently develops in the region of the coccyx after injury. Coccydynia is characterized by a severe distressing pain which is aggravated by walking, coughing, sneezing, defaecation, sudden changes of posture from standing to sitting, or any movement which involves the muscles attached to the coccyx. The usual allopathic treatment for this condition consists of administering salicylates and pain-killing remedies. In obstinate cases the coccyx is excised. Such methods of treatment not only fail to remove the constitutional cause at the back of this condition but the surgical removal of the coccyx leads to chronic lifelong irritation of the sphincter muscles of the rectum.

16. **Coccygeal Relaxation.** The same principle laid down for the treatment of other spinal lesions should be followed in case of coccygeal lesions (Vol. 1, Chap. XXXII). The muscles attached to the coccyx should be thoroughly relaxed before any attempts are made at adjustment. In all cases where tenderness is present inhibition should be given. Inhibition in the region of the coccyx exerts a marked beneficial effect on a host of neurotic disturbances that fail to respond to other methods of treatment alone. This is probably accounted for by the fact that such inhibitive treatment exerts a profound relaxing influence on the sphincters, and through these on the entire sympathetic nervous system, by acting upon the ganglion impar situated on the anterior surface of the coccyx. The ganglion constitutes the point of union between the left and the right sympathetic chains and with the end filaments of the cerebro-spinal system.

The sympathetic relaxation is administered by applying externally strong and persistent inhibition on either side of the coccyx as well as on the following nerve centres along the spine: (a) tender spots along the sacrum; (b) the posterior superior spine of the ilium; (c) on both sides of the spinal column on the level with the spine of the scapulae; (d) over the superior angles of the scapulae. This inhibition is given for about five minutes at a time on one or all centres. The treatment is repeated from twice a week to once in two weeks or longer. In many instances vigorous healing crises develop as a result of such treatment. For this reason it is wise for patients to be in an institution when such treatment is administered.

17. **Tonic and Relaxing Effects of Cold Water Treatment.** The cold sitz baths, Kuhne friction baths and the application of cooling compresses and cold packs to the abdominal and pelvic parts undoubtedly have effects upon the sympathetic nervous system similar to those produced by mechanical dilatation and coccygeal inhibition. The cold applications to the lower orifices and glans penis produce temporary contraction followed by relaxation of the parts, flushing of the capillaries, and a decidedly tonic effect upon the nerve endings of the sympathetic and the cerebro-spinal system in and around the orifices. Similar temporary contraction with following dilatation of the millions of tiny cutaneous orifices all over the body, resulting in a general flushing of the capillaries and in profound excitation of nerve reflexes and peristaltic action of the blood vessels all through the body, is obtained by the various cold water applications, such as the natural bath, cold ablutions, blitzguss, barefoot walking in the dewy grass, as well as the nude air and light baths.

18. **Dilatation of the Nasal Orifices.** The beneficial effects of cold water sniffing are due not alone to the mechanical clearing of the nasal passages from pathogenic excretions, but also to the tonic effects of the cold water flushing upon the sympathetic and cerebro-spinal nerve filaments in the membranes of the nasal passages. This undoubtedly explains the tonic effect of the cold water sniffing, not only upon the physical functions, especially the respiration, but also upon the mental activities.

These natural methods with their profound effects upon the system make entirely unnecessary surgical dilatation of the orifices, curettements, shortening of ligaments, extirpation of piles and the surgical treatment of fissures, papillae and incipient tumours. Such surgical mutilation is suppressive, not curative, and is usually followed in time by serious chronic after-effects — the "mysterious sequelae" of medical science. We must remember also that the abnormal conditions discussed in this chapter are, in general, secondary effects, that the primary causes lie more or less in food poisoning, in the irritating and destructive effects of poisonous drugs, and in wrong thinking and feeling.

SECTION XXIX

NERVOUS DISEASES

It is safe to say that one half of all the patients who come to us for consultation and treatment have been told that they suffer from nervousness. After having given a long recital of their aches and pains, they usually wind up by saying: "All the doctors I have consulted tell me it is my nerves", or, "it is nervousness", or, "it is neurasthenia". What do these terms mean? Do they actually explain the nature and causes of the patients' ailments? They do not. They are merely convenient terms for covering the doctor's ignorance. A well known nerve specialist in Chicago delivered a lecture before a medical society on the subject of neurasthenia. Addressing the assembled physicians, he began as follows: "A patient comes to you complaining that he is suffering from headaches, physical and mental weakness, pressure on top of the head, ringing in the ears, insomnia, irritability and most of the other symptoms of nervousness known to medical science. After a thorough examination you find that all his vital organs are intact; there is nothing wrong with him physically; in fact you do not know what ails him — that is neurasthenia." There are many other latin and Greek names for diseases which serve the same purpose — to cover the doctor's ignorance. Still, the patient who has consulted the "great specialist" goes home perfectly satisfied so long as he gets a Latin name for his troubles. When he is told he has rheumatism, neuralgia or neurasthenia he thinks he knows what is the matter with him. It does not require a medical education to tell a patient that "it is the nerves" or "rheumatism" or "neurasthenia" when his body is racked by aches and pains and his mind is on the verge of insanity. The brain and the nerves will not give out until there is some good reason for it, and the doctor's diagnosis, in order to be of any value to the patient, should define the causes of the weakness and irritation of brain and nerve matter.

1. **The Chemical Causes of Nervous Diseases.** The diagnosis from the iris and the examination of the spine, as given in our institutes, throw considerable light on the causes and the rational treatment of nervous diseases. In the great majority of cases when examining the eyes of "nervous" and "neurasthenic" patients, the first thing to attract our attention is a darkening or decided discolouration of the areas of the stomach and bowels, which are located directly around the pupil. The brownish, reddish, yellowish and other abnormal pigmentation indicates various forms of drug poisoning which have resulted in a diseased condition of the organs. These signs in the iris mean that the membranous linings of the stomach and bowels are in a sluggish, atonic condition and this is bound

to be followed by very serious consequences. The membranous linings of the digestive organs serve two purposes — elimination and assimilation. Certain cells and glandular structures in the membranes absorb the food materials and after purifying and modifying, transmit them into the blood and lymph streams. Other cells and glands in the intestinal membranes excrete morbid matter and systemic poisons.

From the foregoing it becomes apparent that a sluggish, inactive condition of the mucous membranes lining the digestive tract must have the following detrimental results:

First: The food materials are not properly assimilated and so pass out of the body without being utilized. We must remember that the foods, while they remain in the intestinal tract, are not yet in the body. They do not pass into the body until they are absorbed through the walls of the intestines into the venous and lymphatic circulation. Defective assimilation of this kind is aggravated by the use of mineral oils. While these promote evacuation by creating a slippery condition of the bowels, they do not do anything to clear away the colloid substances which clog the absorbent lining of the intestines — therefore these oily laxatives prevent absorption of the food materials through the intestinal walls into the circulation. In time they aggravate chronic constipation because they obviate the necessity for natural effort.

Second: The elimination of waste materials and systemic poisons through the intestinal membranes is seriously handicapped, which results in systemic poisoning, or, as it is called by the medical men, autointoxication. Furthermore, under normal conditions the membranous linings of the intestinal tract throw off mucoid secretions which lubricate the bowels and facilitate the movement and discharge of the food waste and faeces. Certain cell linings in the stomach throw off secretions containing important digestive ferments on which depend the proper digestion of food materials.

What are the inevitable effects of such abnormal conditions in the digestive organs? If the intestinal membranes do not absorb the food materials the blood and lymph are deficient in nutritive elements and cannot properly feed the brain and nervous system. These, as well as the rest of the body, are starved. Somebody has expressed this in the words: "Nervousness is the cry of the nerves for food." While this is partially true, the nerves are also irritated by the systemic poisons which circulate in the blood stream as the result of the retention of faeces and defective elimination. No wonder the nerves weaken and cry with pain when they are thus starved and poisoned at the same time.

Systemic poisoning is seriously aggravated by a sluggish, atrophic condition of the skin. This is indicated in the iris by a heavy black ring along the outer edge, which is visible more or less distinctly in the eyes of most people. This atrophic condition of the skin is caused largely through warm bathing from the time of birth, the wearing of heavy dense clothing, and through clogging and weakening of the skin with antiseptic powders, salves, lotions, etc., used for the suppression of skin eruptions, and by toilet preparations containing substances injurious to the life of the skin. When the bowels and the cuticle are in a semi-paralysed condition the kidneys have to do more than their own share of the work of elimination and in turn become clogged and inactive. This is shown in the iris by chronic defects in the areas of these organs.

From the foregoing it becomes apparent that malassimilation, malnutrition and defective elimination are the most common causes of nervous diseases. What is the usual treatment in such cases? The weakened nerves are artificially and temporarily stimulated by poisonous drugs and tonics, only to become more thoroughly paralysed, for all artificial stimulation is followed by corresponding weakness and atrophy. The temporary stimulation may be produced by alcohol, coffee, tea or nicotine. Infinitely worse in their paralysing effects upon the system than these food, drink and tobacco poisons are drug poisons like quinine, digitalis, arsenic, strychnine, etc., which constitute the active principles in medical tonics. The diagnosis from the iris proves conclusively that these drug poisons concentrate in certain parts of the body for which they have a special affinity and then become the cause of more serious troubles. In fact, as we have learned in other parts of this volume, the most serious nervous symptoms are due to the presence of drug poisons in the body. Aches and pains, restlessness and insomnia are suppressed with bromides, morphine, coal tar preparations and other sedatives, hypnotics and "pain killers". These poisons merely benumb and paralyse brain and nerve matter into temporary insensibility, leaving them in a still more weakened and diseased condition but doing nothing to remove the underlying causes of the nervous or neurasthenic ailments. The only way this can be accomplished is to build up the blood on a natural basis through proper diet and to make the organs of assimilation and elimination more active through natural methods of living and treatment. A natural diet, well suited for this purpose, is outlined in Sec. I and X. In the treatment of chronic ailments this general dietetic regimen must be modified or interchanged with periods of raw food diet, fasting, etc., according to the individual requirements and changing conditions of the patient. The various methods of manipulative treatment are important.

2. **Mechanical Causes of Nervous Diseases.** Let us now consider the mechanical causes of nervous ailments. The nerves may be irritated or benumbed not only by food and drug poisons but also by mechanical

lesions in the spine or in other parts of the framework of the body. According to physiological law, irritation at any point along the course of a nerve is communicated to all the branches of that nerve, similar to the way in which an electric current introduced at any point of a network of copper wires, if not checked or diverted, will travel over all the wires connected with that system. Thus irritation of a nerve trunk will be transmitted to all the cells and organs supplied by that particular nerve trunk and its branches. In this manner many serious disorders are brought about. Frequently patients come to us who have been treated for many years for "sciatic rheumatism". We find that one or both hip bones are subluxated (slipped innominate). In such cases a few manipulative treatments replace the bones, remove the abnormal pressure and tension and thus cure the "chronic sciatica". Other patients have suffered for years from chronic headaches, nervousness, insomnia, eye troubles, etc. They have swallowed large amounts of poisonous sedatives, anodynes and hypnotics. Upon careful examination we find spinal lesions in the region of the neck. When these lesions are corrected the nervous symptoms disappear. In similar manner irritation of any one of the nerves passing out from the spine may cause pain or abnormal function in the corresponding part of the body. For such conditions there can be but one remedy, namely, the correction of the mechanical lesions in the framework of the body which give rise to them.

3. **Mental and Emotional Causes of Nervous Diseases.** While studying mental and emotional causes of disease we must realize that every mental and emotional vibration is instantly transmuted into the physical, material vibrations of the human body. I would define the fundamental law of mental therapeutics as follows: Vibrations originating on one plane of being — physical, mental or psychical — are by continuity transmuted into the vibratory conditions of the other planes. Thus physical vibrations become mental or psychical vibrations, and vice versa. "As from below so from above; as from above so from below." The trouble with many representatives of the physical and the mental and spiritual schools of healing is that they apply the law in only one of its phases. While it is true that habitual irritability will "sour the bile, poison the liver", it is just as true that an excruciating toothache or any other kind of long continued physical pain will affect the mental and emotional vibrations unless the person possesses superhuman self control. Every mental, emotional and psychical vibration is instantly telegraphed from the seat of consciousness in the physical and spiritual brain centres over the nerve trunks and filaments to every cell in the body, and there transmuted into the vibrations of physical health and well being, or into physical irritation and disease.

In another chapter of this volume I have illustrated this transmutation of mental and emotional vibrations somewhat as follows: It is a well known fact that dry sand on a glass plate placed on the top of a piano will arrange itself into harmonious designs in accordance with the musical sounds elicited from the instrument. Thus purely mental or emotional musical vibrations are transmuted into the material configurations of the sand. The melody produced from the instrument had its conception in the mind of the composer. This musical conception he transmuted into corresponding sound vibrations. These in turn were translated into written notes of paper, thus completing the transmutation from the purely mental and emotional into the physical ink and paper. Then again, the player translates the written notes into musical sounds from the piano and these musical sound vibrations cause the sand on the glass plate to be grouped into orderly configurations of geometrical design. It would be interesting to know what sort of higher and finer vibrations paint the flowers and ferns on the frozen window panes. Another illustration in connection with this theme is the music roll of a pianola. Stretch out one of these sheets and observe the wonderfully symmetrical and geometrical designs in the arrangement of the perforations. The perforations stand for musical notes and these for musical sounds. Musical sounds interpret the emotions of the human soul — "music is the established harmonic relationship of the soul's emotions to the universe of sound". Every musical note expresses some vibration in the gamut of human emotions, from the deepest notes of misery and despair to the highest vibratory expressions of love and happiness.

In the Nature Cure Catechism, I have defined health as "harmonious vibration of the parts and particles composing the human entity on the physical, mental and moral planes of being". Health, self content and happiness constitute the music of the soul; discontent, unhappiness and physical disease, discordant, nerve-wracking noises. With these facts in mind, how can we afford to play the discords of fear, anger, jealousy, revenge, greed and self pity on the harpstrings of the soul?

Let us see how the mental and emotional discords become physical agony and disease.

4. **Fear.** The most destructive of all emotions is fear. It has a benumbing and paralysing effect upon the body. Its physiological effects resemble those of freezing. A person freezing to death and one agitated by great fear and anxiety present a similar appearance. In either case the body is bent, cramped and trembling, the face is blanched, the teeth chattering. Cold shivers chase down the spine and through the benumbed extremities. The blood vessels, nerve channels and cells of the body are benumbed and congealed, causing obstruction to the free flow of

the nerve and blood currents, thus shutting off the influx of the vital force. It is this obstruction to influx of the life force which causes death by freezing and also causes death under the stress of some fear or great anxiety. People indulging habitually and continually in the fear and worry habit may not die at once from the effects of it, but they are nevertheless committing slow suicide through psychical refrigeration. They are effectually reducing the inflow of the life force, thus lowering their vitality and resistance to the destructive influences of systemic poisons and disease taints. Furthermore, as I have pointed out, these vibrations are directly transmuted into the corresponding conditions of physical disease in the tissues of the body. The atoms and molecules of the cells arrange themselves into disorderly configuration and produce inharmonious and discordant vibrations just as surely as noisy racket produced on the piano will throw the sand on the glass plate into disorder.

People affected by these destructive thought habits may answer: "It is easy enough to say these things, but how can I prevent fear and worry thought from entering my mind?" As usual, ignorance is at the bottom of the trouble. People can control their thinking and feeling just as surely as their eating and drinking, but unfortunately they have never been taught self control nor even the possibility of it in these matters. It is the lack of such psychological teaching and training from early youth that accounts for untold suffering, physically, morally and psychically. Fear manifests in many forms and phases, such as fright, terror, despair, apprehension, anxiety, mistrust, alarm, horror, despondency, melancholy, cowardice, doubt, suspicion, etc. These mental, emotional and psychical vibrations differ only in degree of destructiveness. All must be held in abeyance and eliminated by self control. This will become easy when we consider the utter uselessness of fear in its various manifestations. While fear is a natural impulse of the soul and useful in so far as it gives us warning of approaching or imminent danger, weak surrender to this emotion robs us of our strength and clear vision, thus making it easier for the threatened evil to overpower us.

Fear is faith in evil. It is the perversion of the great law of faith. He who fears a thing has faith that it can and will master him; thus he becomes a psychological coward and the thing he fears will surely overpower him. How much better is it to profit by the constructive workings of the law than to be destroyed by its evil effects. As surely as fear vibrations benumb and congeal the channels of life, just so surely will hope, faith and confidence in God and man and in the healing forces within relax the whole system, increasing the influx of vital force, thus invigorating and harmonizing the vibrations on all planes of being. All of us have been at times benumbed and paralysed by sudden fear, and many when weakened by physical or mental disease have experienced the wonderfully tonic effects of sympathy, love and joyful emotions. Cheerfulness is the best of all tonics and love the greatest physician. Increasing health, strength and happiness depend upon higher, more refined and more rapid vibrations on the mental, emotional and psychical planes of being. The highest and finest vibration in the universe is love; therefore is the love vibration the greatest of all healers. Love for humanity and sympathy with its suffering was the secret of the healing power of the Master, Jesus. It is the *modus operandi* of magnetic and spiritual healing.

5. **Anger.** While fear freezes, benumbs and paralyses the organism, anger manifests in the opposite conditions of abnormally increased excitement and heat. As fear corresponds to freezing, anger and its kindred emotions affect the body like a consuming fire. They may well be called psychological combustion. Anger manifests in various phases and degrees of intensity, such as impatience, irritability, ill temper, resentment, hatred, rage, fury, revenge, bitterness, indignation, exasperation, malice and destructiveness. These violently destructive emotions act on the physical body like fire. A person thus agitated presents the appearance of one overheated. The face is flushed, the blood pressure to the brain is greatly increased, which may result in apoplexy or in heart failure. The brain is congested as if by the effects of alcohol. As congestion in the lungs or other vital organs of the body tends to destroy the tissues of the affected parts, so also congestion of the brain, caused by wrath and fury, disrupts the subtle molecular structures of brain and nerve substances. One who is inflamed with anger is as irresponsible as one intoxicated with fiery liquor. The crimes of rage intoxication are as frequent and as deplorable as those committed under alcoholic stimulation. Nothing corrodes and frazzles the nerves so badly and wastes nerve force so wantonly as the consuming fires of anger and kindred emotions.

Excessive stimulation is always followed by corresponding depression, weakness and collapse. He who succumbs habitually to violent emotions slowly but steadily weakens his physical organism and lowers his power of resistance to destructive influences on the physical, mental and spiritual planes of being, thus inviting nerve exhaustion and paralysis. Any and all discordant vibrations interfere with and obstruct the inflow of the life force, lowering the vitality and undermining physical and mental health. This is true of anger as well as of fear and of all other forms of destructive vibration. Furthermore, the physical wireless connects the unhappy victim of wrath and fury with the abodes of the most vicious and cruel beings on the earth plane and on the astral and spiritual planes, thus opening his soul to influx from these hellish spheres of cruelty, remorse and despair, and thereby intensifying his own unhappy condition. The only remedy

162

for these consuming diseases of the soul is self control; the making of new records in the plastic grey matter of the brain, records attuned to the vibrations of patience, forbearance, sympathy and brotherly love. We must either acquire constructive habits of thinking and feeling, or suffer the tortures of alternating nervous and emotional excitation and exhaustion. Thus we create within ourselves our own heavens or our own hells.

6. **Self Pity.** Self pity in its vibratory nature and its effects upon body, mind and soul, closely resembles the ravages of tuberculosis. It is psychological phthisis. A person affected by this degrading phase of emotional self indulgence presents the miserable, haggard, negative appearance of a consumptive. The victim of self pity assumes that he is being unjustly dealt with by Providence, by fortune and by his fellowmen. He considers himself a martyr, enduring undeserved hardships, privations and injustice. This results in resentment, gloom and depression. It effectively kills cheerfulness, ambition and virile initiative. This type of psychical consumption affects those possessed of great wealth and of the most wonderful opportunities in life just as frequently as it does those who actually have to endure the greatest privations. The daughter of one of our best known multimillionaires has been confined for many years in a private sanitorium in France. She is obsessed by the delusion that she is facing extreme poverty and the poorhouse, or that she will die of starvation for lack of means to procure food. What a living travesty this is on the popular belief that great wealth secures happiness. Such cases are not at all uncommon among those possessed of immense wealth. They prove that the cause of this psychological disease does not lie altogether in outward circumstance, but rather in the emotional and psychical life of the sufferer. Such egomaniacs are the product of self-centred egotism. If they had paid a little more attention to the real privations and sufferings of their fellow beings instead of brooding over their own real or imaginary troubles, they would have escaped the ravages of psychical phthisis. Sometimes, indeed, these victims of self pity are aroused out of their miserable mental dejection by some real trouble or misfortune. A splendid illustration of this is Mrs. Gummidge in Dickens' story of "David Copperfield". For many years she had pitied and bemoaned herself as a "lone, lorn Creetur", but when real misfortune struck the family through the elopement of Emily, then sympathy and pity aroused her from her self-centred condition and changed her into a veritable angel of mercy who lightened the gloom of the unhappy family by cheerfulness and unselfish service. Forgetting her own imaginary troubles and lonesomeness, she underwent a truly wonderful psychical chemicalization through the magical reagents of pity and sympathy.

In my lectures I frequently take occasion to remind our friends that the best way to help themselves is to help others — that there is no better way of increasing the influx of the healing forces than by treating others for health and strength and happiness. I say to them: "There are those around you who need help just as much or more than you do — some of them as yet unable to help themselves. Treat these weak ones mentally and spiritually, strengthen them by a kindly look and a word of encouragement. You will be surprised how this will increase the flow of vital energy into your own bodies." These higher and finer forces can be received only as we give. Selfish brooding on our own troubles and self pity effectively shut off the inflow of life force, while sympathy and unselfish service open wide the channels of life and stimulate the flow of vital energy.

A well known ancient legend strikingly illustrates the utter foolishness of self pity. The people of a certain country had become very much dissatisfied with their sufferings. Each one believed his own cross was much larger and heavier than that of his neighbour. An angel of God appeared among them in human form and told them to bring their crosses and deposit them in one great heap, when everyone would be allowed to select a burden which he deemed lighter than his own. The people greatly rejoiced at this good fortune, discarded their crosses and proceeded to choose what they thought were lighter ones. However, their happiness at the change was not of long duration. One after another they soon returned, confessing dejectedly that the new cross was heavier and more painful to carry than the old one and asking to be allowed to take up again the old accustomed burden which a wise providence had adjusted to each one's needs and powers of endurance.

Those who consume themselves in self pity forget that this life is not intended to be a continuous Sunday School picnic; that, on the contrary, it is a school of personal and persistent effort for self development of our latent faculties, capacities and powers, through the use of reason, will power and self control; that only through overcoming evil in its many forms can we educate and strengthen our mental and psychical muscle; that evil on all planes of being is constructive in nature and purpose; and that there is no suffering, disease or evil of any kind anywhere unless the law has been transgressed somewhere by someone. These transgressions of the law may be due to ignorance, to indifference or to wilfulness and viciousness. The effects will always be commensurate with the causes. When we look upon evil from this viewpoint it loses its terrors. Then we look upon it as a healing crisis necessary to eliminate the destructive effects of ignorant or wilful violation of nature's laws. Thus we learn to overcome evil, not through anger, resentment and self pity, but through cheerful compliance with the law. Many pity themselves as martyrs to duty, martyrs in the service of their relatives and friends, martyrs to social conditions. They never stop to consider how far they, themselves, help to create these unfortunate conditions through their own destructive thinking, feeling and doing. A lady remarked to her friend: "I don't understand why it is, but every time I move I find bad neighbours." Her friend answered: "Is it not possible that when you move you take the worst neighbour with you?" If our surroundings and our neighbours do not suit us, it is a sign that we are not much better ourselves. If we were better than they we would probably be now in some higher sphere of life and action. The fact that we are here indicates that we need the lessons to be learned on this plane, and we shall not escape to more refined surroundings and better society until we become fit to maintain more refined and more sympathetic associations with our fellow beings. It is safe to assume that at each new birth, or as we now call it, at death, we gravitate to those spheres of life and action for which we are best suited. What would be the use of transplanting a drunken sot from his haunts of degradation and squalor to a home of culture and refinement? Unaccustomed to such intelligent surroundings, he would soon return to his filthy dive. The beautiful home would be hell enough for him. We may rest assured that life will sooner or later place us where we belong.

If you suffer from great physical weakness and nerve exhaustion, find out whether it is not caused by psychological phthisis. If you cannot determine this for yourself, have a good psychologist give you a thorough examination. The trouble with many people who are seriously affected by mental, emotional and psychical disease is that they are unable or unwilling to diagnose their conditions. Frequently they resent vehemently the intimation that they may be suffering from such psychical disorders.

7. **Envy.** Envy represents a combination of the moods of anger and self pity. Anger may be inspired by the thought that somebody else possesses the thing that we covet, and self pity because we are deprived of the thing we desire to possess. Envy, therefore, consumes and wastes the body, mind and soul of its unhappy victims by the combined effects of psychological combustion and psychical phthisis.

8. **Jealousy.** Jealousy is a mixture of fear, anger and self pity. We fear that somebody may take from us that which rightfully belongs to us, and anger results from such real or imaginary injustice. Such fear and anger in turn provoke self pity at the thought of the real or imaginary loss or injury. Thus we are torn alternately or all at once by the most powerful destructive emotions of the human soul. No wonder the victims of the "green monster" suffer the tortures of hell, that overcome by passionate resentment and the desire for revenge they commit unjust and cruel crimes

165

against the innocent as well as the guilty. These terribly destructive emotions, even when seemingly justified, will never right a wrong, but only magnify its destructive effects on ourselves.

That which rightfully belongs to us can never be taken away from us. The majority of people do not distinguish between their real and their imaginary possessions. Quite frequently the things which they believe they possess or do desire to possess are, in reality, their greatest burdens and their worst enemies. That which we have earned through faithful exercise of our natural capacities and powers, that is, our mental, moral and psychical characteristics, can never be taken away from us. They are the only possessions that will remain with us after the great transition. Nothing else besides this really belongs to us. We may enjoy the use of money, property and treasures of art for a day, a year or a lifetime, but they never become part of ourselves and sooner or later we shall leave them behind us. If a friend deceives and deserts us, it simply means that he was not our friend and the sooner we are rid of him the better for us in the long run. Our real friend, the one who belongs to us, is waiting for us somewhere. It is the same with all material possessions. The greater our possessions the more extravagant our wants and needs. People do not possess wealth, but are possessed and obsessed by wealth. The more simple the life, the less the wants and needs, and the less the fear of loss and deprivation. Those who are used to simple and economical ways of living rejoice in them. Those deprived of great wealth and comfort are appalled and discouraged by the loss of it. When we possess a thing we do not appreciate its value, but the moment we lose it we are overcome by unhappiness and resentment. Then why not do without it in the first place? Instead of wasting our vitality in spiteful resentment at our neighbour's prosperity let us rejoice in his possessions and thereby make them our own. If these things be true, then why allow ourselves to be torn by the destructive emotions of fear, anger and self pity because of real or imaginary loss of some ephemeral, or at any rate transient, possession, which after all is not essential to the well being of the real man, the soul man; especially so when these discordant and destructive psychical emotions invariably result in mental and nervous breakdown and physical weakness, disease and premature death?

Diseases of the soul, created by perverted mental vision and lack of self control, continue after death, afflicting the soul in the spiritual life just as heavily as on this side of the "Great Divide". While diseases of the physical body may terminate at death, abnormal conditions of mind and soul continue on the spiritual planes of life. Therefore our spiritual salvation, as well as physical health, depends upon the correction of our perverted mental vision and upon overcoming our lack of self control.

Self control is the master key to the solution of all our troubles and of all higher development on the mental, moral and spiritual planes of being. How to strengthen the power of will and how to overcome evil habits and to develop good habits I have described in the last chapters of this volume.([1])

SECTION XXX

INSANITY OR MENTAL, EMOTIONAL AND PSYCHICAL DISORDERS

In the discussion of this subject I shall not follow the official classifications given in standard scientific works. These orthodox classifications are of little value to us, as they are based on outward manifestations or symptoms of mental disorders, while they do not take into consideration their underlying causes and true nature. In most instances they are merely Latin or Greek names for outstanding symptoms. It is lack of understanding of the true nature and causes of mental and psychical disorders and lack of their rational treatment that accounts for the progressive increase of insanity, which keeps pace with advancing civilization in spite of the most determined efforts of medical science to stem the tide of this great danger that threatens the civilized nations. A prominent physician at the head of one of the largest sanitoria of this country, in a public lecture, made the statement that at the present rate of increase in insantiy all the inhabitants of this country would be insane at a certain future date. Happily this gloomy prediction will not come true, thanks to the rapidly increasing popularity of the Nature Cure idea.

I shall endeavour to treat the subject simply, as it has presented itself to me in actual experience, including under the term insanity all prolonged

([1])
    In his discussion of Nervous Diseases Lindlahr seems to make two points. The first is that nervous disease is for the most part simply a form of physical disease in which the functioning of the nervous mechanism of the body is impaired by bad chemical or mechanical conditions in the body. The second is that there is a constant reciprocal action going on between the mental and emotional life of an individual and his nervous system. Thus, while the first thing to be considered in the treatment of so-called nervous diseases is the creation of a condition of positive good health of the body as a whole, it is also essential in many cases to teach the patient to control his thinking and his emotions so as to eliminate mental and emotional causes which are having an effect on the nervous system and the functioning of the physical body.

departures from normal standards of thinking, feeling and acting. The following table may help to elucidate this complex subject. It will be seen that I divide all forms of insanity into two main groups, the physical and the psychical. By physical mental and emotional disorders I mean all those morbid mental conditions which originate in abnormal functioning or organic degeneration of the physcial organism and particularly of brain and nerve matter.

GROUP I. MENTAL AND EMOTIONAL DISORDERS DUE TO PHYSICAL CAUSES

A. Hereditary and Congenital Disorders

These may be functional or organic; they may result from abnormal prenatal influences of a mental or emotional nature; also from prenatal malnutrition, drug poisoning or traumatism. For example, a few days ago I examined a child four years old who had not yet learned to talk. The thyroid gland seemed to be well developed and the general physical condition to be normal. The frontal region of the head, however, was very low and the sides and the parietal parts of the skull above the ears were somewhat caved in. The brown eyes of the child revealed three fully developed, heavy nerve rings, an extraordinary condition for a child of that age, indicating serious disorder of the nervous system. Both parents were in good physical condition before the conception of the child and have been ever since. The mother told me that during the pregnancy from beginning to end she had been tortured by great homesickness, mental depression and melancholia. This was the only adverse influence I was able to trace in the case. Possibly it had a harmful effect upon the intellectual brain area of which the speech centre is primary and basic. Significant also in this respect is the depression in the parietal bones over Brocha's convolution, the location of the speech centre. In another case a grown cretin and idiot whose eyes I examined showed in the brain region a very heavy scurf rim. The mother, during pregnancy, had taken enough calomel for liver trouble and constipation to produce the symptoms of salivation several times. The mercury sign was distinctly visible in her eyes. In all cases of so-called hereditary syphilis it is the mercury, salvarsan, arsenic, iodine, potassium or other drug poison, not venereal disease, which produces the congenital defects in the offspring. It is a fact that syphilis is not communicated to a nursing child through the milk. Much less is it possible that the disease is conveyed from mother to child prenatally. Nature does her best to protect the young life against adverse influences, but nature is powerless to prevent the introduction of virulent

168

Mental and Psychic Diseases—Varieties and Causes

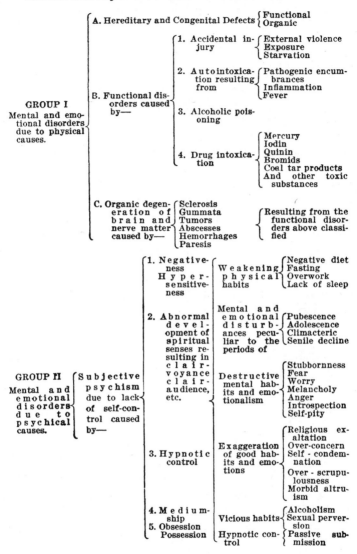

GROUP I
Mental and emotional disorders due to physical causes.

A. Hereditary and Congenital Defects { Functional / Organic

B. Functional disorders caused by—

1. Accidental injury { External violence / Exposure / Starvation

2. Autointoxication resulting from { Pathogenic encumbrances / Inflammation / Fever

3. Alcoholic poisoning

4. Drug intoxication { Mercury / Iodin / Quinin / Bromids / Coal tar products / And other toxic substances

C. Organic degeneration of brain and nerve matter caused by— { Sclerosis / Gummata / Tumors / Abscesses / Hemorrhages / Paresis } Resulting from the functional disorders above classified

GROUP II
Mental and emotional disorders due to psychical causes.

Subjective psychism due to lack of self-control caused by—

1. Negativeness Hypersensitiveness — Weakening physical habits { Negative diet / Fasting / Overwork / Lack of sleep

2. Abnormal development of spiritual senses resulting in clairvoyance clairaudience, etc. — Mental and emotional disturbances peculiar to the periods of { Pubescence / Adolescence / Climacteric / Senile decline

Destructive mental habits and emotionalism { Stubbornness / Fear / Worry / Melancholy / Anger / Introspection / Self-pity

3. Hypnotic control — Exaggeration of good habits and emotions { Religious exaltation / Over-concern / Self-condemnation / Over-scrupulousness / Morbid altruism

4. Mediumship
5. Obsession Possession — Vicious habits { Alcoholism / Sexual perversion / Hypnotic control { Passive submission

poisons into human bodies by the disciples of pseudo-science. Again, serious injuries to the abdomen of a pregnant woman may also cause congenital nervous and mental derangement or physical deformity of the offspring. A few weeks ago we examined in our open clinic a child a few months old whose lower ribs on one side were badly caved in. The mother had a serious fall during the last month of pregnancy. A deformity of this kind can be dealt with by manipulative treatment.

Congenital Deficiency of the Ductless Glands

Congenital deficiency of the thymus and thyroid glands is responsible for most cases of cretinism, idiocy and backward development. Allopathic medicine endeavours to overcome these defects by administration of thymus or thyroid extract. This, however, is only palliative. While these animal extracts may serve to a certain extent as a substitute and may stimulate the physical and mental development of the child, still the administration of these artificial preparations tends to retard the natural development of the glandular structures. Whenever the administration of the thyroid extract is interrupted, the improvement ceases and there is a strong tendency to retrogression. After all, these extracts artificially prepared from animal bodies are not congenial to the human organism and their constant administration tends to create abnormal conditions. This has been observed in many instances. Much better and more permanent results are obtained by natural management and treatment. All the tonic influences of the various methods of natural treatment, especially massage and neurotherapy — manipulation of the nerve centres which supply the ductless glands — tend to develop the defective organs in a perfectly natural manner. We have thus treated and cured many little patients suffering from congenital malformations, backward development, cretinism, defects of the sensory organs and idiocy.[1]

[1]
Since Lindlahr's time there has been a great deal of thought and research directed towards the endocrine glands and various methods of influencing them have been elaborated. It would appear that some of these may be useful and constructive but that others can be very harmful and should be used, if at all, with great caution or as a temporary expedient. Lindlahr is undoubtedly right in pointing out that substitution therapy involving the use of artificial or animal endocrine extracts tends to prevent rather than to encourage the natural functioning of the patient's own endocrine system, which is the object to be attained. He claims to have had excellent results by applying all-round natural treatment to cases in which there is endocrine deficiency or imbalance and he lays particular stress on the importance of manual procedures designed to improve the blood and nerve supply to the glandular structures. The exponents of yoga also claim that many of the yoga exercises or postures have a very specific and powerful effect on endocrine glands. There can be little doubt that the system of Endogenous Endocrinotherapy advocated by Dr. Jules Samuels has made an important contribution to our understanding of the endocrine system and has shown how it can be influenced and balanced when it has gone wrong, although it would seem that his method could and should be simplified and improved in respect both of diagnosis and of treatment. On the other hand, the endocrine system being a very delicate, complicated and far-reaching mechanism affecting body metabolism, the functioning of the brain and nervous system and the emotional life and the whole personality, it is impossible not to regard with great suspicion the wide use of steroid and hormonal preparations for all sorts of purposes, including contraception and the control of fertility, which is now in fashion. The long-term and side effects of such preparations are at present little understood and their use may lead to very serious consequences and to a condition in which they cannot be dispensed with for life.

B. Functional Disorders

1. **Accidental Injury.** Functional disturbance may be caused by external violence such as concussion of the brain from blows on the head or from falls, etc. Spinal analysis frequently discloses lesions, particularly of the cervical region. The impingement on the blood vessels and nerves by such bony displacements or contractions of connective tissues may produce mental and nervous disorders which will abate or disappear when the lesions are corrected by proper manipulative treatment. When mental or nervous disorders result from fractures or indentations of the skull, the fractured bones or splinters pressing upon the brain matter must be removed by surgical treatment.[1]

2. **Autointoxication.** Many forms of functional mental disorders are caused by systemic poisoning resulting from the accumulation of morbid matter and poisons produced in the system, such as acids, alkaloids, ptomaines and xanthiness, which we designate collectively as pathogen. These morbid materials circulating in the blood may unduly exalt or depress the normal activities of the brain and nervous system. For instance, the acids of phosphorus have a powerful irritating and stimulating effect upon the brain and nerve matter, giving rise to nervous irritability, insomnia and hysterical manifestations, while carbon dioxide has a benumbing, depressive effect. The normal structure and functioning of brain and nerve cells depends upon the quantity and quality of the blood supply. Therefore the normality of mental and emotional functions depends to a large extent upon the purity and normality of the vital fluids. If the blood stream which feeds the brain and nervous system is saturated with gluey, mucoid and gaseous materials, the mental and emotional activities will be sluggish and phlegmatic, resulting in impairment of memory and of the reasoning faculties.

Excessive acid formation in the system may result in earthy deposits in

---

A treatment which should be specially mentioned in this connection is the injection of living cells according to the ideas and methods of Drs. Niehans and Henry. Undoubtedly this method of treatment is capable of producing very wonderful results in certain cases, though it is not easy to reconcile with the idea of "Natural Therapeutics" as set forth by Lindlahr and it does seem open to objections apart from the fact of its great expense. The introduction of animal extracts directly into the human tissues by injection does not appear to be a natural procedure and may well be accompanied with risks and long-term effects of which we are not fully aware. Personally I find it hard to accept the idea that the same or better results cannot be obtained by simpler, cheaper and more natural methods. It is interesting to note that, according to exponents of this method, it works not so much by substitution as by stimulating the patient's own cells to function properly by a sort of homoeopathic action. This leads to the thought that homoeopathy of the traditional kind may have a very important role to play in the treatment of endocrine disorders in combination with other natural forms of treatment.

[1]
    The new cranial technique which is now being practised by many osteopaths may well be capable of reducing the role to be played by surgery in cases of this kind.

the walls of the blood vessels, narrowing their lumen and obstructing the circulation, thus causing so-called hardening of the arteries with its attendant depressive effects on brain functions, tendency to haemorrhages, embolism, etc. As we have learned in our study of dietetics, practically all pathogenic materials are formed by excessive intake of starchy, protein and fatty foods because the elements composing these foods are electromagnetically negative and therefore pathogen-forming substances. These foods at the same time are very deficient in the positive acid binding and eliminating alkaline mineral elements. The prevention and treatment of this class of disorders is, therefore, largely dietetic and must consist in reducing the protein, starchy and fatty foods and substituting foods rich in the positive alkaline salts of sodium, potassium, calcium, magnesium and iron. Other efficient methods for eliminating pathogenic materials are hydrotherapy, massage, neurotherapy, air and sun baths, proper breathing and curative exercises, homoeopathic remedies, etc.

3. **Alcoholism.** Alcoholism is another prolific cause of functional disorders of a toxic character, producing gradually degenerative changes in the tissues of the body, especially in the liver, spleen and kidneys. In advanced stages it causes degeneration of brain and nerve matter and may result in various forms of delirium and mania. The symptoms of alcoholic poisoning cover a wide range from simple nausea to violent delirium, coma and death. Alcoholic poisoning may result from the use of distilled liquors, such as whisky and alcohol, or of fermented liquors, such as wines, beer, ale, etc. Many patent medicines and medicinal tonics owe their stimulating effects to the large percentage of alcohol which they contain. Meat eating, coffee drinking, smoking and the use of habit-forming drugs all create a craving for alcohol and vice versa. We find in our work that we cannot permanently break our patients from the use of one stimulant unless they give up all other stimulants. Many times we have weaned patients from meat eating, smoking, coffee toping, the use of alcoholic liquors and habit-forming drugs, and after their systems had been thoroughly purified from these poisons all craving for them disappeared, but occasionally one would again fall victim to the old destructive habits. Enquiry into the cause for backsliding usually brings out confessions like the following: "Oh, doctor, I felt so fine that I thought just a cup of coffee" or "just one or two cigars a day would not hurt me, but I find that my will power once weakened, I could not resist the temptation of indulging more freely. Every time I used a stimulant it seemed to create a craving for another one. When my system was in a purified condition, a piece of meat seemed to stimulate me more than once did a glass of whisky, but the taste of meat created a craving for a cup of coffee or a

cigar, and so on until I became once more a slave to all the old habits and now I seem to be deeper in their bondage than ever before." "Give the devil your little finger and he will soon have the whole fellow in the bargain." When the body is thoroughly saturated with meat poisons, caffeine, uric acid, drug poisons, etc., a dozen drinks or cigars a day, more or less, make little difference; but when the system is purified of these poisons and in normal condition, even small amounts of any kind of stimulant will affect the nervous system profoundly and excite a craving for yet stronger stimulation. That alcoholism is an hereditary disease has been proved beyond a doubt. This should be a matter of grave consideration for those who intend to assume the responsibilities of parenthood.

The symptoms of alcoholism, like those of other diseases, manifest in the acute and chronic forms. The light drinker awakens in the morning in a morose and irritable condition. He has no desire for food and is unfit for the work of the day until he has had his "eye opener". At a later stage of the disease the nausea develops into vomiting and the indigestion becomes more pronounced and chronic. Constant hyperaemia of the stomach, liver and spleen are followed by gradual atrophy. The drinker of whisky develops the shrunken, hobnailed liver; the liver of the habitual beer drinker becomes greatly enlarged, sometimes weighing from twenty to forty pounds, but later on it shrinks. The last stages of alcoholism are marked by malnutrition, emaciation, the loss of memory and intellectual faculties. Alcoholic poisons gradually benumb, paralyse and destroy the best qualities of body, mind and soul, until the victim falls to the depths of physical, mental and moral degradation.

All drug cures for this terrible disease are of questionable value. They may create a temporary revulsion for alcohol, but at best this is another case of Beelzebub against the devil. The drugs used in these cures have a bad effect upon the system and when the sedative effects of the drug treatment have lost their hold on the patient, he relapses into the old, destructive habits.

Exactly the same is true of hypnotic treatment for destructive habits. It is at best only temporarily suppressive. Hypnotic control still further weakens the will of the subject. He temporarily abstains from liquor, not of his own accord, but compelled by the dominating will of the hypnotist. When this begins to wane he has less control over his cravings than before. In this connection it must be remembered that a person cannot be hypnotized unless his own reason, will power and self control are temporarily suppressed and completely in abeyance. If this takes place repeatedly, paralysis of these highest faculties and capacities of the mind and soul become permanent and the victim of hypnotism degenerates into the

173

abject slave of every stronger influence. He becomes a negative weakling and drifter, frequently ending in the insane asylum.

The only possible and permanent cure of alcoholism and of drug habits lies in a complete regeneration of the individual through natural methods of living and of treatment. If the patient is in the advanced stages of alcoholism, afflicted with organic diseases of the stomach, liver, kidneys or heart and subject to attacks of delirium tremens, it may be necessary to wean him gradually from the effects of the poison by allowing him graduated doses of alcohol, morphine or whatever the habit-forming poison may be. An attendant must administer gradually decreasing doses at increasing intervals of time. The strength of the poison at the same time may be reduced without the knowledge of the patient. In many instances we have given such patients injections of pure distilled water when they imagined they were getting strong doses of morphine. In such cases the powers of suggestion frequently show us its wonderful effects. Not long ago a patient came to us from a neighbouring hospital. An operation had been performed on one of his limbs. It was then kept in a plaster cast for four months. The only remedy they had in the hospital for the terrific pain following the operation was morphine. When he was brought to our institution he was using as high as ten grains a day. Under the natural treatment the pains gradually abated and within a few weeks we succeeded in reducing the morphine to minimum doses, but whenever we refused to give him an injection he would yell at the top of his voice, claiming that he could not stand the pain and could not sleep. Pains did not trouble him and he was able to sleep when we injected distilled water. The water did the work just as well as the morphine as long as he was under the impression that morphine was being administered. We had to keep up the deception for three weeks, gradually decreasing the number of injections until he became convinced that he could do without the "morphine".

The active treatment of alcoholism must include everything that is good in natural methods. Of primary importance is a strict vegetarian diet, alternating between raw food, milk diet, and fasting regimen. Tonic cold water applications, massage, Swedish movements, neurotherapy, curative gymnastics, air and sun baths and everything else conducive to a thorough regeneration of the system must be applied systematically. Such patients require constitutional treatment. During the first stages of treatment while the victims of drug and liquor habits are helpless and without will power and self control, they need constant attendance and careful nursing day and night. The poison to which they are addicted must be administered in gradually diminishing doses at lengthened intervals and, unless confined in a padded cell, they must be guarded against escape or self-inflicted injury or suicide. When the system of such a patient has been thoroughly purified and regenerated, when he has become accustomed to and thoroughly enjoys a vegetarian diet, the craving for liquor, tobacco or drugs will have disappeared and will not return unless he wilfully indulges in former habits. We have proved in many cases that such a thorough purification and regeneration of the system is a much better guarantee against relapses than all the poison cures in existence.

Not the least potent among the regenerative influences of the Natural Therapeutic treatment are the daily lectures and private consultations through which the patient becomes acquainted for the first time in his life with the natural laws underlying the processes of health, disease and cure, which he must obey in order to attain perfect health and the greatest possible capacity for enjoying the pleasures of life and the highest efficiency in the performance of his share of the world's work. He now becomes aware that these highest and finest achievements of human life cannot be attained through any form of self indulgence. Having learned his lesson through the great contrast between utter misery and degradation and the enjoyment of perfect health, he is willing to pay the price of self control in the future.

The best of drug treatment, while it may break the alcohol or drug habit more or less permanently, never leaves the system in the purified and regenerated condition such as results from natural treatment, which alone ensures perfect health and the complete enjoyment of the good things of life.

4. **Drug Intoxication.** Alcoholism has been made the scapegoat for the increase of insanity among civilized nations and for the major part of defective heredity. Its influence, bad as it is, has been greatly overrated. Fully as destructive have been the effects of poisonous drugs, especially of mercury, iodine, quinine, arsenic, strychnine, bromides and coal tar preparations. Alcohol is in a way congenial to the human organism. It is manufactured in small quantities in most human bodies as a product of sugar fermentation in the intestines and is burned up in the system like other fuel materials. It is probably for this reason that alcohol is not shown in the iris by a characteristic sign of its own. Nicotine and caffeine do not show in the iris because they are chemically closely related to the uric acid group and are therefore not entirely uncongenial to the system. This indicates that these xanthiness are eliminated with comparative ease. Whenever an habitual alcoholic quits taking the poison its effects are without great difficulty overcome by natural methods of living and of treatment. Poisonous drugs, however, have a strong tendency to accumulate in those tissues of the body for which they have a special affinity, there to act as powerful irritants and poisons, creating many of the most

destructive chronic diseases. The destructive effects of drug poisons are fully described in "Iridiagnosis", Vol. IV of this series. Mental disorders caused by poisonous drugs are more difficult to cure than any other forms because they readily result in organic degeneration.

C. Mental and Emotional Disorders due to Organic Degeneration of Brain and Nerve Matter

All functional mental disorders if prolonged by neglect or intensified by suppressive drug treatment may result in organic degeneration of brain and nerve matter, creating such conditions as paresis (softening of the brain), sclerosis of the spinal cord, anterior poliomyelitis, etc. It is evident that cures are much more difficult or may become impossible when the stages of organic degeneration have been reached. A few cases of organic insanity are caused by injury to the brain, but the great majority are due to the action of morbid matter and paralysing or destructive poisons on the brain. These poisons may have been generated in the body by unnatural methods of living. They may be alcohol, nicotine, caffeine or destructive acids and paralysing alkaloids which are the waste products of faulty proteid and starch metabolism. Morbid encumbrances and organic decay are frequently due to the suppression of scrofulous, psoric and syphilitic diseases. About 60 percent of all organic cases, however, are due to the ever lengthening array of destructive poisons such as mercury, iodine, quinine, arsenic, bromine, acetanilid and other coal tar products.

Organic defects may be created in the following manner: Earthy waste matter forms deposits in and clogs and hardens the minute blood vessels of brain and nerve centres. Xanthiness and alkaloids of the uric acid type, or destructive drug poisons, cause obstruction, abnormal changes, decay and actual destruction of nerve and brain matter. To this group of organic insanity belong all nervous and mental disorders classed by the old school of medicine under locomotor ataxia, paresis, dementia paralytica, senile dementia, etc. This entire range of diseases is looked upon by the medical profession as incurable. Nevertheless, we constantly prove in our practice that all of these types of disorders can be alleviated and a large percentage of them cured by natural methods of treatment, provided there is sufficient vitality left in the organism to respond to treatment and provided also that actual destruction of brain and nerve matter is not too far advanced.

The medical treatment of these disorders consists almost universally in the administration of mercury, iodine, arsenic, strychnine, salvarsan and coal tar products. Diagnosis from the iris, however, and the history of cases of this type, reveal the fact that almost without exception these diseases have been produced by the absorption of these same poisons earlier in life. How, then, can such cases be cured by the poisons which produce them? Is it any wonder that medical science calls them "incurable" when too much drugging is all that ails them? Is it any wonder that they improve under Christian Science or any other non-suppressive treatment? Every case of locomotor ataxia, paralysis agitans and paresis which has come under my observation has revealed the signs of drugs, and enquiry into the history usually confirms the drug records in the iris.

It takes mercury from five to sixteen years to work its way into the brain and spinal cord — then its destructive symptoms begin to manifest. What is commonly called secondary and tertiary is nothing but mercurial and iodine poisoning. Syphilis and gonorrhoea in themselves are easily curable by natural methods of treatment. If properly treated, without poisonous drugs, these taints can be completely eradicated from the system within four or five months' time. Not a single case treated by us from its incipiency, that is before suppressive treatment had been given, ever developed any secondary or tertiary symptoms or hereditary diseases in offspring.

GROUP II. MENTAL AND EMOTIONAL DISEASES DUE TO PSYCHICAL CAUSES

The second main division of our diagram deals with psychical disorders. Under these we classify forms of insanity due to mental, emotional and psychical influences. All mental and emotional disorders may finally result in various forms of abnormal psychism such as hypersensitiveness, negativeness, clairvoyance, clairaudience, hypnotic subjection, mediumship, obsession and possession. Every form of perverted mentalism such as stubbornness, fear, worry, hypochondria, anger, fury, rage, jealousy or self pity may become permanent forms of destructive emotionalism. In our practice we are daily more and more impressed with the fact that any form of abnormal thinking and feeling may easily develop into the most terrible depressive or emotional insanity. Mania is frequently merely a natural tendency exaggerated through loss of self control. If parents could be made to realize that their fond indulgence of a child's selfishness, indolence, wilfulness, irritability and temper may develop into the worst forms of nervousness, hysteria and insanity, they would employ the best means at their command to stimulate, educate and strengthen the will power and self control of the child. In the weakening and loss of

177

self control lies the root of psychical disorders; in its restoration, the cure.

Paranoia, Monomania, Fixed Idea

Forms of mental diseases classified by medical science under these heads are largely the result of destructive autosuggestion. I have not been able to find a better illustration of mental and emotional processes than the phonograph and kinematograph. The grey matter of the brain corresponds to the record in the phonograph or to the film in the moving picture machine. These plastic materials receive, register and retain impressions of sound and passing scenes and reproduce them automatically. So, also, the grey matter of the brain receives, registers and retains impressions from the outside world coming through the sensory organs and also impressions of thoughts and emotions generated in the mind of the individual. After those records in the brain matter have been established, they repeat themselves spontaneously or at the call of the will.

All our distinctly human physical and mental capacities and functions have been created in that way. We had to make the centres or records in the motor or Rolandic area of the brain before we could walk or use our limbs for any other purpose. We had to create the centres in Brocha's convolution in the frontal brain for every word we learned to speak in our own or in any foreign language. In like manner we had to create molecular groupings or brain centres for everything we have gained in the acquisition of knowledge or in the execution of manual labour or artistic productions. Before we can solve a problem in arithmetic, acquire dexterity in the handling of a tool, play the violin or any other musical instrument, we must first establish the necessary centres in the grey matter of the cortex. After these molecular groupings in brain matter have been created, they work almost spontaneously and may control the physical organism and the mentality through what we call habit. It took many months of laborious effort to create in Brocha's convolution the molecular groupings for the pronunciation of the words "papa" and "mama" and of other words in an infant's vocabulary. But after the centres were once established, speech flowed freely at the slightest volitional impulse. Many months of laborious and persistent efforts were required to develop the centres in the brain area for muscular movement and coordination before we could make the first tottering steps, but after these centres in the area of Rolando and in the cerebellum were established, the legs responded to the slightest impulse of the will. In similar manner all thinking and feeling impresses its paths, grooves and records in the plastic grey matter of the brain, and after having been firmly established these records

178

of thought, ideas, feelings and memories repeat at the volition of the ego, or they may play their tunes spontaneously. Memory, habit, character, individuality, the subconscious or subjective mind, are made up of these records in the grey matter of the brain. Whether our memories and our habitual states of thinking and feeling are of a pleasant, cheerful and happy nature, or whether they are discordant, irritable, morbid, melancholy, unhappy, spiteful, critical, jealous or destructive in any other way, depends upon the kinds of records we have made in the past, that is, the kind of thoughts and feelings we have entertained and allowed to impress themselves upon the plastic grey matter of the brain. Our future mental, emotional, moral, spiritual and psychical characteristics will depend upon the records we make from this moment on.

When I explain these fundamental principles of psychology and mentalism, people ask: "How can I prevent unpleasant thoughts and feelings from entering my mind?" There lies the root of the trouble. People have never been taught that they have the power to control their thinking and feeling, as well as their eating and drinking. If these fundamental laws and principles of mentalism and emotionalism were impressed on the child mind from the awakening of understanding, what an amount of unhappiness, mental degeneracy and insanity might be prevented. While conversing with a friend about the terrible fate of the victims of autosuggestion, hypnotism, mediumship, obsession and other forms of subjective psychism, she remarked: "It seems incomprehensible why a kind Providence allows innocent and naturally good people to drift into these terrible conditions which must lead to indescribable suffering and final extinction of the individuality." I answered to this: "Somewhere, some time in the history of these individuals they drifted into abnormal ways of thinking and feeling, brooding over real or imaginary troubles, fear of impending poverty, of persecution or misfortune, fear of eternal damnation, of having committed the unpardonable sin or of other religious delusions. These fear records multiplied until they filled the mind to the exclusion of everything else and then played their direful tunes incessantly day and night, creating a living hell for the unfortunate victim of his own mental obsession. Others in similar manner drift into negative conditions of thinking and feeling, which make possible control and obsession by external influences and vicious intelligences in or out of the body."

These victims of destructive autosuggestion begin to fear, worry and brood about something. There may be some reason for it, or the thing dreaded may be entirely imaginary — nine times in ten it is. This occurs usually among people who have not enough real work in their lives but too much time to think and brood. Every time they indulge in this sort of fear thought they impress it more deeply in the plastic grey matter of the brain. One idea sown in the subconscious mind keeps on growing and multiplying until it crowds out everything else. Thus arises the fixed idea, or monomania. The unhappy victim of his own delusion is no longer capable of thinking or feeling anything else. It fills his mind entirely, shows in his behaviour and in his gloomy, melancholy features. Hundreds of thousands of people in this United States are thus slowly but surely creating for themselves the worst hells in the universe without realizing their danger, and nobody raised the danger signal because people do not understand the laws of destructive mentalism.

I have come into contact with many of these unfortunates whose minds were filled with just one kind of discordant, destructive records playing their dismal tunes by day and night, without relief of intermission. Just now I have under observation a man of twenty-eight years of age who has worked himself into such a deplorable condition. He belongs to a wealthy family, is well educated and has had every possible opportunity to make life a success. A few years ago he began to brood and worry over an unhappy love affair. His friends tell me the severing of this attachment was in reality most fortunate, because the object of his affection was not of good moral character, and according to her own confession tried to marry him only for his money. Notwithstanding this, he allowed the matter to occupy his mind to the exclusion of everything else. He imagined that he had wronged the young woman beyond the possibility of atonement. This brought up the idea that he was unworthy of respect and unfit for association with his fellow beings, and this in turn led to more introspection and seclusion, until these melancholy, morose and self-accusatory ideas filled his mind so completely that he tried in various ways to end his misery by suicide. In spite of all this the man is endowed with splendid intelligence. Even during this mental obscuration he was able to vanquish some of the best draughts and chess players in Chicago. Only a few days ago he mentioned to me from memory the telephone numbers of a dozen firms he dealt with two or three years ago. The telephone book proved his memory to be absolutely correct. Still, long continued and persistent explanations and persuasion have so far proved inadequate to lift his dismal mental obsession. His trouble undoubtedly originated by making the wrong kind of brain records.

People do not realize that this sort of fear and worry thought is a form of destructive self indulgence just as surely as is overindulgence in alcoholic liquors or in habit-creating drugs. They have never been taught that destructive mentalism and emotionalism may be prevented by the exercise of will power and self control just as easily as alcoholism or the cigarette or drug habits.

Treatment of Monomania

These forms of fixed idea or monomania cannot be successfully treated at home. Old surroundings, relatives, friends, and accustomed scenes and objects constantly call up the old brain records and cause them to play their dismal tunes. Change of environment — new people, new sights, new ideas — is absolutely necessary to create new brain records and to throw the old ones into disuse and oblivion. We endeavour to hasten the mental regeneration by arousing interest in new ideas and higher ideals, by instilling new faith and the will to be well in place of the old doubt and despair thought. We have found that the best way to accomplish this is through daily health talks in which we explain to our patients how physical and mental ills are created through violation of nature's laws of thinking, feeling, breathing, eating, drinking, bathing, etc., and how they must learn to help themselves by complying with nature's laws in their habits of living. Nervous and mental patients who would resentfully reject any helpful suggestion in private consultation will allow the ideas propounded in a public lecture to sink into their inner consciousness without arousing antagonism and repulsion. Hand in hand with change of surroundings and suggestive treatment must go the purification and upbuilding of the physical body, as outlined in this volume.

About a year ago a woman came to us for treatment who was firmly convinced that she had committed the unpardonable sin against the Holy Ghost, that she was damned to hell for all eternity and that there was no possibility of salvation for her. The unhappy condition of her mind may be easily imagined. For four months she exerted all her strength to refuse my helpful arguments and suggestions. Like most of these people she argued with the ingenuity of an accomplished lawyer trying to prove that she was indeed utterly depraved and lost, while in reality she had been the best and kindest of human beings all through her life, until these unfortunate delusions overwhelmed her. About two months after she had left for home I received a letter from her which contained the following passage: "Toward the end of my sojourn in your institution I began to realize that you were right and that I was altogether wrong in my foolish imaginings through which I had created for myself the worst imaginable hell, of mental and emotional suffering. But through long continued habit and stubbornness of mind I was not ready nor willing to acknowledge my fault. But after I arrived home and had time and leisure to think things over I became fully conscious of the absurdity and terrible consequences of my mental aberration. Now I have found my old self again and the dreadful delusions which obsessed and threatened to destroy me seem like a bad dream or dreadful nightmare."

Psychic Insanity or Abnormal Psychism

The majority of psychical mental disorders are induced by negative, sensitive conditions on one or more planes of being. I mean by this that physical, mental and moral vigour and resistance have become weakened in some way or another and that as a result, reason, will and self control are benumbed and paralysed to such an extent that the individual comes into abnormal contact with the lower spiritual planes of existence and lays himself open to hypnotic control by other intelligences in or out of the physical body.

The paranoiac, the delusional maniac and the true medium are frequently hypnotically controlled by vicious intelligences on the physical or spiritual planes of being. The drunkard in delirium tremens actually sees things. The snakes and other horrid creatures which terrify him are not altogether hallucinations of a distorted imagination. In his case the physical organism and its sensory organs, under the deadening influence of alcohol, have become so benumbed and paralysed that the senses of the spiritual body are abnormally active. In other words, the victim of alcohol becomes clairvoyant on the lowest planes of spiritual life — the hell of the theologians. Our physical material plane of life corresponds, as far as location in space is concerned, to the lowest spiritual plane, the astral plane of the theosophists, and therein lies the awful danger of premature and abnormal psychical development through negative, subjective processes. All such experiments are extremely dangerous as long as the individual is bound by his heavy physical body and by heavy spiritual gravity to the lowest plane of spirit life. The doctors who have lately "weighed the soul" by observing and recording the loss of weight at the point of death were right in their conclusions. The spiritual body, mentioned by Paul and visible to the seer, is material just as is the physical body, and although this spiritual counterpart of the physical body consists of matter in a very rarefied form, still it occupies space and has some weight. Those who, by a weakening of will power and subjective, negative processes of psychic development, rashly expose themselves to psychic control and abnormal quickening of the spiritual organs of sense, come in contact with the slums and vicious inhabitants of the lowest planes of spiritual life.

To the religiously inclined who doubt these statements I would say that if these things are untrue, then the New Testament is false from beginning to end. If abnormal psychism and obsession was a fact in nature nineteen hundred years ago, it is a fact today. To the materialist, sceptical scientist, I would adapt the quotation and bid him remember "there are really more things in heaven and earth, my medical Horatio, than have been dreamed of in thy philosophy". Only he who has sincerely and earnestly investigated and tested these subjects has a right to speak and judge.

When I took "incurable paranoiacs" from a state asylum, the doctors in charge smiled at my presumption and informed me that never yet in the history of the institution had a case been cured. Yet we have permanently cured several such cases within four to twelve months' time. It is not to be wondered at, however, that these patients are incurable under the conventional treatment when we stop to consider that insane asylums are veritable "hells on earth", where ignorant and vicious spirits congregate to obsess and vampirize defenceless victims. The latter are rendered more negative and subjective by idleness, improper diet, solitude, confinement, constant communication with other insane, by the vicious spiritual atmosphere, and by the paralysing influence of sedative and hypnotic drugs which are negative in their effects on the human organism.

There are those who endeavour to restore lost self control by "hypnotic suggestion", which however is a misnomer. An able writer on this subject draws the following distinction between suggestion and hypnotism: "It is safe to say that in its most common acceptance the word suggestion is intended to mean a deferential method of calling the attention of one person to the subject matter in the mind of another and inviting favourable consideration of the same. For some reason, quite inconceivable at this time, the word has become inseparably connected and associated in thought with the subject of hypnotism. By a sort of tacit agreement, as it were, among writers and students generally, it has come to include almost, if not quite, all the means and methods by and through which a hypnotist impresses his own thoughts, impulses, desires and will upon the consciousness of his subject. But it must be borne constantly in mind that in exact proportion to the depth or intensity of the hypnotic state the hypnotist controls the will, voluntary powers and sensory organs of his subject. Under these conditions the subject, to the extent that hypnosis exists, is deprived of the power of independent choice, without which the word suggestion is entirely meaningless to him. Indeed, every thought, every impression, every impulse of the will projected by a hypnotist upon the consciousness of his subject during the hypnotic relation has, just as far as the hypnotic process is able to carry it, the force and binding effect of a definite and inviolable command. It is not presented to the subject for his consideration as an independent, self-conscious and rational intelligence possessing discretionary powers. It is not submitted to the rational judgement of the subject at all. It is not offered upon the theory that it may possibly be rejected. On the other hand, it is forced upon him under conditions which, according to the laws of nature, make its rejection an impossibility. And yet, notwithstanding all this, it is called "suggestion" by learned men who are wise enough instantly to discover many a less conspicuous error."

Careful scientific investigation has demonstrated that hypnotism may not only produce insanity and physical death, but that it seriously interferes with the normal development of mind and soul and entails evils far greater than mere physical debauchery. If fact hypnotism is debauchery of mind and soul.

It is not to be questioned that hypnotism practised in a helpful spirit may produce temporary results which seem in a measure to justify its use, but if these be observed in their unfolding it will be found that there has been no actual cure; that the results were merely the effects of a brain paralysis and the substitution of the will of the operator for the will of the victim. In other words, hypnotic treatment, like that by drugs, is suppressive, not curative. There is a single consideration which of itself should deter any self-respecting and prudent person from submitting to hypnotic control. This process involves the temporary subjection and abeyance of reason, will power and self control of the subject. With each repetition, these highest attributes of the soul become more benumbed and paralysed. This not only prevents the development of the higher faculties, capacities and powers, but starts the victim of hypnotic control on the downward road of mental and moral deterioration and retrogression. Such a person becomes an easy prey to any outside influence that may desire to control him for good or evil. Those who are regularly experimenting with this dangerous power, believing that they are accomplishing beneficial results, should ask themselves if they have a right to extinguish self consciousness and to usurp absolute control over the mind and soul of another individual when this means criminal intrusion upon the sacred rights of individual consciousness and personality for the sake of merely temporary and doubtful benefits.

It is our highest and most solemn duty to maintain the waking consciousness and to guard the citadel of our being at all times against intrusion and control by outside intelligences. Any process which progressively weakens the victim's control over his own acts is in violation of the primary law of individual life — the law of moral and personal responsibility. Reason, will power and self control are the attributes which distinguish the human from the animal. Take these away and there is nothing left but an idiot or a lunatic. When these highest qualities of the human soul are permanently benumbed and paralysed through the hypnotic process, the individual sinks below the animal plane, because he has not even animal instinct to guide him. This is soul murder.

I began to realize the destructive nature of hypnotism and mediumship when I was studying Nature Cure in Berlin. At that time I also took a course in "Suggestive Therapeutics" under Jacques Groll, at that time the most celebrated hypnotist in Germany. My fellow students appeared to enjoy the abject submission and helplessness of our clinical subjects when under hypnotic control, but from the beginning the pitiable condition of these wretches, deprived of reason, will and self control, was revolting to me. Although endowed to a marked degree with the power to exert hypnotic control, I decided there must be other less harmful methods of curing human ailments and resolved never to employ subjective methods in any form whatsoever. There is no delusion more fatal than that encouraged by certain church organizations engaged in the work of psychic healing, namely, that will power can be restored and strengthened by hypnosis — the very process that destroys it more surely than any other known agency, a process which is the greatest crime which can be committed against a human being.

We now come to the consideration of subjective psychism, in its various phases closely related to hypnotism. These states all have their incipiency in negative physical and mental conditions. By a negative condition we mean weakness, lack of resistance, susceptibility and submission to outside influences. Prominent factors in producing negative physical and psychical conditions are hereditary tendencies, debilitating diseases, drugs which exert a negative hypnotic influence upon the organism, a negative diet, vicious habits, such as alcoholism, sex perversion, etc. Habits not vicious, but which have been indulged in to the extent of jeopardizing self control, may lead to subjective psychism. Among these are religious emotionalism, overscrupulousness, concern about the future, morbid altruism, in fact any good habit exaggerated to a degree involving loss of equilibrium. Again and again physicians hear from the patient this complaint: "It is not that I like doing these things; I abhor and detest the very thought of them. A foreign influence seems to come over me and to control me. I feel as if it were another person." Indeed, it often is. All habits carried to a point producing loss of self control open the door to control by outside intelligences having the same tendencies. Yet, even so, hypnotism and the seance room may accomplish more harm in a few "sittings" than evil habits during a lifetime. Hypnotic control depends upon the temporary paralysis of reason, will and self control. If persisted in it may result in the permanent loss of these capacities and powers which distinguish man from the brute. Under abnormal psychism I include all phases of psychism, from mere sensitiveness and awareness of conditions on the spiritual planes (clairvoyance, clairaudience, etc.) to actual obsession, which is the hypnotic control of an individual in the body by an intelligence outside the body. Such control by a spiritual intelligence may result in complete possession of the physical organism by the obsessing influence.

185

Not long ago I received from a distance a manuscript describing the author's experience in developing mediumship, from the time when she began to receive strange vibrations and to be impressed by peculiar sensations until she heard voices and came in actual contact with her "controls". These experiences became very annoying and interfered with her daily occupations as well as with rest and sleep. She begged her tormentors to leave her and threatened to disclose her true condition. They laughed and told her if she did she would be adjudged insane and would be confined in an asylum. When her condition became unbearable she related these experiences to her husband and to the family physician; the latter shook his head and left a prescription for her "nerves". A few days later, her husband took her for a walk and with her entered a large building. Presently she found herself before an assemblage of physicians and nurses and was asked to tell her story. After she had done so the doctors agreed that she was suffering from delusional insanity and committed her to the institution. In the manuscript she tells a piteous story of her experiences. During two years she was confined in three different asylums. "All this time," she says, "I was as sane as ever in my life, but the mere mention of my psychic experiences was sufficient to commit me."

People no more insane than we are have been tortured by experiences which in many instances they are afraid to tell their nearest friends, lest they be committed to the insane asylum.

Psychic exposure is brought about by a weakening of the physical body and its magnetic envelope, sometimes called the aura. The physical body and its magnetic envelope form the protecting wall dividing us from contact with the astral plane and the lower spiritual spheres. If between the room where I am sitting and the adjoining one there were a heavy brick wall, I should be unconscious of what is transpiring on the other side; but if the partition consist merely of wood and glass, I apprehend every sound and can hear distinctly the conversation in the other room. Thus it is with a person whose protective physical and magnetic envelopes have been weakened and attenuated to such an extent that the spiritual senses have become abnormally active on the lowest spiritual planes co-existent with our earthly plane.

From what I have said it becomes apparent that the cure of abnormal psychism cannot lie in solitude, confinement, idleness, sedatives or hypnotics, either in the form of drugs or of "suggestion", but in the application of natural tonic treatment. Fundamental is the right diet, rich in positive dairy foods and in positive vegetable foods which grow in and near the ground. Massage and neurotherapy are important because they stimulate in a natural manner the dormant nerve centres. Hydrotherapy and open-air baths stimulate and invigorate the circulation and the vital activities of the skin. Daily physical culture drills, particularly the psychological exercises, not only strengthen the body but teach coordination of mind and muscle, thereby exercising in a most effective manner will power and self control. Medicinal treatment, if administered, must be tonic, never depressive. Suggestion also plays its part, but it, too, must be tonic, not depressive. That it must not be administered in the hypnotic trance, but directed to the waking consciousness, in order that the patient may accept it and respond to it by the exertion of his own will, not through coercion by the will of another. This is the danger line. Let the psychotherapist beware that he does not cross it.([1])

([1])
   Lindlahr's approach to Insanity and to mental, emotional and psychical disorders is very different from that of orthodox specialists in the subject, both in the matter of classification and in treatment. In classification he recognizes two groups of diseases, namely those which are due to physical causes and those which are due to psychical causes. Obviously the prognosis in cases in the first group will very much depend on the extent to which the physical condition can be improved by natural living and treatment, and will be very much less good in those cases in which there has been organic degeneration of brain and nerve matter. In cases in the second group it is clear that some kind of psychological treatment is indicated, though Lindlahr firmly maintains that all treatment of mental conditions should begin with a thorough toning up and purification of the physical body as this will often of itself be sufficient to enable the patient to live through or overcome his mental or emotional troubles. It is interesting to note that there does now seem to be a tendency among psychiatrists to make use of physical and chemical methods of different kinds in the treatment of mental conditions rather than relying altogether on psychological techniques. Among such treatments are such things as the use of drugs in various ways, shock treatment and leucotomy. These treatments all aim at doing something to the mind of the patient through something which acts upon his body and particularly upon his central nervous system either in a physical or chemical way. Much of this kind of treatment has been developed since Lindlahr's time, but it can be said with certainty that he would have disapproved of nearly all of it, though he would have approved of the idea that mental states can and should be approached by way of the body. For instance, there are techniques of physical treatment and relaxation which are capable of normalizing nerve and brain function and of producing the kind of "abreaction" which can release subconscious fixations and tensions without the use of drugs or hypnosis. There is also, it would seem, some place for the use of shock in the treatment of certain mental conditions, but there are obvious dangers in the kind of shock treatment which is now commonly given, especially when it is carried on frequently or for a long time. It is also clear that very little is being done at present to explore to the full the possibilities of homoeopathy in the treatment of nervous and mental conditions, and yet the fact that so much importance is attached by homoeopaths to symptoms of a psychological or emotional type when prescribing their remedies points to the conclusion that homoeopathy should be of great value in dealing with mental states. Homoeopathy is, after all, a form of shock treatment. Electroconvulsive therapy, as now generally applied, is most crude in its dosing and timing, and the site of application needs more consideration. For instance, the giving of mild shocks through the feet is capable of giving much quicker and better results than the sort of shocks now generally used.
   The proper functioning and balance of the endocrine system is another thing which has a special bearing on the treatment of nervous and mental diseases.

187

SECTION XXXI

MENTAL AND SPIRITUAL HEALING

1. **Telepathy, the Language of Impulse.** Telepathy means the transmission of words and ideas from mind to mind through vibrations in the ether. That this is possible is now a matter of common experience among those who are physically and mentally sufficiently refined to become sensitive to such etheric vibrations. A few years ago materialistic science would have dismissed telepathy as "another evidence of hysterical self delusion or as tricks of pretenders and fakirs". This is hardly possible now in the days of wireless telegraph and telephone. If it is possible for metal instruments to transmit messages through thousands of miles of open wireless space, why should it be impossible to send mental vibrations from mind to mind and brain to brain through the all-pervading ether? What is now possible to a comparatively few physically and mentally refined and sensitive individuals will in the course of evolutionary development become the common capacity of all mankind. Those who have attained the power to travel to foreign lands — that is, in the spiritual planes of life — assure us that in the higher spiritual spheres telepathic communication, the language of impulse, becomes the common mode of expression. Though we may not be aware of it, it is a fact that all of us are more or less sensitive while waking, and possibly more so while sleeping, to thought vibrations from our physical and spiritual surroundings.

Every human brain and the consciousness back of it is a wireless telegraph with its sending and receiving apparatus. We live in a great sea of mental, emotional, spiritual and physical vibrations. All of us are constantly sending forth our own vibrations and receiving those of other minds. Much of that which appears to us as our own thinking and feeling is thus inspired or forced upon us from without. This becomes particularly apparent in what has been called mob psychology. Our mental and physical wireless connects us with all the planes of earth and heaven, of hell and purgatory, and with their inhabitants. The nature of the vibrations which we receive, whether they be cheerful or of a depressing nature, helpful or harmful, constructive or destructive, depends upon the quality of our own vibrations. In order to make communication between wireless instruments a possibility, the sending and receiving apparatus must be attuned to the same rate of vibration. So also the human wireless receives and registers those vibrations only which are nearest in vibratory quality to its own. Thus the brain habitually attuned to the vibrations of hopelessness, fear, despair and melancholy will receive and register like vibrations from the earth plane and the lower and lowest spiritual spheres which are the abodes of gloom, remorse and despair. In like manner, vibrations of greed, jealousy, revenge and cruelty will attract and register like vibrations from other depraved and cruel minds. From this it appears that those who indulge in destructive mentalism and emotionalism intensify their own unhappy or depraved conditions through the operation of the law of spiritual attraction and repulsion. I use the word "indulge" advisedly because destructive mental and emotional habits are just as much forms of self indulgence as are the drug or liquor habits. The person who indulges in fear and worry thought is just as much a victim of intemperance as the drunkard and drug fiend.

Lack of self control is the cause of all vices; the exercise of self control the only remedy. The preacher of temperance may be surprised to learn that his fear and worry mania or his irritability and nervousness is just as much a matter of lack of self control and of intemperance as the liquor or cigarette habit of those whom he tries to reform by force of law. The trouble is that people have not been taught that they can and must control their thinking and feeling just as strictly as their eating and drinking. They grow up under the impression that they cannot help what they think or feel — that thought and feelings come and go "as the wind listeth"; they think of the brain and mind as an aeolian harp which is played upon by the passing breezes. They do not realize that the brain is a musical instrument under the absolute control of the will of the ego, that the will is the artist who may elicit harmony or discord from his instrument as he desires. Fortunately the laws of spiritual attraction and repulsion work just as accurately in the constructive as in the destructive way. Just as surely as we can connect our mental, spiritual and psychical wireless with the astral planes and the deepest hells, just so surely can we connect them with the higher spiritual and celestial spheres and their inhabitants, with the invisible helpers and angels and with the all-pervading spirit of the universe whom we call God, the Father, the Logos, the Great Spirit, Brahm, and by innumerable other names. Just as surely as wireless connection with the lower spheres will fill our souls with the discords of unhappiness, remorse and despair, just so surely will connection with the higher spheres bring us an influx of more life, love and happiness, of "peace that passeth all understanding".

To illustrate the foregoing, think of a hall in which an orchestra is performing a great symphony. The audience, instead of listening quietly and attentively, creates loud and disturbing noises. Naturally the beautiful music is drowned in the general clatter and merely serves to increase the nerve-racking noise. In similar manner the influx of peace, harmony and healing power from the higher spheres of spiritual and celestial life cannot fill the soul, cannot have a harmonious effect upon the physical,

189

mental and psychical conditions of a person if mind and soul be agitated by discordant and destructive mental and emotional vibrations.

2. **The Secret of Spiritual Healing.** Mind and soul must be in a condition of perfect serenity and peace before they can receive the wireless vibrations of healing power from the source of all life. This is the *modus operandi* of true spiritual healing. It means the opening of our souls to the influx of almighty love from the source of all life and love in the universe. Life and love are identical in nature. Love is the highest vibratory activity of the human soul as well as of the universe. Why should we depend upon spiritual healers when within ourselves we have the shortest wireless connection between the human soul and the oversoul? A spiritual teacher cannot help us more effectively than by showing us how to establish this wireless connection and how to operate it.

A sufferer, confined to bed for many years, said: "You ask me to make myself receptive to the healing currents coming from the innermost source of life and power within me; you say I must relax and fix my attention and desire on the spiritual and celestial ranges of vibratory activity. I fail to understand how I can come into living contact with heavenly vibrations while confined in this hell of ignorance, sin and suffering." Smilingly, she added: "Don't you think it is a far call from Chicago to heaven?" To this I replied: "It is within your power to receive as you desire — the discords of hell or the peace and harmony of heaven. Though the planes of mundane, spiritual and celestial life differ greatly in locality, the vibrations of the higher and highest spheres penetrate to the lower and lowest. Even the denizens of hell may catch glimpses of heaven. You fail to understand how it is possible for you to be in heaven and hell at the same time, yet, in this great city all spheres are represented in the souls of its inhabitants — the highest and celestial spheres as well as the lowest abodes of hell. It is possible for you to be at the same time in closest touch with these varying places and conditions. Suppose your sickbed was surrounded with telephones, phonographs and kinetoscopes which transmitted to your eyes and ears the sights and sounds of these varying localities and conditions. What impressions you would receive would depend upon your desire, the direction of your attention and upon the refinement and receptivity of your physical and spiritual sensory organs. So your psychical wireless connects you with all the spheres of our planetary universe."

The invalid to whom I allude — a woman of about thirty-five years of age — had been confined to her bed for four and a half years, unable to turn from side to side, her physical body being slowly eaten away by cancer — the result of five surgical operations. When I first called to see

190

her she had been suffering with the dread malady for two years. Christian Science had been of no avail to ease her suffering. Morphine and other opiates brought only temporary relief. From the day I first met her until the day she died, she never took another dose of pain killers or hypnotics. The simple, natural methods of treatment and her own serene and exalted mental and spiritual attitude made her suffering bearable and enabled her, under the most distressing circumstances, to remain in a cheerful and even happy frame of mind. Her relatives and friends frequently assured me that instead of their having to console and cheer the sufferer, she was the sunshine of the home. As she became acquainted with the laws of constructive psychism and learned to control the higher and finer forces of mind and soul, it seemed that the spiritual predominated over the physical. Towards the end her consciousness was as active on the spiritual plane of life as on the physical. While her poor body was racked with pains, her spiritual eyes delighted in rapturous spiritual visions. It was undoubtedly the supremacy of the spiritual life over the physical which helped to keep her alive and which harmonized the physical vibrations sufficiently to ease her suffering and make it bearable. She had learned to connect her mental and psychic wireless with the highest vibratory ranges of spiritual and celestial activity. This experience more than any other disclosed to me the marvellous possibilities of constructive mentalism and psychism as a healing power.

PART IV

THE BABY BOOK

Natural Therapeutics can claim to have solved the problem of treating human ailments. All other schools and systems will in time have to adopt the natural way. It is the hub of the healing art; all therapeutic methods radiate from it like spokes from a wheel. Natural Therapeutics, however, has something better to give than treatment of disease, and that is prevention of disease. If children were brought into this world in the manner ordained by nature and reared in harmony with the teachings of natural philosophy, disease would soon be a thing of the past. Human beings would then enjoy good health and be as beautiful and perfect in their kind as are animals, which live in the freedom of nature, guided by instinct, and therefore in harmony with the laws of their being.

We must begin, then, with prevention, for prevention is always easier and cheaper than cure. But where must we begin to study the prevention of disease? Some will say, "At birth, because that is the beginning of life." Not so; that would be too late. The mould is made and the foundation laid for health or disease, for happiness or suffering, for efficiency or deficiency, before the human being in process of creation sees the light of day. "Then", it may be said, "we must begin with prenatal influence, for the physical, mental, emotional and moral habits of the mother influence powerfully the development of the new life she is carrying." True — but we must start earlier than that. The making of the human being begins with mating and conception. All subsequent development depends upon a right start.

SECTION XXXII
Heredity

Editor's Introduction

I have had some hesitation in including this section in its original form in the present edition. Lindlahr undoubtedly had many ideas on the subjects of race and of eugenics which are now extremely unfashionable and which might appear to have some affinities with the kind of racialism which infected the German people in this century and which led to such terrible consequences. It is clear that Lindlahr was intending further to develop his ideas in a volume which never appeared but which seems to have been in a state of preparation at the time of his death. I have, however, decided to include the section because it does seek to face up to a number of problems which undoubtedly exist and to contain much which is very stimulating to thought in connection with matters which are ignored and problems which are unrecognized. For instance, in connection with the subject of "Correct Mating", the tendency now is to regard all races as being essentially the same with the same capabilities and potentialities and to deny that race has any real meaning or purpose. The idea that one race is superior to another or more developed or evolved than another is looked upon with the greatest suspicion. The corollary of this is that there is no harm in mixing everyone together socially and sexually provided that they are all subjected to the same kind of education and upbringing to turn them into good world citizens without a thought of what race they belong to or what colour they are. Presumably this would finally result in a world population of very mixed origins and of a sort of beige colour. Lindlahr was obviously opposed to this kind of thought. I believe that his ideas were largely theosophical in origin and that he looked upon the planet and all that is on it as going through a process of development or evolution. Races, according to these ideas, have appeared, developed and divided into subdivisions, and, like individuals, they have a youth, a maturity and an old age. When new races appear they must doubtless develop or evolve from those which have gone before. Lindlahr is in fact arguing that man could and should consciously co-operate with the evolutionary process which is going on. This implies that we must seek to do our mating in a manner which is sound and constructive for the future of race, and also that there is such a thing as miscegenation which is to be avoided.

Again, in connection with "Use Heredity" and "Pernicious Heredity", Lindlahr would appear to be out of tune with views which are now generally held. It is not now generally believed that acquired characteristics are inherited or passed on and when changes or improvements take place it is thought to be due to natural or artificial selection working on the basis of chance variations. Lindlahr, however, was a firm believer in the transmission of acquired characteristics, both good and bad, and on this belief he founds his argument in favour of late marriages, especially for the male.

It is clear that the views which are expressed in this Section and in other places in Lindlahr's works are the result of much thought, observation and reading and it would be of interest to see them further developed: a thing which was evidently intended by Lindlahr. Certainly these views deserve respect and could form the basis for useful research and observation, but, as Lindlahr himself appears to recognize, there do seem to be some arguments against them, at least in some circumstances, which also require consideration. For instance, in connection with mating, it does seem that to a limited degree or occasionally an infusion of new blood from another race or subrace can enrich or improve a family or national strain, while there are great dangers in too high a degree of inbreeding. In connection with use heredity, there are in many societies considerable dangers and difficulties in encouraging late marriages or too great an age discrepancy between the parties to the marriages.

---

1. **Importance of Correct Mating.** Of primary importance in the sacred rite of procreation, as already intimated, is mating. This should take

place only between descendants of the same subrace, or of closely related subraces such as the Indo-Caucasian and Celtic. If the racial descent of the marriage partners is so far removed that it has produced pronounced differences in racial characteristics — as in the case of the swarthy Mexican and white-skinned Englishwoman, or the dark-eyed Magyar and blue-eyed Scandinavian — then procreation becomes miscegenation and degenerates into mongrelization of the offspring. Everywhere in the animal and human kingdoms nature has set the mark of disapproval on the mongrel. The offspring of miscegenation is doomed to deterioration and extinction unless assimilation of the elements of a lower race by a higher takes place sparingly and gradually. The law of racial purity may be summed up as follows: When a member of a higher race cohabits with a descendant of a lower race, the offspring of the union loses more or less the characteristics of the higher race and reverts in physical, mental and moral traits to the level of the lower race. The constructive results of racial purity are evident in Hindus of the higher castes; in that portion of the Jewish race which in mating has faithfully adhered to the law of Moses, and in the blond and blue-eyed remnants of the Indo-Caucasian and Celtic races in northern Europe and North America. The destructive results of miscegenation are plainly evident in the mongrelized population of Mexico and everywhere in the half breed and many kinds of mixed breeds. These naturally fall below the physical, mental and moral standards of the parent stock, and almost invariably revert to the customs and habits of the inferior race.

2. **Use Heredity.** Use heredity deals with the transmission to offspring of acquired physical, mental and moral characteristics of the parents. According to this law as it has been formulated, the chances of the offspring for long life, health, mental efficiency and moral stamina, other conditions being favourable, are better in direct ratio to the advancing age of the parents at the time of conception. While this is contrary to popular opinion, which assumes that younger parents produce more perfect offspring than older ones, the fact of use heredity is proved, both in the animal and human kingdoms, by common observation and statistical evidence. The working of the law is based on the fact that the procreative elements of the parents, or rather the microzymes of those elements, cannot contain the impression of physical, mental and psychical characteristics which at the time of procreation were not developed in the three-fold organisms of father and mother.

The age of the father at conception is called the "birth age" of the offspring and determines its birth rank. While the father and previous male ancestors, for reasons hereafter explained, seem to exert greater control over the mental and psychical characteristics, the mother furnishes

194

the nutrient soil for physical growth. This does not mean that she exerts no control over the mental and psychical characteristics of the offspring; in addition to her influence through use heredity she has added opportunities through prenatal influence and postnatal training. According to this law, then, the chances of the offspring for excellent physical, mental and moral development become better as the age of the father at the time of procreation advances beyond thirty-five; while the physical condition of the mother for reproduction is best below thirty-five years. But we must not overlook the fact that too great a discrepancy of age beween the man and woman may become the cause of physical and mental incompatibility, of aversion and great unhappiness, especially on the part of the younger woman.

Extensive statistical evidence seems to prove that the birth age of the mother has been of less importance than that of the father. It seems that the majority of famous men in all lines of human endeavour had old male ancestors, while the mothers and previous female ancestors were of much younger age at the time of conception. This may be accounted for by the following reasons: The man is usually considerably older than the woman at the time of marriage. Men, as a rule, devote much more time and effort to acquiring a scientific, professional or business education than do women. This has been true in the past more than it will be in the future. Thrown early into the competitive struggle of life men generally have had to make greater mental and physical effort than have women. These points are of considerable importance because it has been proved that it is not inherited brain mass and mental capacity but strenuous and persistent effort that intensifies use heredity. The earlier this begins and the longer it continues before procreation takes place, the better the chances of the offspring for physical, mental and moral capacity. The reproductivity of the mother has usually ceased at thirty-five. Though she be capable of child-bearing a few years longer, usually conception has been avoided after that age. Men under favourable conditions remain reproductive to an advanced age. Some of the world's greatest men descended from fathers over sixty years old.

That intellectual and creative capacity has followed the male line of descent rather than the female line is indicated by the fact that the high intellectual capacity of many eminent men has skipped their daughters to reappear in male descendants. This may be partly accounted for by the fact that the daughters in their limited spheres of activity have not had the opportunity to unfold inherent intellectual capacity to any conspicuous degree. There has been a tendency in some quarters to criticize the general entrance of women into professional and commercial life and to dilate upon the adverse influence this will have upon womanly characteristics and family life. In the light of the knowledge we possess upon the subject of use heredity, it is safe to say that any such problematical drawbacks will be far outweighed by the general postponement of the marriage age. This will ensure not only better physical fitness but also higher intellectual development and greater moral stamina on both sides of parentage. The tremendous benefits which this increased hereditary endowment will confer upon future generations cannot be overestimated. Greater intellectual and economic equality between the sexes will emancipate women from degrading sex subserviency. Under the old order, sex appeal was too often her only stock in trade by which to attract and hold the male and thus secure a living. Economic independence will ensure greater consideration and higher esteem for the woman on the part of the man. It will go a long way towards solving the problem of birth control in a natural way, by leaving it more in the judgement of the mother.

We find the law of use heredity according to birth age verified in the intelligence and moral development or obliquity of nations and tribes all over the earth. The lower average birth age of a race or nation, the lower, other things being equal, the intellectual and moral development. The greatest development and efficiency is found among those nations where marriage is delayed to a later age through custom, economic necessity, professional or military training. The following quotation from "Control of Heredity", by Casper Lavater Redfield, is of interest in this connection: "In general it may be said that wherever there are no restraints upon the sexual propensities, as with the Digger Indians, the Fuegians, the Andamanese, the Wauraus of the Guianas, the Bushmen and the tribes along the Gabbon river, there we find reproduction taking place at the earliest possible age, and the lowest grade of intelligence. Where we find some special circumstances or customs that delay the age at which reproduction takes place, as with the Patagonians, the North American Indian and the Polynesians, there we find considerably higher grade of intelligence. Where we find the custom of marrying late in life, as was customary with the Greeks and the Romans, there we find a very high grade of intelligence. And where we find a fortuitous succession of very late births, there we find the very great men of the world's history. In other words, the longer the time in which the individuals have to use, develop and strengthen their brains before reproduction begins, the greater and more powerful are the brains of their descendants."

The book by Redfield mentioned above contains elaborate and highly interesting statistics which reveal the effects of the various birth ages on physical, mental and moral characteristics. It appears that, with few exceptions, the great artists, scientists, philosophers, statesmen and philanthropists were born from fathers whose ages ranged from forty to

196

sixty-five years at the time of the procreation of their famous offspring. The existence of these laws and principles as facts in nature is very evident in the training of race horses and of other animals along certain lines of proficiency.

3. **Pernicious Heredity.** The effects of deteriorating and destructive heredity, prenatal and congenital influences have been traced and commented upon in so many different ways that I do not believe it necessary to enter deeply into this phase of the subject. Various authors have filled entire volumes with the unsavoury family histories of the descendants of the Jutes, Ishmaels and other drunkards, prostitutes, degenerates and criminals, which prove positively the transmission of morbid and pernicious traits through successive generations. It has been proved statistically beyond the shadow of a doubt that youthful delinquency, pauperism and criminality are the aftermath of immature marriages. The laws of use heredity and prenatal influence, like all other natural laws and principles, manifest along opposite lines of expression. It remains for us to determine whether we shall align ourselves with their destructive or constructive activities. The effects upon ourselves and our offspring will show accordingly.

If I succeed in arousing the consciousness of prospective fathers and mothers to the glorious privileges and enormous responsibilities which these laws of nature confer upon them, then my labour will not have been in vain and I shall feel deeply gratified.

SECTION XXXIII

THE CREATIVE ALCHEMY OF LOVE AND AFFECTION

1. **Procreation** — as in the case of everything else pertaining to the constituents and functions of the human entity — takes place on three planes of being, the material (physical and spiritual), the mental and the psychical planes. Which of these elements shall predominate in the offspring depends upon the mixture and adjustment of qualities in the triune make up of the mating couple. In order to fulfil the law and to draw the divine blessing upon themselves and the fruit of their union the partners in the procreative function must be united by the bonds of love, or at least by the ties of true affection. The source of creative genius is love and

197

wisdom, and the essence of intelligence and power is sincerity and good-ness. Without these, intelligence degenerates into selfish cunning, power into self-destructive brute force. The spring cannot rise higher than its source; its water cannot be pure and wholesome when contaminated by impure admixtures from filthy surroundings.

It is not generally known that use heredity pertains to intellectual and psychical qualities, as well as to the physical material. Animalism breeds nothing but selfish animalism. The vampire who craves and absorbs the love of its victims and robs them of vital energy, without being capable of feeling or bestowing affection, is the child of a discordant union — of brute animalism on the part of the man, of secret aversion and hatred, usually, on the part of the woman. These bestial and degrading tenden-cies on the one side, and unrequited love craving on the other, breed sex perversion, and propagate the harpies who delight in the seductive power of superficial beauty, while gloating over the weakness and ruin of their victims.

True love and affection, paired with intelligence and goodness, liberate the creative elements necessary to the production of prefect offspring. The finer qualities of mind and soul open the fountains of life on the higher planes, liberate and harmonize the male and female procreative fluids, and charge them with the purest and most potent intellectual, spiritual and psychical elements. The divine fire of creative genius burns only in the love aura of truly mated couples. It is true that these are rare under our artificial, unrighteous social institutions, and that accounts for the rarity of complete manhood and womanhood. Perfect off-spring, endowed with beauty and power of body, mind and soul, destined to shed through life a radiance of health, happiness and helpfulness — to love and be loved — issue only from the union of love and affection with intelligence and goodness. "Love lieth at the foundation" (of all that is). "Love is passion, enthusiasm, affection, heat, fire, soul ... God."

To the extent that love enters into the holy rite, to that extent its attributes will be absorbed in the three-fold organism of the woman and become active in the child building in her womb. While she loves her man more than ever, her most passionate affection is centred in the new being in process of development. On it she bestows the purest and best in her food and drink, in her thoughts, emotions and secret desires. Fear, worry, anxiety, jealousy and hatred are strangers to her soul; these are the emanations of the lower spheres — she lives in heaven. Somebody en-dowed with deep insight into these matters has said: "Whatever male and female shall truly will for, hopefully pray for and earnestly yearn for, when love pure and holy is the nuptive ascendant, in form, passional, affectional, divine and volitional, that prayer shall be granted, and the boon be given — but the prayer must precede."

What are the direct effects of the marital rite upon the participants? If the sex attraction operates on the physical material plane only, if lust instead of love presides at the matrimonial feast, then temporary gratification of erotic craving will be followed inevitably by monotony, satiety, gradual revulsion and aversion, culminating in a morbid craving for change and variety. The partners in carnal self-indulgence are intuitively aware of these tendencies to marital unfaithfulness, and, therefore, easily dominated by distrust and jealousy. The procreative function is attended by complete satisfaction, buoyancy of body and mind and lasting happiness only when sex attraction operates on the higher and highest planes of being, as well as on the lower; when desire and impulse are operative on both sides. Thus only will the generative function fulfil its sacred purpose and confer the highest possible benefits upon parents and offspring. The woman, being the more highly sensitized, must be responsive to the call of holy passion. To force unwilling compliance will ruin the woman, kill her love and curse her offspring. Balzac says: "He who begins with his wife by a rape is a lost man." It is impossible for a wife to love unless she is won, not forced to compliance.

2. **Sexual Intercourse during Pregnancy.** Sexual intercourse should be considered the most sacred function of the human entity. From the highest and best viewpoint it should be exercised only for the propagation of offspring. However, considering the present stage of ethical and moral development, temperate indulgence may not be wholly condemned. Excessive intercourse is always weakening and harmful to both participants. We must remember that the sex fluid is the carrier of the life force. It is that which constitutes strength, resistance to disease, initiative and genius. During abstinence from intercourse the sex fluids with their creative energy are absorbed through the inguinal glands into the organism and increase physical, mental, moral and spiritual capacity.

Set rules for frequency of intercourse cannot be given This must depend entirely upon individual conditions. One safe rule is that after indulgence there should be no feeling of satiety, weakness and exhaustion. The more frequent the indulgence the stronger will grow the power of habit and of passion and the greater will become the abnormal craving. It is the same with all other appetites and passions. The more frequently they are indulged, the stronger they grow, until they attain complete control and develop into destructive habit. A free and confidential understanding in regard to these matters between those who contemplate matrimony would go far to prevent marital misery. A great deal of unhappiness arises from the fact that mates in the matrimonial union often labour under misapprehensions concerning the attitude of each towards the sex relation, and are prevented by excessive sensitiveness and delicacy from frankly discussing it. There is no problem of married life that needs more thorough mutual consideration and understanding than this one. Lack of it accounts for a great deal of "incompatibility", loss of love, revulsion, hatred, and the final tragedy of the divorce court.

Among animals, no female allows intercourse after conception. In this respect, as in many others, man has sunk below the natural standards of the animals. No greater crime can be committed against the woman and the unborn life. It is a sad commentary on our system of education, scholastic as well as religious, that our young people are not instructed before and after marriage in these all-important laws of nature. To do this should be the province of the priest who unites them in marriage, or of the family physician, if the parents have failed in their duty. It is well known (notwithstanding the denials of medical sceptics) that the unborn infant may be "marked" by transitory impressions, especially by strong emotions; that even insignificant parental characteristics are reproduced in the offspring. Is it any wonder, then, that the most powerful of human emotions should leave its impress on the growing brain and sex centres of the foetus, causing abnormal and precocious sex consciousness? All too often is sex perversion born and bred in bone and flesh, before the child sees the light of day. The mother cannot be blamed for this "slaughter of the innocents"; she has not been instructed on the subject. Though she intuitively senses the horror of it, she submits, in order to maintain her hold upon the man — and many a life is thus cursed before it is born. The fault lies primarily with those of the medical profession who teach our young men that the free indulgence of sexual passion is not only legitimate, but a necessity to manly vigour. This dictum of pseudo-science is almost universally concurred in by spiritual guardians. No greater lie was ever promulgated from the blackest abyss of Hades. If our young men were taught that greater happiness is to be attained by the exchange of tender affection than by the indulgence of the coarser animal appetites, that the creative forces thus preserved develop and strengthen their own finest capacities of body, mind and soul, they would wisely and chivalrously protect mother and child, at the same time conserving their own physical and moral integrity. In no other way is it possible to call forth the deepest gratitude and unfailing esteem of a true woman. Many a man whom we have thus advised has become a lifelong friend in consequence.

3. **Limitation of Offspring.** I believe that the unlimited production of offspring, encouraged in some quarters for swelling the ranks of religious bodies or for increasing tax-paying and cannon-fodder material, is a misfortune, both to the family and to society. Limitation of offspring, in

accordance with the means and circumstances of the parents, is not only justified but should be encouraged. In any case, the production of off-spring entails great responsibility upon the parents, and if they cannot properly comply with the needs and rights of their children, they fail in their responsibility and duty.

Any method, however, which interrupts intercourse or prevents concep-tion in an artificial way is absolutely to be condemned, because this has very harmful and positively destructive effects upon the physical, nervous and mental organism of those who thus try to cheat nature by the suppres-sion of a natural process. In our professional work we frequently meet the victims of such pernicious practices. The ordinary contrivances for prevention make of intercourse something akin to masturbation. This is also true of intercourse without orgasm which is strongly advocated under various guises. The use of poisonous antiseptics and germ killers in warm water douches is not essential for prevention, and is highly inju-rious. These chemicals have a tendency to poison the sexual organs and to produce in time atrophy, many kinds of female disorders, and tumours. Undoubtedly the greater number of so-called female troubles and malig-nant tumours in later life are caused by curettements, antiseptic douches and the use of poisonous drugs, for producing abortion. The only legiti-mate methods of birth control are abstinence or common cleanliness.[1]

There is nothing more conducive to the physical, mental and spiritual health and development of a woman than child-bearing and child-rearing in harmony with nature's laws, as outlined in these volumes. Under favourable conditions it is not a thing to be dreaded, but to be looked upon as the greatest of blessings and opportunities in the life of a woman. Natural philosophy and practice takes these problems of progeniture, child-bearing and child-rearing out of the domain of uncertainty and haphazard management with its dire consequences, and makes eugenics the most exact of all sciences and the sublimest and most enjoyable of all the arts.

4. **Determination of Sex.** Numerous theories have been advanced con-cerning this interesting subject. Many attempts have been made to wrest from nature the secret of sex determination and numerous more or less ingenious methods have been recommended for sex control. I know of one method only which seems to have a rational basis and which has proved of practical value. Observations seem to prove that the right ovary liberates male ova only, while the left ovary discharges female ova.

[1]
It must be assumed that what Lindlahr here means by "common cleanliness' is the use of the warm water douche with, at most, some salt added. He says nothing at all here or elsewhere about birth control by the use of the so-called "safe" periods. This is a matter which is discussed in an Appendix to this volume.

The two ovaries discharge ova only at alternate menstruations. With this data at hand, it is possible to determine the sex of a child after one birth has taken place. Suppose the first child was a boy. By consulting our pregnancy table we can determine when the last menstrual discharge took place. This menstruation liberated a male ovum; the next menstruation would liberate a female ovum, the next a male, etc. Thus, using the last menstruation period before the last conception as a fixed point, it would be possible, figuring from period to period, to determine the sex nature of the ovum to be discharged at each following menstrual period. Account is taken of all regular periods during the time menstruation is suspended in pregnancy. Thus conception may be timed in such a way as to impregnate at will a male or female ovum. This theory also seems to solve in a simple, rational manner another of nature's riddles, namely, the reason for the practically equal division of the sexes.([1])

SECTION XXXIV

PRENATAL INFLUENCE

1. **Medical Science Denies Prenatal Influence.** Medical man, as usual cock-sure of the correctness of their theories and hypotheses based on the "latest discoveries", deny and ridicule the possibility of prenatal influence, and relegate it to the rubbish heap of popular superstitions. They base their judgement on the fact that no nerves pass from the body of the mother through the umbilical cord into the growing foetus in the placenta, which forms the soft protecting nest of the new life within the womb. They claim that since no direct nerve connection exists between the two, mental and emotional vibrations cannot be transmitted from the brain of the mother to the brain and nervous organism of the foetus.

Are there no other means of communication between the mind of the mother and the brain of the unborn? Cannot the universal intelligence and creative will become individual intelligence and personal will? Cosmic

([1])
  The determination of sex by the method here outlined has been thought to be possible by a number of people for some time and there is a certain amount of literature on the subject and a certain amount of evidence that it can and does work. The idea is, however, quite contrary to the general view now held by geneticists who consider that the sex of the embryo is determined entirely by the male, there being male and female spermatazoa but all ova being the same. This question is further discussed in an Appendix to this volume.

vibrations do not flow into the grey matter of the human brain over coarse physical nerve tracts. They come over the psychical wireless which connects the human soul with the world soul, the individual intelligence with the universal or cosmic intelligence, the human will with the divine will. Since, as proved by modern brain and nerve anatomy, immaterial cosmic intelligence and "power to will" fashion the brain of the mother into physical material centres for the expression of human intellectual faculties, capacities and powers, why cannot these cosmic vibrations act in like manner over the psychic wireless through the soul and mind of the mother on the brain and nervous system of the foetal organism? Why should the wireless, which transmits impulses of intuitive intelligence and creative energy into the soul of the mother, cease to operate at that point, and fail to transmit its message to the brain and nervous system of the foetus which is most intimately related and connected with the organism of the mother?

What about the phenomena of hypnotism? Absolute control of the subject's mind through the intelligence and will of the hypnotist does not depend on the existence of an umbilical cord and physical nerve connection between the two. The hypnotist, by silent command, may call his subject from distance, far beyond the reach of his voice. People telepathically attuned may communicate in like manner, spontaneously, or by conscious intent. Why then should we doubt the possibility of vibratory correspondence between the mental and emotional conditions of the mother and the plastic nervous organism in process of development within her womb?

If a complexity of sound can impress itself permanently upon the wax cylinder of a phonograph, or what is still more marvellous, if the photographic rays of passing scenes can be fixed and retained in the picture film, why should it be impossible for the mental and emotional vibrations of the mother to impress and modulate the molecular and cellular constituents of the foetal brain and nervous organism? I have compared this creative power of the mother mind to the process of electroplating. As the particles of metal in suspension in the fluid adhere to the spoon that is to be coated with silver, so the atoms and molecules in the grey matter of the brain of the foetus group themselves in harmony with the thought forms and emotional vibrations of the mind and soul of the mother. While this mental and psychical electroplating takes place automatically, the mother's brain and nerve moulding power can be greatly strengthened and intensified by the conscious and voluntary operation of the psychical wireless that established vibratory oneness between her and the human entity in process of development within her own body.

Thus it is revealed how the brain prenatally refined, organized and

203

fashioned may endow the nascent individuality with certain aptitudes and talents along established paths of cerebration. There surely will be less resistance along such lines of physical, mental and moral endeavour than along other lines not prenatally influenced and moulded. Therefore I strongly advise mothers, pregnant with new life holding marvellous possibilities for good or evil, not to be influenced by the superficial reasoning of materialistic science, but to follow the sacred intuition and impulse of their own creative genius in this, the most holy function of their being. Every normally constituted mother is intuitively aware of this wonderful power, and is willing and anxious to exercise it when her consciousness has been aroused to the great possibilities and responsibilities which the divine privilege of motherhood confers on her. It is natural for us to admire the great artist who portrays the human form, true to life, on the painted canvas, or who fashions it from inanimate stone, metal or marble; how much more grand and godlike is the creative power of truly mated parents whose privilege it is to bring into the world, and to fashion according to their highest ideals, a human being endowed with life and intelligence, with the infinite possibilities of a new centre of creative activity.

Yet many mothers, totally ignorant of their divine creative privileges and possibilities, victims of physically and morally degrading marriage relations, and often filled with secret aversion or open hatred for their marital companions, pass unwillingly through pregnancy and not infrequently seek to destroy the new life. When the unfortunate victim of such marital incompatibility, conceived in passion and developing under the worst possible influences of mental and emotional discord, comes to arouse the maternal instincts of affection and devotion, then fear, anxiety and worry, like a continual nightmare, haunt the unhappy mind of the mother and impress their discordant vibrations upon the sensitive films of infant consciousness.

Compare this condition of fear, apprehension and gloom in the mind and soul of an unhappy and unwilling mother with the joyful and ecstatic state of mind of a mother conscious of the creative power of her intelligent will, who, from the time of mating and procreation, with accurate prescience prepares the most favourable conditions, astrologically, prenatally and postnatally, for the finest development of the physical, mental and moral characteristics of the future world citizen. The loftiest exaltation of a creative genius working in dead clay and cold marble cannot approach the ecstasy of a mother who has acquired a knowledge of the great laws which make possible the development of a perfect human being — the embryo of a master, an angel, a being destined to be godlike in its faculties, capacities and powers. In place of fear and anguish of soul, what joy to the mother who knows that it lies within her power to prevent disease and degeneracy in her offspring; that the development of the child depends solely upon her own intelligent effort. Nothing is left to accident. Child-bearing becomes an exact science, the most beautiful and inspiring of all arts and professions. Under such conditions motherhood, instead of being the greatest of hazards and hardships, becomes a divine privilege and the highest achievement of human existence and endeavour. It falls short only of the creative work of the great Universal Intelligence whose instrument of creation is the mother.

2. **An Example from History.** Let us consider the oft quoted example of Napoleon Bonaparte. His mother, Lutitia Bonaparte, while pregnant with future military genius, accompanied her husband on a military expedition, sharing with him the hardships and excitement of camp life, and the marches and battles of a military campaign. If there be nothing in prenatal influence, is it not singular that Napoleon should have become one of the greatest military geniuses of all ages, while not one of his brothers ever exhibited enough military ability to make an efficient corporal? What was it that favoured or determined the birth of the great military prodigy under these circumstances? The ancestors of Napoleon's father were not professional soldiers, nor was the father especially interested in military matters before the conception of his gifted son. The dominant influence, therefore, must have operated through the singular occupation and surroundings of the mother during this particular pregnancy.

Many similar striking examples have been cited in works on prenatal influence. I myself might add many convincing proofs from an extensive experience in medical practice; but time and space do not permit. Contributory evidence may be secured from many excellent works dealing with this vital problem in human life. I may be permitted to say that use heredity and prenatal influence are distinctly manifest in the physical and mental characteristics of our three children who were born at intervals of seven and five years. Each one of them clearly mirrors in his or her physical, mental and emotional peculiarities the predominant mental tendencies, occupation and surroundings of the parents during the respective prenatal periods. Similar manifestations of prenatal influence may be observed in almost any family.

3. **Birthmarks.** Medical men of late deny also the possibility of "marking" the offspring by sudden fear or shock in the mother during pregnancy. Incidents of this kind, however, are of such common occurrence that it is waste of time to refute these flippant denials. There are good reasons for believing that marking is more likely to occur during the periods when the menstrual flow should take place, but is suspended. It may be argued that to mention the possibility of marking to a pregnant

woman will greatly increase the probability of "electrotyping" violent emotions upon her offspring; in other words, that the fear of the thing will help to materialize it. This may be true to a certain extent, but we must remember that sudden shock through fear or disgust may cause the mischief anyway, whether or not the expectant mother is aware of the possibility. Understanding a danger and being prepared for it seems the best protection. The pregnant woman should study carefully Sec. XXX, dealing with mental and emotional causes of nervous diseases, and should learn to relax to any sudden surprise and thus neutralize unpleasant and fear-arousing impressions. Self control is the royal remedy, and the key to mastership.

4. **Physical Influence.** Now that we have studied some of the more important hereditary mental and psychical prenatal and postnatal influences, let us see how the physical condition of the mother's organism influences the brain and nerve matter of the foetus in its last stages of development, and after birth. Materialistic science teaches that brain matter exudes thoughts and feelings, as the liver excretes bile, or the stomach pepsin. Natural science proves that mind is superior to matter, that the newborn ego, by the power of intelligent volition, must fashion in the grey matter of the brain the molecular groupings or centres for the expression of intellectual and emotional activities, such as language, music, numbers, scientific and philosophic speculation. This means that active cerebration and brain moulding do not begin until after birth. But it stands to reason that the work of the nascent intelligence may be greatly facilitated or impeded by the physical condition of the brain. It is reasonable to assume that intellectual and emotional vibrations will more easily shape the grey matter of the brain into new configurations when it has been prenatally refined, organized and developed along certain lines of cerebration by use heredity and by constructive prenatal influences.

There exists a remarkable similarity between the brain-moulding and memory-building activities of the intelligent ego and the making of phonographic records and moving picture films. Lifelike impressions of sounds and passing scenes can be made upon the phonographic and photographic media only when wax and film are in a highly refined and plastic condition. When impure of substance and coarse of texture they are not sensitive and plastic enough to register and retain the subtle and highly complex vibrations of sounds and passing scenes. In order to receive and register a great variety and complexity of sounds, the wax on the phonograph cylinder must possess a certain degree of refinement, softness and plasticity. If it is too hard and coarse it registers the loud and coarse sounds only Such a record cylinder, exposed to a beautiful symphony executed by a great orchestra, would register and reproduce only the shrill cries of the trumpet, the rattle of the snare drum and the booming of the big horns and bass drums. The softer sounds of string, wood and wind instruments and finer shadings of tone and rhythm would be lost. With increasing refinements and plasticity, more subtle and delicate sound vibrations will be retained and reproduced.

In like manner the sensitive grey matter of the cortex of the brain must be in a pure and plastic condition in order to receive and register the impressions and impulses coming through the sensory organs, the psychic intuition and the intellectual and emotional activities of the mind. Anything in the way of physical impurity or foreign matter that tends to clog the brain, or to feed it with waste and morbid materials, or with corroding poisons, will lessen the atomic and molecular motility of brain and nerve matter, and will interfere with, or impede, the groupings and subtle transformations involved in the fashioning of brain centres through mental and emotional influences. If the nutrient blood which feeds the brain substance of the foetus be saturated with CO_2, the benumbing, paralysing carbon dioxide, with clogging uric acid or the destructive acids of phosphorus and sulphur, the grey matter cannot respond to the subtle and complex impressions and impulses from without and within. The purity or impurity of the plastic matrix of the cortex depends upon materials absorbed from food and drink. If these are so constituted as to create in the system excessive amounts of clogging and corroding substances, then these food and drink poisons will have a benumbing and deteriorating effect upon the sensitive grey matter of the brain, as well as upon the coarser tissues in the joints, muscles and vital organs. There is a rheumatism of the mind as well as of the joints.

A brain asphyxiated and clogged with pathogenic materials cannot be alert and active; it is too dull and lazy to think; it would much rather sleep than work; it is incapable of doing its best when its tiny blood and lymph vessels are obstructed with waste and morbid deposits which prevent the oxygenation and drainage of its delicately organized cellular tissues. This, of course, is true postnatally as well as prenatally. A brain originally capable of the highest and finest achievements of the human mind may become utterly worthless, and may degenerate into idiocy through food, drink and drug poisoning.

Medical men tell mothers they need not worry over prenatal feeding, because the placenta, the vascular bag which forms the nest of the new life, acts as a filter which purifies the blood before it reaches the foetus. Common sense and everyday experience tell another story. Even the best in the blood of many mothers is not good enough to serve as food for the new life. The placenta does not filter out of the blood of the mother all food, disease and drug poisons. This is proved by the wretched condition

207

of many infants, suffering from malnutrition, anaemia and rachitis, after delivery. If the vital fluids of the mother are deficient in the mineral elements, or in other important nutritive substances, how can they deliver them to the foetus?

Occurrences like the following, quite common in our institutional practice, prove positively that the placenta is not a perfect filter for systemic poisons and for disease taints circulating in the blood of the mother. One of the most pitiable cases of eczema in a little child less than one year old we traced to the fact that the mother, during her first year of marriage, had travelled with her husband through Eastern European and Asiatic countries, and during her pregnancy had been vaccinated five times while passing through localities where smallpox was prevalent. Both she and her husband had always enjoyed perfect health. The family record was excellent as far as traceable; still the body of the infant, soon after birth, was covered with open bleeding sores, presenting a revolting sight. We could find no explanation for this strange phenomenon other than the many vaccinations during pregnancy. These had contaminated the blood of the mother, and through her the body of the foetus, with a filthy scrofulous taint. The baby suffered terribly. For many months it slept but little because of the excruciating pains. The eczematous eruptions were of a very stubborn nature; they broke forth again and again. Finally, however, after eighteen months of natural treatment, we succeeded in purifying the little body of the horrible infection. The child is now a little over three years old, in perfect health, and during the last twelve months has shown no signs of the morbid taint.

Under another section I shall describe the influence of food upon character and sex life.

To recapitulate: Purity, plasticity and motility of the highly refined and sensitive materials which make up the grey matter of the brain depend upon pure food, plenty of fresh air and exercise, and upon all other natural methods of living described in these volumes.

SECTION XXXV

CONCEPTION AND PREGNANCY

1. Conception takes place whenever the male spermatozoon joins the female ovum within the woman's womb. Normally the female organism

liberates from its ovaries but one ovum each month, while the male discharges millions of spermatozoa at each orgasm. Conception does not always follow copulation, but when the male and female germs merge into one another conception or impregnation takes place. As soon as this has happened, the impregnated ovum becomes attached to the inner lining or mucous membrane of the womb and begins its new life as an embryo. The period comprising the time from the impregnation of the ovum until the beginning of labour or childbirth is called pregnancy.([1])

2. **Exercise During Pregnancy.** Unfortunately a great many expectant mothers labour under the idea that they must rest and be relieved from work and exercise. This of course is a great mistake. Light housework is good exercise. There is nothing more harmful during pregnancy than nursing "that tired feeling" by lounging idly about the house and coddling one's real or imaginary aches and troubles. Of great benefit to the pregnant woman are all outdoor sports such as tennis, golf and other games which require vigorous exercise without straining or overworking the body. The great benefit of walking and other outdoor exercises, aside from their general invigorating effects, lies in the strengthening of the abdominal muscles and ligaments, which at delivery will greatly facilitate expulsion of the foetus. The walk should be brisk and rhythmical, body erect, head thrown back, chest forward; the breathing at the same time should be deep and regular. These walks should be continued as long as time and endurance permit. Nothing, of course, must be pushed to the point of exhaustion. One good long walk every day is necessary; two are better.

We all understand the necessity for a plentiful supply of oxygen under ordinary conditions, and especially in time of illness. During pregnancy the demand for oxygen, as well as for mineral salts, is doubled or trebled on account of the needs of the rapidly developing organism in the womb of the mother. These extra demands for oxygen and ozone must be

([1])
    I have taken the liberty of omitting from the text a number of the sentences at the beginning of this section, because Lindlahr has here made some statements which can hardly be sustained in the light of researches and observations which have been made since his time. Though there are often irregularities and abnormalities in connection with ovulation and menstruation, and though our knowledge is still far from complete, it now seems to be clearly established that the cycle starts with ovulation rather than with menstruation and that ovulation normally occurs between the sixteenth and the twelfth day before menstruation is due to take place. Also it seems to be established that the ovule is only fertilizable for a very short time after ovulation, probably not more than forty-eight hours, and that the spermatozoon loses its power to fertilize within three days of being discharged. Lindlahr seems to have believed that ovulation takes place at the time of menstruation or very soon after it, and that ova can live for a number of days and spermatozoa for a week or more within the female, genital tract. These matters are obviously of great importance if conception is to be encouraged or avoided by the regulation of coition to the appropriate time in the cycle. This is fully discussed in an Appendix to this volume.

supplied by systematic deep breathing, cold bathing, outdoor walks, etc. If circumstances do not permit the taking of outdoor exercise, deep breathing should be practised as often as feasible, at the open window. Next in importance among gymnastic exercises is the internal massage described under Sec. XXI, No. 16. Those exercises are especially valuable which bring into play the abdominal muscles and the muscles and ligaments of the genital organs.([1])

3. **Clothing.** Clothing and the manner of wearing it profoundly influence the normal or abnormal development of the foetus, the health of the mother, labour and delivery. At no time should the waist-line be constricted by a corset or even by the ordinary skirt band. All clothing should be as loose and light as possible — one-piece under and outer garments, with the weight suspended from the shoulders, are best. If skirts are worn they should be fastened to skeleton waists of some thin cotton material. The close, heavy texture of the material from which the corset or so called "reform waist" is made is injurious because it interferes with the free circulation and the normal blood supply to the abdominal organs, which is of especial importance in pregnancy; it also hinders the free expansion and movement of the uterus during the various stages of pregnancy. Within the waist-line are located a dozen or more important vital organs of the body. Any sort of constriction compresses these organs and pushes them out of their normal position. While this is extremely injurious to the body of a woman under ordinary conditions, it is doubly so to the pregnant mother and to the rapidly growing foetus. Undoubtedly many deformities and monstrosities are produced by unnatural constriction of the blood vessels and vital organs in the abdomen and pelvis of the pregnant woman.

If due attention is paid to the foregoing influences, labour and delivery will be brief and easy. This we have proved in hundreds of cases which have come under our management. The reason why women of civilized countries spend many hours and sometimes days in dreadful agony of childbirth, while those of primitive and savage races, as we call them, produce their young easily and painlessly as the animals do, is that primitive women live more simple and natural lives, while "civilized" mothers violate practically every law of nature in their daily habits of living. Civilization unfortunately stands in many respects for that which is artificial, unnatural and therefore productive of disease and suffering in all domains of life, not only as regards physical health, but social and political health as well.

([1])
The name of Grantly Dick Read is associated with the great development in recent years of prenatal exercises to prepare mothers for childbirth and to make the process relatively easy and painless.

SECTION XXXVI

DANGER SIGNS DURING PREGNANCY

1. **Dropsical Swelling.** Swelling of the limbs and distension of the veins of the legs during pregnancy may be caused by a tendency towards varicosity, intensified by obstruction of the circulation due to the enlarged uterus. Such a condition requires, aside from the natural regimen, careful and competent treatment. Swelling of the limbs or other parts of the body may also be caused by incipient or advanced Bright's disease. The urine should be examined from time to time, especially if there is a swelling of the feet and ankles, or if there are dropsical symptoms in other parts of the body. Such dangerous conditions are usually brought about through the excessive intake of starchy and protein foods which overwork the liver and kidneys and cause pathogenic clogging of the capillary circulation. This may result in uraemia attended by violent and sometimes fatal convulsions.

2. **Uraemia.** This is the result of retention in the system of waste materials and poisons that should be eliminated through the kidneys and skin. Medical treatment for such conditions, aside from the administration of stimulating drugs, consists in hot bathing with the idea of opening the pores of the skin. We understand that all hot water treatment gives only temporary relief and is followed by greater enervation and inactivity of the skin. The best water treatment for systemic poisoning of any kind consists in the application of wet packs followed by cold ablutions as described in Sec. XV. In addition to the packs, dry friction rubs, air baths, good massage and neuropathy treatment will aid in restoring the normal activity of the skin, bowels and kidneys.

Whenever the urine contains sugar or albumen, fasting alternating with raw food diet is indicated.

The idea of giving heavy food to the mother with the idea of increasing the flow of milk is all wrong. We have found in all cases that the diet outlined in Sec. X will produce a more copious flow of rich milk than the "nourishing" meat diet. The best remedy for a scanty flow of milk is slow and thorough mastication of a few spoonfuls of raw crushed wheat every day.

3. **Morning Sickness.** One of the common disorders experienced during pregnancy is that known as morning sickness. One suffering from this ailment, though following a natural diet, should sip a cup of hot postum while remaining in bed. If this does not have the desired effect, half a cup of black coffee with a few drops of lemon juice will quiet the irritated nerves. It is necessary after taking the hot drink to remain in bed

211

for at least thirty minutes. It is understood that this is only an emergency measure. If continued, it will lose its good effect and work injury.([1])

SECTION XXXVII

LABOUR AND DELIVERY

At about forty weeks, or nine solar months, from the time of conception the foetus reaches full maturity, and labour begins.([2]) Labour is divided into three stages. During the first stage the neck of the womb becomes slowly and gradually distended and the orifice of the womb opens widely. When this has taken place, the foetal membranes burst and the amniotic liquid surrounding the foetus escapes. During the second stage the foetus emerges from the womb. After expulsion of the foetus, the placenta is expelled from the uterine cavity. This constitutes the third stage of labour.

The first stage usually begins with more or less radiating pains in the abdomen, accompanied by dull pain in the small of the back and a drawing pain in the limbs. Sometimes women with the first baby feel these

([1])
It should be noted that sacro-iliac lesions have a very special connection both with the tendency to swelling of the legs and with morning sickness. They are also a very common source or contributory cause of nearly all the troubles which are apt to take place during pregnancy, and during and after parturition, such as backache, haemorrhage, miscarriage, difficulties and excessive pain during delivery. It should be a matter of routine for a check to be kept on the pelvic joints up to the time of delivery and after it.

([2])
As Lindlahr here states, the normal length of gestation would appear to be 280 days from conception to delivery. This is forty weeks or ten lunar months. Though this may be the normal, some modern physiology text books state that the average is about 270 days. It is obvious that when an obstetrician wishes to calculate the expected day of birth he should ideally do this from the day of ovulation or conception. However, as this is often not known with any accuracy, it is common for the calculation to be made from the first day of the last menstruation before conception and to look upon nine calendar months as the length of the period of gestation. Nine calendar months is about 274 days, the average length of a calendar month being between thirty and thirty-one days. It is usual to add seven or more days to the nine calendar months when calculating from the first day of the last menstruation. (Thus if the first day of the menstruation was on January 1st the birth could be expected on October 8th.) The use of the formula of nine calendar months and seven days makes calculation easy and gives a good rough idea of when the child is to be expected, but it would seem likely to lead in many cases to the child being expected a few days sooner than it is actually due and to be considered as overdue when in fact it is not so. It would seem probable that the formula came to be used at a time when ovulation was thought to take place earlier in the intermenstrual period than in fact it usually does and it might therefore be that greater accuracy could be obtained by adding ten or even fourteen days instead of seven to the nine calendar months. This would allow for the fact that the usual time of ovulation would seem to be about two weeks from the onset of menstruation.

212

pains weeks in advance of the actual commencement of labour. At first they occur at long intervals and are of short duration, but gradually become more prolonged and more frequent. The pains are due to a cramp-like contraction of the muscular apparatus of the uterus forcing its contents downwards. Under this pressure from above, the neck and mouth of the uterus distend to their limits, and the walls become thinner and thinner. First the inner, then the outer orifice of the neck of the womb opens and the foetal membranes protrude and finally rupture, allowing the amniotic fluid to escape. Shortly after this the part of the foetus nearest the orifice, normally the head, makes its appearance. At the present time the average duration of the first stage of labour is six hours, but it may last twenty-four hours or longer, depending upon the plasticity and elasticity of the bony structures of mother and infant, the rigidity of the cervix, and the vigour or lack of vigour of the muscular apparatus of the uterus.

While the foregoing is true of the average delivery under ordinary ways of living, we find that after the enforcement of a natural regimen of living during and, better still, before pregnancy, the entire period of labour and delivery does not cover more than half an hour, or at the utmost from one to two hours. Even the disadvantages of slight build and smallness of pelvis can be overcome by the natural regimen outlined in Sec. X. When our youngest child was born, the mother gave the first sign of pain at about midnight. I rose from bed instantly, but had no time to finish clothing when the membranes broke. Within twenty minutes after the commencement of labour the infant was resting in my hands.

The wife of a prominent lawyer in a western city had experienced three difficult deliveries. Each time surgical instruments had to be used and she had suffered untold agonies lasting from twenty-four to thirty-six hours. When she became pregnant the fourth time the most prominent physicians in her home city assured husband and wife that it was not safe for her to go through another delivery, that the womb was in worse condition than ever before; therefore they recommended surgical removal. For conscientious reasons, however, the husband and wife did not follow the advice of the doctors, but decided to try natural methods of treatment. The lady placed herself under our care during the fifth month of pregnancy. From that time on she followed strictly the natural regimen of living and received daily the usual hydropathic and manipulative treatments. This was continued until a few weeks before delivery. In this case the baby was born within an hour from the first contraction, and the mother of the patient, who was in an adjoining room, had not heard a sound. Many similar experiences refute the idea that it is unsafe and injurious for pregnant women to undergo the ordinary natural treatment, such as hydropathic sprays, sitz baths, massage, Swedish movement and other forms of manipulation.

1. **Preparation for Delivery.** The diet during the last week before the beginning of labour should be very light, consisting mostly of fruits and vegetables. From the commencement of labour no food at all should be given, until at least twenty-four hours after delivery — a three day fast is better. In addition to a competent physician, a nurse or midwife should be engaged. If a good neurotherapist, who has had sufficient experience in obstetrical work, can be found, he should be preferred, because he can assist delivery and make it much safer by manipulative treatment. The nurse will make the necessary preparations and provide the various supplies needed in labour. With the first sign of approaching labour, the physician in charge should be summoned. A rectal enema of one pint or more of warm salt water (Sec. XVIII, No. 4) should be administered. The woman should be given a vigorous cold rub and her genitals thoroughly cleansed. She may then remain on her feet and walk about, comfortably dressed, until actual labour commences.

2. **No Anaesthetics.** The attending physician should not be impatient to hasten delivery with drugs or instruments. The use of anaesthetics should be avoided in so far as this is possible. They should be employed only when absolutely necessary — that is, when excessive pain must be allayed or when surgical delivery is unavoidable.

3. **Breaking of Water Bag.** When the bag of waters is about ready to break, the patient is placed in bed. Premature discharge of the amniotic fluid must be guarded against. An escape of the liquid at an early stage means difficult and prolonged labour. Usually the membranes burst when the orifice is fully dilated. A large sponge is held in readiness to catch the outflowing liquid.

3a. **Umbilical Cord.** When the infant has been delivered, the umbilical cord should not be severed at once. Plenty of time should be allowed for the blood to transfuse itself from the body of the mother to that of the child. This is important. If the connection is severed too soon, the child begins life in an anaemic condition. The newborn baby usually greets the world with a lusty cry. It should be placed on its right side with its face turned away from the mother, care being taken that the cord is not stretched tight. As soon as the cord stops pulsating, plenty of time being allowed for blood transfusion, it is tied about two inches away from the baby's abdomen and cut a little above the ligature. The baby is now wrapped in a warm blanket and put in its crib.

4. **After Delivery.** Immediately after the baby is born, the nurse or attending physician gently compresses the abdomen and womb of the mother, kneading and rubbing it occasionally in order to secure complete

contraction and thus prevent haemorrhage. After delivery the mother enjoys a period of rest and recuperation which usually lasts for about half an hour.

5. **Afterbirth.** Meanwhile the placenta becomes detached, and when pains set in again a few contractions usually suffice to expel it with all the membranes. The attending physician must make sure that none of it is left in the body, since this might result in putrefaction of the remains and blood poisoning. The woman's genitals should now be washed with clean sterilized water. The exhausted woman should now enjoy a deep, wholesome sleep and awaken from it in a few hours refreshed and strengthened.

In the foregoing I have not gone into the details of obstetrics and of technical management because this must be left to a competent obstetrician. I have called attention only to those points which are of special importance from the viewpoint of Natural Therapeutics and to the differences in treatment between the conventional and natural methods.

6. **The Lying-In Period.** The lying-in period varies from five to twelve days, according to the constitution of the mother and the care that she has taken during pregnancy. The greatest danger of the lying-in period is puerperal sepsis or blood poisoning. This condition is the result of infection occurring during labour, or it may result from the retention of parts of the placenta. The only way to prevent this is by observing the most scrupulous cleanliness during the entire process of childbirth and during the lying-in period. When blood poisoning has developed it must be treated the same as all other acute inflammatory diseases (see Sec. IX).

7. **Care of the Newborn.** The child should begin to breathe immediately after the cord is cut. If it fails to do this, the physician should lift the baby by its feet to facilitate the escape of mucous from the trachea and throat. If necessary, the mucous must be removed from the trachea and throat by the insertion of the little finger, or by means of a tiny stick covered with gauze. Breathing may be accelerated by a few sharp taps on shoulders and buttocks. If this fails to bring the desired result, artificial respiration must be resorted to at once. The attendant grasps the child by its shoulders, its head resting between his palms and the two index fingers being hooked under the child's armpits. It is now swung between the physician's legs and lifted high above his head so as to be turned upside down. This is repeated from fifteen to twenty times, after which it is placed in a basin containing a few inches of warm water. Its body should then be rubbed briskly with cold water. Father Kneipp used to take the newborn baby by the nape of the neck and the feet and submerge it quickly in cold water. This, a few times repeated, is probably the quickest way of resuscitating an asphyxiated baby.

215

In order to soften the cheesy deposit which frequently covers the body of the newborn, it is well to rub the skin with warm olive oil. After the greasy covering has sufficiently softened it may be removed with bits of gauze. This is followed by a cleansing bath with warm water and Castile soap. After the warm cleansing bath, the little body should be quickly rubbed down with cold water, wrapped in a soft, warm blanket and laid away to sleep until it wakens of its own accord. A normal baby should sleep for about twelve hours, and must not be disturbed to force food on it before it is ready to take it.

8. Bathing. From the first day, the baby must have a morning and evening bath. This consists, as before described, in a quick, cleansing bath of warm water and Castile soap, followed immediately by a brisk cold rub. In the course of a few weeks the baby can be placed, for the cleansing bath, in a small bathtub containing a few inches of warm water. Immediately after the cleansing bath the warm water is replaced by cold water. This is taken up in the hollow of the hand and briskly applied to the little body. In this fashion the child, within a few months' time, will enjoy its cold rub just as much as an adult. I have seen several such Nature Cure babies, but a few months old, object most vigorously to a warm bath. The cold rub is the best preventive of chilling; but care must be taken that the temperature of the room where the bath is taken is not below 70°F.

The olive oil bath or rub, often recommended for premature babies or infants suffering from malnutrition, is very injurious, because it occludes the pores of the skin and prevents the elimination of poisonous gases and other morbid materials from the body. The skin is not an organ of digestion. Olive oil, like all other foods, must enter the body through the alimentary canal where, under the action of digestive ferments, it is broken down into its component elements which are then assimilated through the intestinal membranes. Oil absorbed through the skin is not digested, and it circulates in the body as foreign matter which in this state cannot be assimilated and utilized in the system.

9. Powdering after the bath is fully as injurious as the rubbing with oils or massage creams. Powders and creams tend to clog the pores, and most of them contain poisonous antiseptics which lower the vitality of the skin and prevent or suppress elimination in the form of skin eruptions, eczemas, etc. For chafing use nothing but cold water. In case the chafing should become unusually severe and painful, through neglect, a soothing and healing lotion composed of one part lemon juice and two parts olive oil may be applied a few times, until the irritation is under control.

10. Air Baths. Next to cold water, there is nothing that will invigorate a baby's skin and nervous system as will the air and sun bath. If the season will not allow the outdoor air bath, the baby should be allowed to lie nude several times during the day, for thirty minutes or more, in a warm, well ventilated and sunny room.

11. **Constipation.** Glycerin and suppositories should never be used; neither laxatives nor cathartics. Oat extract and cooling sitz baths will produce natural movements.

12. **Diarrhoea.** This is a form of morbid elimination, and must never be suppressed by drugs. If it is habitual, barley or wheat extract prepared in the same manner as oat extract is a good remedy. If the diarrhoea is persistent and of a violent nature, no food at all must be given, except water with dilute acid fruit juices, until the purging ceases. Even then plenty of time must be allowed for the rebuilding of the sloughed intestinal membranes.

13. **Bandages.** Until the umbilical cord dries up and falls off, it is necessary to cover the navel with a gauze compress dipped in olive oil. This is held in place by an abdominal bandage made of soft cotton material. These strips should not be hemmed, merely torn or cut. They should be drawn just snugly enough to hold the compress in place, but not tightly enough to interfere with circulation. The navel must be cleansed and the compress renewed twice a day. After the abdominal cord has dropped off we no longer apply the abdominal bandage. This is contrary to common usage, but it is the best practice. The abdominal bandage overheats the body and interferes with the free movement of the diaphragm and the circulation of the blood.

14. **Clothing.** The clothing of the infant should be loose and light and as simple as possible. Freedom of movement is very important; binding or pressure upon any part cannot help but interfere with the circulation, and otherwise produce injurious results. The clothes should be short, in order to allow the feet and legs free play. Lightweight, porous cotton materials are best for both under and outer garments. A lightweight wool petticoat may be worn when absolutely necessary to provide sufficient protection. Cotton hose and bootees may be used, but under no circumstances should such articles be of wool because it prevents free elimination from the skin. The baby's head should not be covered out of doors, except in severe weather. At no time should a veil be placed over the face, as it will cause the infant to reabsorb the poisonous exhalations from its own lungs. All clothing should be changed every day. No garments should be starched — such a practice is not only useless but harmful.

15. **Diapers.** These must be provided in sufficient numbers to allow thorough cleansing and drying. The wet diapers should be scalded in hot

water and very thoroughly rinsed in several waters after. They should then be dried in the open air and sunshine. Soiled diapers must be well washed and boiled. Washing powders, soda, ammonia and other chemicals should never be used. They have an extremely irritating effect upon the delicate skin of the baby. In order to save labour and to facilitate the cleansing of the diapers, small squares of clean old linen or muslin rags, or pieces of absorbent gauze, may be placed inside. These inserts will absorb all or most of the bowel movement and may then be burned. If the skin is irritated or chafed, the parts should be sponged off with cold clean water at each change, paying especial attention to cleansing the genitals. Oils or powders must not be used to soothe the sore places, because they clog the pores and interfere with natural elimination.

16. **Nursing.** A wet nurse is to be preferred to artificial feeding. She should be thoroughly healthy, not over thirty years of age, of equable temper, not excitable or nervous, and her diet should be that prescribed for the mother.

17. **Care of the Nipples.** These should be thoroughly cleansed before and after nursing; not with carbolic acid, but with water and dilute lemon juice. The lemon juice tends also to harden the nipples. Treatment of the nipples may begin before the birth of the child.

18. **Care of the Eyes.** The baby's eyes, whether awake or asleep, should always be shielded from strong light, either sun or artificial, and from dust and wind. The eyes should be washed with cold water after every cleansing bath. If they show any tendency to weakness or disease, slight vibratory massage over the closed eyelids should be given after the cold eye bath.

19. **Care of the Mouth.** A healthy baby's mouth needs no cleaning before the arrival of teeth. As a matter of fact, the teeth of a perfectly healthy adult would not need cleaning any more than do those of an animal living in the freedom of nature. The saliva is a sterilizing fluid, under normal living, intended by nature to keep the mouth clean and healthy. Cleansing the mouth of an infant with the finger or with a cloth may injure its delicate membranes. If the mouth must be washed, in case of disease, a swab made by twisting a piece of sterilized absorbent cotton-wool on the end of a smooth stick should be used. The swab should be dipped in warm boiled water, and the interior of the mouth washed thoroughly, the cottonwool being then burned.

20. **Care of the Ears.** The external ear should be cleansed with a soft rag or swab as before described. Never use a hard instrument inside the ear.

21. **Care of the Nose.** A baby's nose should be cleansed as part of the daily toilet, in the same way as the ears. A swab may be made by twisting

a piece of gauze to a cone. As soon as the child becomes old enough, it should be taught to sniff up cold water through the nostrils and nasal passages. This is the best way to keep the nasal membranes in a clean, healthy condition.

22. **Care of the Genital Organs.** The genital organs of both sexes must be kept scrupulously clean with as little handling as possible. The foreskin of the penis of the male baby should be drawn back at bathing time and the organ thoroughly cleansed, always finishing with cold water.

23. **Phimosis.** The treatment of phimosis is fully described under Sec. XXVIII, No. 1.

24. **How to Lift the Baby.** The best way to lift a young baby is to slip the left hand under the back beneath the shoulder, spreading out the fingers in such a way as to support the neck and head. Then lift the feet and legs with the right hand. Never lift an infant without first supporting the spine. When a baby has grown strong enough to hold up its head and has gained considerable strength in the muscles of the back and neck, he may be lifted by grasping him with outspread fingers under the armpits; the body must be held firmly so that the entire strain does not come on the shoulders. A baby should never be lifted by the arms. This may dislocate the shoulder joints.

SECTION XXXVIII

PRENATAL FEEDING

1. **Effects of Diet During Pregnancy.** The problem of infant nutrition begins before birth. Prenatal feeding determines the physical start in life. On it depends not only the condition of the mother's health during pregnancy, but also the size and weight of the foetus, pliability of the bony structures, ease or difficulty of delivery, and the quality of the mother's milk.

The fleshier and heavier the newborn infant, the prouder and happier are the parents and the doctor. Yet, excessive size and weight of the child constitute the most prominent cause of difficult and painful childbirth and frequent necessity for instrumental delivery. The biblical saying: "In sorrow thou shalt bring forth children", has led many to believe that woman's dreadful suffering is a necessity ordained by God; but is not man's ignorance, rather than the cruelty of an avenging God, to blame? This latter view is confirmed by the fact that other mammalia literally cast

219

their young, without pain or difficulty; and the labour pains of primitive mothers are insignificant, their delivery presenting little more difficulty than that of the lower animals. A squaw on the Western Plains stops a few hours by the wayside to deliver her papoose and then resumes her journey as though nothing had happened. Women among the European peasantry, who wear no corsets, live on black bread and vegetables, and have plenty of exercise in the fields and in the house to the last day of pregnancy, have their babies without help of midwife or physician and resume their usual routine of work within a few days after delivery. Thousands of mothers who have adopted natural ways of living have learned to dispense with anaesthetics and the surgeon's instruments; they now bring forth their offspring without excessive pain.

2. **Results of Faulty Diet.** It is significant that the offspring of the lower animals, at birth, consist of little more than skin and bones, while the newborn human is often abnormally large and fat. This is especially true of babies born of weak and anaemic mothers. As before stated, excessive size and weight of the infant is not a matter for congratulation, but is a pathological condition. It indicates fatty degeneration of the foetus, due to the anaemic watery condition of the blood of the mother, and the cause of this hydraemia of mother and child lies in the faulty dietetic habits of the former.

The ordinary diet of American women consists almost entirely of meat, fish, fowl, potatoes, white bread, pastry, coffee, tea and refined white sugar. The few vegetables which enter into the daily dietary are first deprived of all their important organic salts by faulty cooking; fruits are looked upon as luxuries and frequently are regarded as harmful. The anaemic, watery condition of the blood of mother and child is not due to a lack of starchy, proteid and fatty materials in food and blood, but to a deficiency of organic mineral elements. Neither is the anaemic condition, as the regular school of medicine assumes, caused by lack of iron. Any ordinary food mixture, as well as the blood and milk of anaemic mothers, usually contains a sufficient amount of iron. The actual cause of the anaemia is a deficiency of other mineral elements. As I have explained in Vol. 3 of this series, carbonic acid poisoning and the resulting sluggishness of the surface circulation, coldness of the extremities and congestion of the inner organs are not caused so much by a lack of the oxygen-carrying iron as by a deficiency of the carbonic acid neutralizing and eliminating sodium and magnesium. If the blood is deficient in lime, phosphates, silicon and fluorine, rachitic conditions, softening of the bones, deformed spines and legs, and decay of the teeth are inevitable results.

It is an easy matter to supply the daily needs of the organism for proteids, starches, fats and sugars; the difficulty lies in supplying a sufficient amount of the organic mineral elements. The deficiency of sodium in human blood, Dr. Lahmann proved in the following table of comparative blood analyses. In a hundred parts of ash he found as follows:

In the blood of	oxen	12.41 to 31.90	per cent of sodium
,, ,,	sheep	13.33	,, ,, ,,
,, ,,	cows	10.40	,, ,, ,,
,, ,,	hogs	5.33 to 7.62	,, ,, ,,
,, ,,	dogs	2.02 to 5.78	,, ,, ,,
,, ,,	humans	2.03 to 6.27	,, ,, ,,

The percentages of lime and of other positive mineral elements in the human blood are also much lower than in the blood of cows, oxen and sheep. While the blood of cattle and sheep raised on pasture is very uniform in composition, hardly any two samples of human blood are alike. It is for this reason Dr. Lahmann adopted cow's milk instead of human milk as the standard elementary food combination. In the following table, he compares the percentages of minerals in the ash of cow's milk with the percentages of mineral elements in the ash of various other food materials.

	Sodium	Calcium	Iron
Cow's milk	4.73	10.66	0.26
Lean beef	1.47	1.15	0.28
White flour (wheat)	0.04	0.13	—
Rye meal	0.34	0.20	0.50
Potatoes	0.99	0.97	0.45
Peas	0.26	1.36	0.16
Spinach	0.16	19.58	5.52
Apples	3.76	0.59	0.20
Strawberries	9.68	4.83	2.00

A daily dietary consisting largely of meats, eggs, white bread, potatoes, peas and beans, though excessively rich in proteids, fats and starches, will, on account of its deficiency in sodium, lime and magnesium, inevitably result in carbonic acid poisoning, anaemia, rachitis, premature decay of teeth and a multitude of other acute and chronic ailments. If, however, the daily dietary contains a liberal amount of green vegetables and fruits, a normal food mixture resembling that of cow's milk can easily be obtained. It must be remembered that fruits and vegetables are not only rich in the most important mineral salts, but that they are relatively poor in proteids and carbohydrates. For this reason fruits and vegetables facilitate the establishment of an equilibrium between proteids and carbohydrates on the one hand and organic mineral salts on the other.

3. **Excessive Fat Fomation.** We can now understand why the ordinary faulty diet of pregnant mothers causes anaemia, softening of the bones, sluggish circulation, carbonic acid poisoning and fatty degeneration in mother and offspring. Lack of sodium causes excessive accumulation of carbonic acid, and oxygen starvation. This results in the defective oxidation of food and waste materials; in other words, in fat formation. Defective draught prevents consumption of coal, and chokes the furnace with the products of imperfect combustion. Similarly, lack of oxygen in the tissues (due to carbonic acid poisoning) causes an incomplete combustion of food materials and waste products, resulting in fat formation and in the generation of poisonous by-products. Lack of sodium also prevents the neutralization and elimination of uric and other acids and ptomaines (pathogenic matter) which accumulate in the tissues, block the circulation and assist in the smothering of the vital processes. In order to eliminate these pathogenic materials, there arises an abnormal craving for water — "the anaemic thirst" — which is closely related to the thirst of fever patients and of diabetics. Excessive water drinking is encouraged by the popular "flushing" fad. To make things worse, the anaemic, for reasons before stated, usually suffers from weak heart action and sluggish circulation. This means defective elimination of water through the skin and kidneys, resulting in a watery (dropsical) condition of the tissues and fatty degeneration.

Not all anaemic, carbonic-acid-poisoned mothers, however, develop the tendency to obesity. On the contrary, under certain constitutional conditions, they may become exceedingly lean, like the anaemic, carbonic-acid-poisoned consumptive. Briefly stated, sluggish heart action and weak kidneys favour retention of carbonic acid and water in the tissues and thus make for fatty degeneration. Good circulation and normal activity of the kidneys may keep the system free from excess of water and carbonic acid, but excess proteid in the diet may result in sulphuric and phosphoric acid poisoning. These destructive acids break down the tissues, rob them of their mineral constituents, and thus cause excessive loss of flesh and fat.

In both types of dysaemia the blood of the pregnant mother is overloaded with poisonous gases, waste matter and the debris of broken-down tissues. The oxygen supply to the foetus is therefore very much impeded and we find that both fleshy and lean mothers produced babies of abnormal size and weight, ranging from eight to twelve pounds, while the normal weight of the newborn should not be more than six pounds.

4. **Advantages of Natural Regimen.** We know of many instances where mothers, after having given birth to heavy, fleshy babies, in subsequent

births have reduced the weight of the newborn to normal, and the pain of delivery to a minimum, by the adoption of a natural diet, plenty of exercise in the fresh air and systematic deep breathing. The effects of a natural regimen are manifested in various other ways. The bony and muscular structures of mother and child are much more pliable and elastic, making parturition and delivery much easier. Pure blood, normal nutrition and abdominal exercises, walking and special gymnastics, greatly strengthen the abdominal and uterine muscles, thus facilitating expulsion of the foetus. The morning cold rub, systematic deep breathing and general exercises, everyday outdoor walks and right mental and emotional attitude are all of paramount importance in the regimen of pregnancy. The Regimen of Wholesome Living, Sec. I, is admirably adapted for all the needs of the pregnant mother.

SECTION XXXIX

POSTNATAL FEEDING

Thanks to the educational influence of Nature Cure propaganda, a decided change for the better in baby feeding has taken place during the past ten years. Up to that time the "top cream mixture" was universally recommended by allopathic physicians and given to babies by trained nurses. While in the meantime many physicians and nurses have adopted more natural methods, the "top cream mixture" is still too common and must be entirely abolished in order to safeguard the health of our little ones.

1. **Bottle-Fed Babies.** Our food analyses disclose the interesting fact that the elementary composition of the ash of the milk of an animal is about the same as the composition of the ash of its body. They also show that good cow's milk when normal comes closer to the requirements of the infant body than does inferior human milk. Our analyses tables show that chemically the composition of cow's milk and of human milk is very much the same. Human milk contains a little less proteid and a little more sugar than cow's milk, and the latter is much richer in organic salts than the former. There is much more of the all-important sodium in cow's milk than in human milk and about twice as much calcium and iron. This explains why rachitis is so common among babies, while never found among calves. As we have learned, the elimination of poisonous acids

from the body depends on sodium. The building of the bony structures depends on lime; the oxygenation of the blood, on iron.

Many years of practical experience in the care of babies has convinced me that milk fresh from a healthy cow is greatly to be preferred, as nourishment for infants, to the impoverished milk of scrofulous mothers.* In this connection it is significant that one half of all "civilized" mothers, thanks to unnatural food and drink, vaccination and poisonous drugs, are incapacitated from nursing their offspring. To one who has studied the comparative analyses of cow's milk and human milk, it is incomprehensible why the former, when given to infants, should be diluted and spoiled by large quantities of water, salt, soda and inorganic mineral lime (in the form of lime water). This procedure, however, is still frequently recommended by physicians of the regular school. Undoubtedly, the great frequency of anaemic and rachitic diseases, the darkening of the iris, the appearance of a scurf rim, and the signs of catarrhal conditions in stomach and bowels are caused by such unnatural feeding. Physicians would never think of giving such advice as this, if they were acquainted with natural dietetics founded on exact and complete analyses made by food chemists of the Nature Cure school. I have already called attention to the fact that food chemistry, whether practiced in allopathic colleges, in great sanitoria or by vegetarian food reformers, deals with proteids, starches, fats and sugars only, and leaves entirely out of consideration the all-important mineral elements or organic salts of potassium, sodium, iron, lime and magnesium.

On these five positive mineral salts, as we have shown, depend all the important vital functions of the human organism, while proteids, starches, fats and sugars serve only as building and fuel material. The digestion of the proteid and carbohydrate foods, as well as the elimination of the waste matter resulting therefrom, depends upon the positive organic mineral salts. Study carefully the recipes for baby feeding recommended by some of the experts on child care and compare these mixtures with the analyses of cow's and human milk which we have been discussing. For instance, in the "top milk" or "cream" mixtures the mineral elements, which remain in the skimmed milk, are practically excluded. Moreover, when the "top milk" or plain milk formulae are used it is common for them to be diluted with barley water, for bicarbonate of soda, salt and sugar to be added and for the milk to be pasteurized. Where in six ounces of cream and twenty-four ounces of barley water is the baby to get the necessary amount of sugar for fuel material, of lime for bone-building, of iron for oxygen-carrying, and of sodium, magnesium and potassium for the processes of elimination?

* This may not be true in the future if our milk cows continue to be regularly subjected to tuberculin tests. (Author's note.)

It would seem that the deficiencies in feeding formulae of this kind are, if considered at all, intended to be overcome by the baking soda, mineral table salt and lime water, so generally prescribed by physicians. Many times I have demonstrated that inorganic salts, with the possible exception of a little table salt, should not enter the animal or human organism, that these salts must first be organized, made alive in the plant or animal cell, before they are wholesome food for animals or human beings. I have shown that, taken habitually in the mineral form, these salts accumulate in the human body, act as irritants and poisons and reveal their presence in the iris of the eye. I fail to understand why the tender and sensitive organism of the newborn infant should be encumbered with inorganic minerals while cow's milk contains them in ideal form, made alive first in the grasses and grains, then still more highly organized and magnetized in the body of the animal. It is bad enough to give mineral sodium, lime and table salt to an adult, but it is little short of criminal to give them to babies under the guise of foods and medicines.

The cream mixtures are readily digested, because there is not much to digest. The fact that infants thus fed cry for food continually is good evidence that their needs are not satisfied. Babies fed with this sort of slop grow fat for a while. The watery food inevitably produces fatty degeneration. This for a season swamps the little body with unhealthy fat. But the first crisis which happens often takes away not only the unnatural fat, but the baby also. The artificial mixtures contain entirely too much water in proportion to nourishing elements. The resulting malnutrition and the constant irritation caused by the inorganic minerals result in chronic diarrhoea or constipation.

The Right Way

The best food for the newborn and growing infant is undoubtedly the mother's milk, provided that she is in fairly good health. Unfortunately, many mothers are unable to nurse their offspring, and if a healthy wet nurse cannot be secured, other food must be provided. The best substitute for human milk, without question, is cow's milk, fresh, pure and undiluted as it comes from the animal.[1] "Why," indignantly exclaims the trained nurse, when we give these instructions, "undiluted cow's milk is altogether too rich, it is indigestible for a baby; if the milk is not boiled or pasteurized, germs and bacilli will surely create infectious diseases." To this we answer: Our analyses show that the difference in composition

[1]
It is contended by some that good goat's milk is better for small children in composition and digestibility than cow's milk.

between cow's milk and human milk is not enough to affect the infant. The danger lies not so much in overfeeding on "rich" cow's milk as in underfeeding on watery milk and cereal dilutions, and in poisoning the young body with inorganic minerals. As regards germ infection and the necessity for pasteurizing the milk, the menace to health and life is greater through malnutrition than through germs and bacteria. Germs we cannot escape, not even if we were surrounded on all sides by walls of air-purifying and antiseptic materials.(¹)

One of the foremost French bacteriologists claims that in the mouths of infants shortly after birth he has found almost every disease bacillus known to medical science. Sir William Osler, to whom the English language is indebted for the verb "to oslerize", says in "The Principles and Practice of Medicine", 10th edn., on page 65, in the chapter on Diphtheria: "The presence of the Klebs-Loeffler bacillus is regarded by bacteriologists as the sole criterion of true diphtheria, and as this organism may be associated with all grades of throat affections, from a simple catarrh to a sloughing, gangrenous process, it is evident that in many instances there will be a striking discrepancy between the clinical and the bacteriological diagnosis." In the first part of this sentence he states that bacteriologists regard as the sole criterion of diphtheria the Klebs–Loeffler, or diphtheria bacillus; in the last part of the sentence he admits that this bacillus is found in even slight catarrhal conditions, and he might add that it is found just as frequently in the mouth and throat of healthy infants and adults. This is a good example of "orthodox" scientific reasoning.

If germs and bacilli of themselves could destroy health and life, the human race would in a short time become extinct. Disease germs are omnipresent. They permeate the tissues of our bodies and in the intestinal tract swarm by millions. Whether they prevail depends upon natural resistance, or reserve force, and upon the disease soils in the system. The air we breathe is saturated with all sorts of disease germs or their microzymes. Since a baby cannot escape germ invasion, the real problem is how to increase the resistance of the little organism and how to purify it of morbid matter, so that disease germs will not find anything to feed on. Resistance depends largely upon proper nutrition. Diluted, watery milk contaminated by inorganic minerals is not a good nutrient; its nutritive value is still more reduced by pasteurizing or boiling. Heating milk or any other proteid food above 150°F. coagulates the albumen, disorganizes organic compounds, precipitates salts and dissipates the life elements. Nature does not provide the

---

(¹) We have now learned that low vitality and morbid soil will develop perfectly normal microzymes into so-called disease germs. [Author's note.]

226

young animal with boiled or pasteurized milk, and we should not lower food values by such methods.([1])

I do not wish to intimate, however, that scrupulous care and cleanliness should not be exercised in the selection and handling of the milk. Wherever possible, secure the milk of a single healthy cow which grazes on green pastures or is fed on normal clean food mixtures. Milk from cows kept in stables and fed on brewery and distillery slops and other refuse should not be used. Every vessel and utensil with which the milk comes in contact must be carefully scoured, submerged in boiling water, drained and kept in a light airy place. The nursing bottle, after each feeding, must be taken apart and carefully scrubbed, inside and out, in hot water with the addition of a little soda. It should then be left in pure, cold water, until the next feeding time.

2. **When to Feed.** Physicians quite generally recommend feedings at stated hours, in fixed quantities. This is altogether wrong. It establishes at once the stuffing habit, does not permit the development of natural desire and its regulation. The infant very soon becomes accustomed to eating at certain times, whether it really needs the food or not. Food should not be given until there is an actual demand for it, which will express itself in real hunger. By careful observation and experiment the mother will soon learn to distinguish the ordinary crying of the baby and the desire for food expressed by it. If this practice of feeding only when there is a natural desire for food is strictly followed, the infant will soon establish its own regular feeding times, usually at intervals of about three or four hours in the daytime. The stomach digestion of a feeding of milk will require about three hours, therefore a minimum of that much time should be allowed between feedings after the first few weeks.

If the mother can nurse her baby, it should be put to the breast upon awakening from its first sleep, either before or after bathing and dressing. The first secretion of the breasts (colostrum) is not really a food, but performs an important function in cleansing the intestinal tract and preparing the digestive system properly to digest and assimilate the milk when it comes, usually about the third day.

3. **How to Feed.** If artificial feeding must be resorted to, no food at all should be given, except a few teaspoonfuls of water, during the first twenty-four hours after birth. During the next few days, cow's milk should be given, well diluted — about one half milk and one half filtered or boiled water. From week to week the water should be reduced until at the end of the second month the baby takes cow's milk undiluted.

[1]
It is now admitted that pasteurization and boiling kills vitamins which are the "life elements" constantly referred to in my early writings. [Author's note.]

4. **Night Feeding.** In the night time feeding should not be encouraged. During the first four months it is advisable to feed not more than once during the night. After that the child should be weaned from the habit entirely. This will be facilitated by giving a drink of water instead of milk.

5. **Amount of Food.** Discretion should be observed in determining the amount of food. Do not induce the baby to take as much as possible, rather as little as possible. Its welfare does not depend upon the amount of food consumed, but upon the amount it can easily digest and assimilate. When more food is given than the digestive organs can take care of, the entire mass may ferment and sour.

6. **Grain Extracts.** If undiluted milk proves too rich, grain water may be added. In order to prepare this, take clean grain as it comes from the field, crush it in a hand grain mill or new coffee mill, take three tablespoonfuls of crushed grain to one pint of cold water, and boil on a stove for one hour; or in the fireless cooker for two or three hours, in which case use a little more water at the start. While the gruel is boiling over the fire, add enough water to allow for evaporation and absorption. When thoroughly cooked, strain the gruel through a fine cloth or sieve. Add one tablespoonful, or more if necessary, to each milk feeding.

When the baby is constipated, add to the milk, grain extract made from oats, and frequently cool the bowels with cold water. This will cure the most stubborn constipation. If the bowels are too loose, add to the milk, extract made from barley or wheat. The small particles of hulls in the grain extracts improve digestion and evacuation, in a mechanical manner. They permeate the curds and keep them from coagulating too solidly, thereby facilitating the penetration of digestive juices; they also exert a mild stimulation on the walls of the intestines, thereby increasing the peristalsis of the bowels and evacuation of faeces.

7. **Natural Medicines.** Fruit juices and scraped raw pear or apple and the pulp of cooked fruits such as prunes or figs, without addition of sugar or sweetening of any kind, are the finest medicines for a baby. They increase the supply of organic salts for blood, nerve and bone building and for purposes of elimination. They are nature's own cholagogues, laxatives, tonics and antiseptics. They keep the little body sweet and wholesome. All babies under our care receive fruit juices, beginning with the second week. During the first two months, give one teaspoonful of orange juice, grapefruit juice or prune juice, one hour before or after each nursing. After the second month, gradually increase the amounts of fruit juices and begin to add raw pear or apple scraped with a spoon or dull knife, or the mashed pulp of fully ripened peach or grapes.

8. **Weaning the Baby.** Nursing infants should be weaned from the

breast after the eighth or ninth month. From the sixth or seventh month, both nursing and bottle-fed babies should begin to take some solid food. The best of these to begin with are whole grain cereals, gruels, raw and cooked fruits and tender vegetables in small amounts. Mealy baked potato is one of the best foods, better than the cereals.

9. **Feeding After the First Year.** After the lapse of the first year, the solid foods are gradually increased and the milk reduced in quantity. Eggs should not be given before the eighteenth month, then soft boiled or poached. During the second and third year half an egg twice or three times a week is sufficient; after that an egg at a time may be given once or twice a week.

Meat and all other foods prepared from the dead animal carcass are bad enough for adults, but it is inexcusable to give them to tender infants and children. Well informed physicians now generally advise not to give meat to children before the fifth or sixth year. They have learned this much from the Nature Cure people.

Foods undoubtedly have a powerful influence, not only on the physical body, but also on the mentality and the emotions. These problems will be interesting subjects of investigation for the food chemist and psychologist of the future. In general, we may say that flesh foods are stimulating and feed the passional nature, while fruits and tender vegetables refine and stimulate brain and nerve matter as well as the intellectual, emotional and spiritual activities. Cereals, nuts and pulses build and repair the physical body and supply the body with heat and muscular energy. The majority of animals adhere strictly to one kind of food, and therefore faithfully exhibit in their mental and emotional characteristics the effects of different food materials. Ferociousness we find personified in the carnivorous bulldog, lion, tiger and panther; gluttony and omnivorous voraciousness in the hog, chicken and hyena; cold-blooded cunning in the fox, and cruelty in the cat. The intelligence of the carnivorous animals displays itself mainly in the cruel cunning with which they stalk their living prey. It resembles in quality the low intelligence of the human criminal. Personifications of great physical strength, intelligence, endurance, patience, gentleness, fidelity, affection and self control, we find among the vegetarian animals. The beaver, the arboreal ape and the elephant are especially noted for their intelligence; deer, antelope and sheep for gentleness; the horse for its almost human intelligence, affection and fidelity; oxen, elephants and camels for their great strength and endurance.[1]

[1] What Lindlahr says here seems to be borne out to a great extent by the writings and researches of Sir Albert Howard, Sir Robert McCarrison and Dr. C. T. Wrench on the health, agriculture and diet of the various races of the Indian sub-continent. McCarrison showed very convincingly that the health of these races, including their psychological and

[continued overleaf

Meat is detrimental to the child in every way, physically, mentally and morally. The poisonous acids and alkaloids which it contains clog the capillary circulation, causing anaemia, coldness of the extremities and defective elimination through the skin. This results in congestion in the interior organs, high blood pressure in brain and heart, headaches, nervousness, irritability, tendency to fevers, inflammations and catarrhal conditions. With the meat the child often absorbs the eggs of worms, tubercular bacilli, and other parasites and disease germs. Certain forms of epilepsy, St. Vitus' dance and hysterical conditions are due to uric acid poisoning and other pathogenic materials and ptomaines contained in flesh foods. Such patients, in times of crisis, frequently emit pronounced odour of raw meat or uric acid. Strictly vegetarian diet, combined with other eliminative natural methods of treatment, cures the majority of these cases.

Most of these poisonous acids, alkaloids and ptomaines contained in the flesh of dead animals are powerful stimulants. I have frequently noticed that people who have abstained from meat for a long time, when they first partake of it again experience sensations and exhibit symptoms resembling those of alcoholic intoxication. We have learned that these stimulating extractives of flesh foods chemically closely resemble caffeine, theine and nicotine. The use of one or more of these stimulants invariably creates a craving for the others. This explains why a heavy meat eater is usually a confirmed coffee drinker or inveterate smoker, and vice versa; and why we find it almost impossible to wean people from one of these stimulants as long as they persist in taking the others.

The legumes or pulses — peas, beans and lentils — are close seconds to meat in acid-producing qualities. Eggs contain considerable ready-made

---

behaviour patterns, depended very largely on the food which they ate and the way in which it was grown and prepared. He confirmed his findings by feeding rats on the different diets of these different races and producing in the rats the most remarkable similarities to the races. Also a small booklet issued by two Salvation Army doctors called "We are what we eat" relates how 120 delinquent children became of mild disposition and lost all their tendency to delinquency after two years of purely vegetarian feeding and their health was much improved all round.

As regards the feeding patterns of different kinds of animals and their relation to the characteristics of these animals, the dog does seem to be something of an exception. Here is an animal which is undoubtedly carnivorous and which can be very fierce, especially when bred and trained to be so, but which can also show remarkable degrees of intelligence, affection and fidelity. However, some dog fanciers, when they sell a valuable dog, advise the buyer not to give the animal any meat before the second year, lest it become a victim of distemper. Moreover, good vets and breeders are generally in favour of feeding adult dogs to a considerable extent on various forms of vegetables and grains in addition to raw meat and also of using herbs to prevent or overcome disease. It is said to be the tradition among Scottish shepherds to feed their dogs almost entirely on their own diet of oatmeal. No dogs could be more intelligent, faithful and well behaved than these, as well as being remarkably healthy. It would, of course, be undesirable for dogs employed in this way to be encouraged to develop a strong taste for meat.

uric acid and a great deal of sulphur and phosphorus. These may become dangerous to the organism. For these reasons, meats legumes and eggs are always danger foods for the child. Children brought up on such foods will show the effects in nervousness, irritability, lack of self control, craving for cigarette and alcoholic stimulation. The most serious aspect of this matter lies in the stimulative influence of meat poisons on the sex centres. It is a well known fact, verified by close observation, that flesh foods stimulate the sexual passions to a marked degree. This tendency is greatly increased by the use of coffee, tea and alcoholic stimulants — in the form of wines, spirits or medicines. If the sensitive nervous system of a child is overwrought by these powerful irritants, there can be but one result: precocious sexual awakening.

From the third year the child may gradually adopt, with slight appropriate modifications, a diet as outlined under Sec. I, No. 10, and Sec. X, No. 7.

SECTION XL

EXERCISES IN INFANCY

1. **Proper Exercise** is important from the very beginning of life. A baby will follow its natural instincts for exercise if allowed to do so, by working its arms and legs and writhing its body about in all directions, if not unduly hampered by tight clothing and bandages. A few nude air baths every day will afford excellent opportunity for gymnastic stunts. After he is a few months old he may be placed on his stomach, when he will exert himself vigorously by trying to raise his head, to turn around, or to raise himself with his arms. He will soon learn to roll over and to creep. He may now be pulled up gently by his arms and lowered again a number of times in succession. When three or four months old he may be lifted by one or by both arms; by the right arm and left leg; or by the left arm and right leg. When the baby is six or eight months old, he should be strong enough to rise from his back to a sitting position. This may be encouraged by holding down his feet. I have known a number of Nature Cure babies who at six months of age clung tightly to a stick while being lifted a few feet from the bed. Another good exercise which is greatly enjoyed is to roll the baby back and forth on a bed.

The average healthy child will secure ample exercise while learning to walk and run and while playing with simple toys or with other children; but this may be supplemented to good advantage by special exercises devised by the father and mother. Nothing is better for the health and happiness of both parents and children than to join in a merry kind of play. Between two and five years of age the child may be taught more difficult stunts, performed either by himself or with the assistance of the father or mother; but swinging the child high overhead, throwing him up and catching him, and other dangerous tricks should be avoided. They are risky and have very little effect in developing the body of the child. The best exercise at this age consists in outdoor play and games.

From the sixth year, the question of exercise becomes a more important one, especially since the children are confined for many hours in school rooms. If exercise at this time of life, through play and games, and special gymnastics, is neglected, it may affect the health, strength and efficiency of the child for life. Those of good physique and ample strength may gradually take up and practice the exercises for adults outlined in Secs. XXI, XXII, XXIII, XXIV.

2. **High Chair.** A baby should not be put in a high chair until he is quite well able to hold the spine and head erect, and should never be left in a chair for any length of time. If a baby is forced to maintain a rigid, sitting position for a considerable time, before the bones and muscles are sufficiently developed, this may produce deformity of the spine. Maids and nurses, if not properly supervised, sometimes fasten a baby in a high chair and leave him there to take care of himself for long periods.

3. **Toys.** Since most babies have a habit of putting everything in their mouths, toys must be selected that can do no harm. They should have no paint or corners which might hurt the eyes or mouth, and must be of material which can be easily and thoroughly cleansed. Hairy and woolly playthings are unsafe, being unclean and germ carriers. Objects small enough to be swallowed must never be put within a baby's reach. The simpler the playthings the better; a few clothes-pegs, empty spools or other simple objects are better than expensive toys.

SECTION XLI

INFANTILE AILMENTS

1. **Hernia.** As a result of a weakly or sickly condition of the mother during pregnancy and of faulty prenatal management, many children are born ruptured. So far I have not known a single Nature Cure baby that was born ruptured. Such defects are due to weakness of the tissues. This results from mineral starvation. The tissues contain too much mortar (protein) and not enough building stone (mineral salts). Prevention of hernia, therefore, lies mainly in proper diet of the pregnant mother, but all the rest of the prenatal regimen described in these pages is of great importance in preventing this and other ailments and deformities. There are three principal points at which rupture or hernia may take place in infancy — at the navel, in the groin, and at the line between the navel and the lower end of the sternum. Other kinds of rupture are extremely rare.

2. **Umbilical Hernia.** This is a protrusion of the intestine at the navel. It is the most common rupture in infancy. Pulling on the cord during childbirth, urging at stool or violent crying may result in rupture. The umbilical ring first expands and this forms a pouch into which one of the folds of the small intestine protrudes.

Treatment: Of primary importance is the diet, as outlined herein. The baby must have plenty of fruit juices in order to reinforce the mineral salts in the milk. Cold bathing is very beneficial. The rupture itself should be cleansed several times a day with warm water. This must be followed by a wash with cold water mixed with lemon juice. Gentle, passive exercise, such as raising, lowering and twisting the limbs from side to side, also raising and lowering the body while supporting the shoulders and head, is of especial value. The rupture must be reduced and kept from protruding by placing over it a large button or other article of similar shape, wrapped in gauze and held in place by broad strips of adhesive plaster. The adhesive tape is fastened over the button crosswise and must be applied in such a manner as to draw the skin from all sides over the rupture. Instead of the button, a compress made of gauze may be laid over the rupture and held in place with one broad adhesive strip. The covering of the rupture must be removed and renewed every day in order to allow cleansing, as before described. When the child is old enough to exercise by himself, he should be taught special movements of the body and the limbs which develop the muscles of the abdominal region.

3. **Ventral Hernia.** This occurs along the mid line of the body between the navel and the breastbone, sometimes below the navel. The rupture

may not be larger than the size of a pea or small marble, and may disappear on pressure. The treatment is the same as for umbilical hernia.

4. **Inguinal and Scrotal Hernia.** This may occur in infancy or in adult life; sometimes the inguinal canal does not close after the descent of the testes from the abdominal cavity into the scrotum, and the intestines descends through the open canal, thus producing the rupture. These forms of hernia become aggravated by coughing. They can be reduced immediately by gentle manipulation while the patient is lying on his back. This kind of rupture may be distinguished from hydrocele by the fact that in reducing it goes back easily with a gurgling sound. Hydrocele is not affected by coughing. A hernia is opaque to transmitted light; hydrocele, transparent.

These ruptures should be protected with a well fitting truss. This has to be removed daily for cleansing of the parts. Appropriate exercises passive and active, together with cooling sitz baths and washes with cold water and lemon juice, are the best remedies for these, as well as for other forms of rupture.([1])

5. **Congenital Hernia.** This occurs in the form of inguinal hernia and has to be treated in the same way. Ruptures of any kind must be reduced and properly supported. Constipation and consequent urging at stool may cause or aggravate any form of hernia and must, therefore, be overcome by the right treatment described under Sec. XXVI, No. 1.

6. **Colic.** This is usually caused by indigestion due to overfeeding, improper feeding or too frequent feeding. The intestines are distended with gas, giving rise to severe pain. The baby cries sharply, alternately drawing its legs up to the body and kicking them away. One of the quickest means of relief is a small enema of warm water and gentle circular massage of the abdomen from right to left. Food should be withheld until the symptoms have disappeared. The giving of milk or other feed may quiet the attack temporarily, but the pain is apt to return with greater intensity. Warm water may be given if the baby will swallow it. A baby managed in the natural way prenatally and postnatally is not likely to

([1])
Daniel Mackinnon, the disciple of Lindlahr, was firmly of opinion that most cases of inguinal hernia could be cured by manipulative treatment and he claimed to have had success in doing this in a number of cases. This view does not seem unreasonable in view of the fact that so many cases of hernia are produced by some sort of strain of the low back. According to Mackinnon, the first thing to do is to make a careful adjustment of the sacro-iliac joints, but when this has been accomplished it is usually found that there is also a twist or torsion or tilting of the sacrum which is being maintained by tension and imbalance of some of the muscles and ligaments concerned. This condition must be worked on and corrected and it can then be hoped that the hernia will disappear in a shorter or longer time. The particular sacro-iliac lesion which seems to be associated with hernia is the so-called long leg lesion (i.e. the lesion which lowers the acetabulum and causes the extremity to lengthen) on the side of the hernia. This is obviously a matter which requires to be the subject of some careful clinical research.

suffer from this ailment. Constipated babies are more prone to it than others. Colic may also be caused by sudden chilling. In that case a warm bath for five or ten minutes, followed by gentle body massage, will bring about a warm reaction.

7. **Convulsions.** These cause a great deal of anxiety to fond mothers. They are always reflex symptoms of some slight or serious internal disturbance due to wrong management. They commonly result from some form of autointoxication caused by digestive disturbances, and the resulting systemic or drug poisoning. An inactive condition of the skin, bowels or kidneys will favour autointoxication and convulsions. If proper care is taken to keep the system pure, and the organs of elimination in active condition, convulsions will not occur. The best treatment during an attack is a quick, cold rub all over the body; application of a whole body or trunk pack; gentle soothing magnetic massage, and neurotherapy treatment. These treatments draw the blood into the surface and relieve congestion in the brain and nervous system.

8. **Ailments of Teething.** Many ailments of children are laid to teething, but this is a mistake. Well managed, healthy babies go through the teething period without any trouble whatsoever. This is practically always true of Nature Cure babies. When, however, the little body is heavily encumbered with hereditary and acquired morbid materials, food poisons and disease taints, the process of teething will not run its natural course and may precipitate any form of disease crisis. When teething is difficult it is frequently associated with digestive disturbances. Diarrhoea may alternate with constipation and vomiting is of common occurrence. The baby may be restless and fretful. He tries continually to bite on something in order to facilitate the projection of the teeth through the hardened gums.

No teething lotions or soothing medicines of any kind should be given for the relief of pain in teething. They all contain poisonous sedatives which benumb and paralyse the nerves and have serious after-effects upon the system. They usually contain opium in some form, or other narcotic drugs. The only way to prevent these and other infantile ailments is to keep the little body as nearly normal as possible through the natural treatment described in these pages. If this is closely adhered to, it will prevent, in many cases, the development of even measles and other common eliminative infantile diseases. During this critical period in the baby's life the diet must be extra light; starchy food should be reduced to a minimum and replaced by raw and cooked fruits and vegetable juices. Cooling sitz baths will help to keep the bowels active and to abate internal fever.

9. **Acute Catarrhal Diseases.** Acute catarrhal diseases of infancy, such

as croup, cold in the head, acute bronchitis and whooping cough, are different forms of acute elimination through which nature tries to purify the child's body from hereditary and acquired accumulations of morbid matter, systemic poisons and disease taints. In accordance with this conception of acute diseases, as purifying, healing efforts of nature, we would not do anything to check or suppress elimination but would rather cooperate with nature in her purifying, healing efforts. How we do this has been fully explained in other parts of this volume (Sec. VIII). The natural treatment is very much the same in all acute inflammatory ailments. Feeding must be reduced to a minimum. If the baby does not insist upon eating nothing should be given except water with acid or subacid fruit juices, such as lime, lemon, grapefruit and orange. If the temperature does not run high, say not above 100°F., frequent ablutions with cold water at intervals of from one to two hours will be sufficient to promote heat radiation and elimination of morbid matter through the skin and other organs of elimination. If the temperature runs higher, say between 102° and 105°F., wet packs must be applied, and renewed when they become hot or dry.

The wet packs are of especial value in all kinds of coughs, whether it be ordinary cough, croupy cough or whooping cough. A whole body or trunk pack, with or without a throat pack, will give almost instant relief. In many instances where the child is making the night hideous for the anxious mother with its coughing, a well applied whole body pack, or a combination trunk and throat pack, will relieve the coughing almost instantly, and induce restful sleep.

In serious cases it is always advisable to call in a natural therapist or some other drugless physician, if one can be reached. The mother should not forget that all acute diseases, after they have once developed, must run their natural course. She must, therefore, not become impatient and lose faith in the natural treatment if it takes a week or more to cure a common cold in the head or an attack of bronchitis, or if it takes from two to eight weeks to cure a case of whooping cough. Serenity, patience and cheerfulness are the primary requisites of the Nature Cure physician.

PART V

SECTION XLII

FIRST AID IN ACCIDENTS

A person in possession of a clean, healthy, supple body as a result of natural living and treatment is not nearly as likely to suffer injury from accidents or to develop chronic after-effects resulting from them as one whose body has lost its natural elasticity, keenness of sensory organs and recuperative powers through unnatural living habits and the resulting pathogenic conditions. This is well known to physical examiners for accident insurance firms. When a body is in a pathogenic condition a slight scratch may be sufficient to cause serious blood poisoning or a bruise or fracture may result in necrosis or tumour formation.

Natural methods of treatment are as efficient in giving first aid as in the treatment of acute and chronic diseases, though it may be necessary in serious cases to procure without delay the aid of a surgeon or trained manipulative therapist in order to examine for internal injury or to correct sprains, dislocations, fractures or other mechanical lesions. However, any lay person possessed of ordinary intelligence and common sense can apply the first aid methods herein described. In many instances, natural treatment applied in time will greatly ameliorate the suffering and establish the best possible conditions for perfect recovery. The old time drug treatment which was held to be indispensable in case of accident is as useless and harmful under these conditions as in the treatment of acute and chronic diseases. Much experience in all kinds of emergencies has convinced me that this is true. In case of an accident it is of primary importance not to be come excited and thereby to lose presence of mind and self control. It is only by remaining cool and relaxed that one can think clearly and decide quickly upon the best course to pursue.

In first aid as well as in acute diseases the quickest and best results are obtained by hydropathic and manipulative treatment. It is, therefore, necessary for the student of emergency work thoroughly to study the

237

methods and applications described under those headings. In order to facilitate quick and ready reference. I shall treat the various occasions for first aid in alphabetical order.

1. **Alcoholism.** Acute alcoholism may result in complete collapse and stupor. It has frequently happened that a person found in an insensible condition in a public place is mistaken for a drunkard in a stupefied condition, and carted off to a police station, when in reality he is suffering from injury — a stroke of apoplexy, sunstroke, heat prostration or from some other serious physical disorder. In order to prevent such mistakes, which might easily result in the death of the sufferer through lack of proper care, it is necessary to smell the breath, which, in cases of alcoholism, will immediately tell the story.

(a) The best treatment for alcoholic stupor consists in brisk cold rubs, followed by good massage and neurotherapy treatment, calculated to stimulate and to revive the activity of the brain and nervous system. An enema of a warm, normal salt solution is also very beneficial. When the patient revives, half a cup of black coffee with lemon juice will act as a mild heart stimulant.

(b) Delirium tremens is a form of acute mania brought about through temporary paralysis of the brain centres which are the seat of reason, will power and self control. The lower animal emotions are running amuck and in many such cases various forms and symptoms of abnormal psychism prevail. The horrible experience and visions of people in this condition are not always delusions and hallucinations but frequently are the result of clairvoyance and clairaudience on the lowest spiritual or astral planes, the purgatories and hells of the theologians. This abnormal functioning of the sensory organs of the spiritual body is brought about through the temporary paralysis of the sensory organs of the physical body.

In order to prevent complete collapse it may be necessary to give, at increasing intervals and in decreasing doses, alcoholic liquor, coffee, tea or other light stimulants to revive and strengthen the animal magnetism of the physical body. Tincture of passiflora administered every two or three hours in from ten to twenty drop doses is a good non-poisonous vegetable tonic. Meat broth and flesh foods may be given until the patient has recovered from the abnormal psychic condition.

The hydropathic treatment consists of cold rubs and cold douches, wet packs and cooling sitz baths. Massage and neurotherapy treatment is of great importance in such cases, not only for its mechanical but also for its electromagnetic effects. Epsom salt or sea salt rubs also have a positive magnetic effect upon the system. Hot bathing, bromides and other "sedative" measures only aggravate the condition because they have a weakening, benumbing effect. Those who apply such sedative remedies forget that delirium tremens and other maniacal conditions are the result of weakness, exhaustion, and of a benumbed and semi-paralysed condition of the brain and nervous system, and that, therefore, tonic, energizing treatment is required instead of benumbing, sedative remedies and applications.

When the patient has recovered from the effects of acute alcoholism he should undergo thorough systematic natural treatment in order to eradicate completely the craving for alcoholic stimulants. We have treated and permanently cured many victims of the drink habit who had undergone all sorts of drink cures without permanent results. All drug cures for the drink habit work on the principle of "poison kills poison". It is Beelzebub against the devil. While drugs may temporarily kill the craving for alcoholic liquors, the results thus obtained are not permanent. As the effects of the drug treatment pass off, the old craving returns and the drugs themselves have a weakening and deteriorating effect upon the system. Such cures do not influence the moral nature. Natural treatment with its "back to nature" life, its pure food diet, and its educational influences through daily lectures and suggestive treatment, arouses higher ideals, strengthens will power and self control, and thus overcomes in a natural way the desire for alcoholic stimulants as well as habit-forming drugs. It accomplishes this, not by the introduction of other poisons but by the purification of the organism and by the presentation of higher and purer ideals. One who, after such physical, mental and moral regeneration, has tasted the sweetness of the natural life will never again crave the gross, deceptive gratification afforded by indulgence in alcoholic liquors and habit-forming drugs. Strict adherence to a natural regimen for three or four months will take away all desire for alcoholic or drug stimulation. Patients have confessed to me that they did not backslide on account of an irresistible craving but through careless surrender to temptation. Self control must be strengthened by educating the moral nature. (For antidotes see "Poisoning".)

2. **Apoplexy.** Apoplectic stroke and the resulting paralysis are caused by the breaking of one or more blood vessels in the brain. If the haemorrhage occurs in the right brain hemisphere, the left side of the body will be affected by paralysis on account of the crossing of the nerve tracts in the medulla and spinal cord. If the haemorrhage occurs in the left brain, the right side will be affected. The extent of the paralysis depends upon the amount of damage done to the brain centres in the area affected by the haemorrhage. The breathing is laboured and stertorous, the face is flushed and purple in colour, the features are twisted and drawn to one side, the pupils of the eyes are usually dilated.

(a) The head and shoulders should be slightly raised. Quick, cold salt rubs followed by stimulating manipulative treatment will draw the blood away from the brain into the surface and extremities. A lay person can give the extremities and fleshy parts of the body a good, thorough kneading, rubbing and stroking, but a trained masseur or neurotherapist should be procured as quickly as possible to complete the treatment.

(b) Wet packs applied to the body and the extremities will draw the blood away from the congested brain area. A warm normal salt enema (Sec. XVIII, No. 4) will help to establish normal circulation. A hot mustard bath applied to the feet or, better still, magnetic treatment will divert blood into the lower extremities.

(c) After consciousness has been restored, the patient must undergo thorough, systematic natural treatment in order to eliminate from the system the pathogenic materials which have caused high blood pressure and the hardening and occlusion of the blood vessels in the brain and all through the body, and which brought about the haemorrhage and resulting paralysis. No alcoholic or drug stimulants should be given because they increase blood pressure to the brain.

(d) In cases of concussion of the brain, apoplectic stroke, or of haemorrhage from the lungs or stomach, the patient must not be transported in a vehicle because the jolting might aggravate the condition. The sufferer must be carefully carried on a stretcher.

Of the many patients we have treated after a first apoplectic stroke, not one, as far as I can remember, has suffered from a second attack, provided of course there has been strict adherence to natural ways of living.

3. **Artificial Respiration.** In many kinds of accidents such as drowning, strangulation, asphyxiation by poisonous gases, and in serious cases of fainting and stupor, it may be necessary to resort to artificial respiration in order to restore normal breathing. There are several good methods for this purpose.

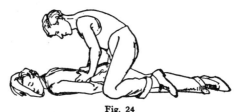

Fig. 24

(a) Quickly remove the clothing from the upper part of the body; lay the patient prone upon his stomach; place a small wad made of clothing, or any other material at hand, under his forehead in order to elevate nose and mouth sufficiently to allow free breathing. The operator kneels athwart the legs of the sufferer and places his spread hands on both sides of the small of the back and then exerts gentle but steady pressure, thus

240

compressing the lower ribs and chest; he then gradually releases the pressure, allowing the lungs to fill with air. This alternating compression and relaxation of the chest must proceed at the same rate as the normal tempo of breathing, which is about fifteen breaths to the minute in adult life and a little more than this in childhood. With adults, therefore, each complete movement in artificial respiration should consume about four seconds including expiration and inspiration, while in children it should consume about three seconds. (Fig. 24, p. 240.)

(b) The same method may be applied with the patient lying on his back. Make a roll of clothing and shove it under the small of the back so that the head lies lower than the chest. Then kneel astride of the hips, place both hands, fingers spread as far as possible, on the lower ribs below the nipples of the breast and count slowly, one, two, three, four; while counting one and two, compress the lower chest gently but firmly, and relax the pressure while counting three and four. Continue this alternating compression and relaxation until normal breathing commences (provided life is not extinct). A sudden trembling and heaving of the chest and flushing of the face will indicate when natural breathing commences. While compressing the chest, the operator should at the same time apply strong vibration. This is accomplished by vibrating the hands loosely and vigorously from the wrist joint. The slow, regular counting corresponds to the tempo of regular, normal breathing.

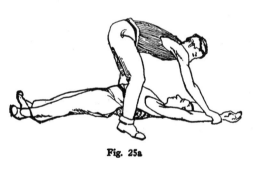

Fig. 25a

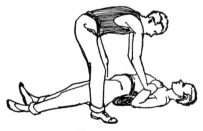

Fig. 25b

241

(c) Another, more commonly applied method of artificial respiration is the following: The patient is put upon his back; a small roll of clothing or other soft material is placed under the small of the back in order to raise the chest and to facilitate expiration. Inspiration is induced by raising the chest through bringing the arms above and back of the head; expiration is produced by returning the arms downward and in an outward, circular movement to the sides of the body, doubling them at the elbows and pressing the forearms on the chest. Compression must be followed by relaxation. This alternating compressing and releasing or raising of the chest should also be continued at the rate of fifteen complete movements to the minute for adults and twenty for children, or it may be regulated by counting as in the operation previously described. (Figs. 25a, b, p. 241.)

The first method (a) is to be favoured because it prevents the falling back of the tongue into the throat and because it facilitates the escape of water, mucus or froth from the mouth. This is especially important in cases of drowning when the lungs are more or less filled with water.

(d) The best method for facilitating the escape of water from stomach and lungs is the following: Lay the victim prone upon his face, stand athwart his body, place your hands under his stomach and raise him at short intervals, thus partially doubling the body upon itself. This compresses the internal organs and facilitates the discharge of fluids through the mouth (Fig. 26).(¹)

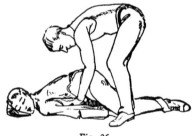

Fig. 26

4. **Asphyxiation.** Asphyxiation or suffocation is a condition of unconsciousness and insensibility resulting from suspended respiration. It is caused by a deficiency of oxygen in the system and an excess of carbon dioxide. This may be produced by strangulation, as in hanging, by smothering or internal obstruction as in choking, drowning, or by inhalation of smoke or poisonous gases.

(¹)
The "Kiss of Life" technique is now very much used. This consists in forcing breath into the patient's lungs and exercising pressure on the ribs to foree expiration.

The treatment consists, first, in artificial respiration described previously; and, secondly, in restoring the circulation of the blood and nerve currents. This is best accomplished through hydropathic and manipulative treatment described under acute alcoholism. The revival of an asphyxiated person may require long continued effort. Cases are known where by three or four hours of persistent effort, people have been revived after hanging or other forms of strangulation or suffocation.

(a) The victims of carbon dioxide asphyxiation die because this gas is heavier than oxygen and therefore does not allow this life-sustaining element to enter into the lungs and tissues of the body. A pulmotor may help to force the oxygen into the lungs and to expel the carbon dioxide.

(b) While rescuing a person from a room filled with smoke or poisonous gases, a wet handkerchief should be tied over the mouth and nostrils. Breathing should be restrained as much as possible. Care must be taken not to strike a match as it may explode the hydrogen gas. The windows should be opened or broken at once. This will enable the life saver to take an occasional breath of fresh air while trying to find and remove the victim of asphyxiation to the outer air.

5. **Bandages.** When bandaging wounds, fractures or other bodily injuries, care must be taken not to apply the bandage too tightly. This might seriously interfere with the circulation, especially if swelling develops in the injured parts.

(a) *Triangular Bandage.* One of the most useful bandages in accidents is the triangular bandage. This may be prepared from any square piece of cloth by folding it diagonally in the shape of a triangle. Figs. 27, 28 illustrate the application of the triangular bandage to a broken forearm. Fold the square piece of muslin or other material into triangular form and place against the body underneath the injured arm. Point A is drawn over the shoulder on the uninjured side; point B is brought up over the injured arm and shoulder and knotted or tied to point A behind the neck.

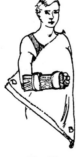
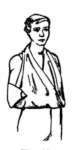

Fig. 27   Fig. 28

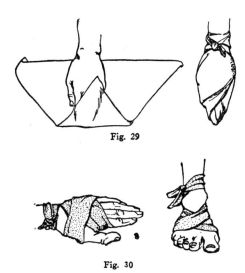

Fig. 29

Fig. 30

The projecting flap D is folded over the elbow and fastened with a safety pin. This supports the arm in a comfortable position. The inner surface of the hand must be turned inward and the thumb upward. Fig. 29 shows the application of the triangular bandage to injured hands and feet.

(b) *Figure of Eight Bandage.* Fig. 30 illustrates the Figure of Eight bandage applied to hand and foot. A long bandage, three or four inches wide is applied with its centre to the injured part. The ends are then drawn crosswise around the wrist or ankle and knotted or pinned with safety pins.

(c) *Roller Bandage.* Figs. 31, 32 illustrate the application of the roller bandage. This bandage may be from a few feet to a few yards in length

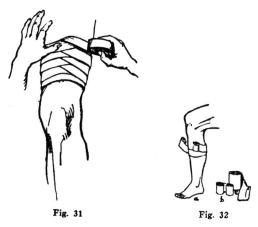

Fig. 31   Fig. 32

244

and of any width best suited for its purpose. The bandage is first rolled in a single roll or in two rolls from each end. The single roll bandage is rolled up from one end and applied by unrolling from one end. It should be applied by winding smoothly and evenly around the injured part, but this is only possible when the part is of even thickness, as in the case of an arm from the wrist upward or a leg from the ankle upward, the bandage in order to be applied smoothly and firmly must be reversed upon itself. This is done by placing the thumb upon the bandage where it is folded back upon itself, as illustrated in Fig. 31.

(d) *Double Roll Bandage.* The double roll bandage is applied with its centre over the injured part; both ends cross in the back and are then wrapped around the part in opposite directions (Fig. 32).

(e) *The T Bandage* has been described under Sec. XV, No 18.

(f) *Head Bandages.* Bandages suitable for injuries to the head or for holding in place compresses to the head are applied as shown in Fig. 33. One bandage is drawn over the head to point C and fastened under the chin at A. The other bandage is drawn over the back of the head and base of the skull, and fastened over the forehead.

(g) When the chin or lower jaw is injured bandage (a), which supports the chin, is knotted on the top of the head. Bandage (b) is applied over the chin and knotted at the back of the neck (see Fig. 34).

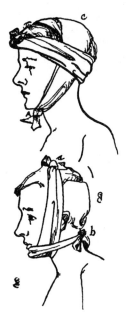

Figs. 33, 34

245

6. **Bites** by snakes, dogs, cats, or by persons in an enraged or maniacal condition, should be sucked out immediately if they can be reached, by either the victim himself or by a friend. The mouth of the one who performs this operation must contain no wounds or abrasions and should be thoroughly cleansed with water after each withdrawal of blood. The wound, if necessary, should be widened by an incision and cleansed with dilute lemon juice. Immediately after this there should be applied a wet bandage or wet pack. The elimination of any possible infection must be promoted through fasting or raw food diet, manipulative treatment and other natural methods described in this volume. Of special importance in this respect is the bed sweat bath followed by cold ablutions.

In cases of snake bites, never administer alcoholic liquors or stimulating drugs. This is not only absolutely useless but decidedly harmful and dangerous. According to reliable statistics, less than 8 percent of people bitten by rattlesnakes or other poisonous reptiles die from the effects of venom even though no whisky is administered. On the other hand, many cases undoubtedly end fatally on account of the whisky treatment. Excessive stimulation is always followed by corresponding depression and frequently by complete collapse. This is more likely to occur when large quantities of fiery liquor are poured into people who are not accustomed to its effects.

7. **Bruises, Bumps and Contusions.** These are treated best by the application of wet packs or clay packs (see Sec. XV and XVI). While bruises and bumps do not bleed externally, the torn blood vessels may bleed internally and cause red or black discolourations. Such internal haemorrhage can be best arrested by firm pressure around the affected area; that is, by pressing some hollow object such as a spoon or a cup firmly around the bruise. The cooling packs or compresses will allay any tendency to inflammation or suppuration. Raw beefsteak applied to bruises acts in a similar manner to wet packs.

8. **Burns and Scalds.** When the clothing is afire one should not run about excitedly, as this will only fan the flames to greater intensity. The best way to extinguish the fire is to throw oneself prone upon the ground and smother the flames by rolling. Rugs, blankets, pieces of clothing or any other material within reach may be used by the victim or by those who are trying to aid him, to smother and to extinguish the flames. Rolling on the floor prevents also the inhalation of the flames or smoke and the burning of face and hair. While removing the clothing from a body injured by burns or severe scalds, do not try to tear it off by force, but cut around the places where the clothing adheres to the flesh.

The best treatment for burns and scalds consists in applying a mixture made of ordinary baking soda (bicarbonate of soda) and ordinary boiled oil (linseed oil) or olive oil.   This simple remedy which can be procured in almost any household is of wonderful efficacy in the healing of burns and scalds.   It allays pain even in severe and extensive sores and prevents the formation of blisters while greatly facilitating the healing process.   The alkaline sodium neutralizes the poisonous acids which form in the sores and the oil keeps the flesh in a softened condition and prevents caking and cracking.   In cases of very extensive burns or scalds, immersion under water of body temperature or slightly below has been found very beneficial.   In such cases the patient may remain suspended under water in a hammock for days or weeks at a time until the sores are healed sufficiently to allow exposure to the air.   Burning of the eyes and face by strong acids, fresh slaked lime, etc., is best treated by the immediate application of the olive oil and baking soda mixture.   For the treatment of shock due to scalds or burns, see "Shock".([1])

9. **Choking.**   Infants and children frequently choke as the result of swallowing small playthings or other foreign objects.   Adults may choke from getting fish bones stuck in their throats or trying to swallow large pieces of meat.   If the patient is a child, place him face downward over your lap, and slap him vigorously between the shoulders.   If this does not remove the obstruction, then compress the nostrils, which forces him to open the mouth and throat widely, introduce the fingers of the other hand quickly into the throat and try to grasp the obstructing object.   If this is not possible, tickle the palate with a feather, or with a handkerchief rolled to a point.   The tickling will cause coughing or hawking which may dislodge the obstruction.   An adult may throw himself over a chair or table, the head hanging downward, while another slaps him vigorously between the shoulders or, if necessary, performs the operations above described.

10. **Convulsions.**   These are due either to congestion of the blood in the brain, to abnormal pressure of gas on the heart, or to excessive irritation of the brain or nervous system by toxic substances.   The treatment must be adapted to the individual condition.

(a) For first aid the patient should be placed in a recumbent position with the head slightly raised.   Alternating hot and cold fomentations are most effective for drawing the blood or irritating toxins from the affected area to the surface.   The patient should sip hot water mixed with a little

([1])
Daniel Mackinnon, the disciple of Lindlahr, in his book "The Conquest of Pain" gives details of a treatment which was discovered by D. P. Ghadiali, a colour therapist.   Burns, such as sunburn, are the result of the exposure of the body to too many highly concentrated rays from the red and orange red areas of the spectrum.   If the burnt areas are then exposed to blue light from a bulb passed through a proper shade of blue glass, this will counteract the effects of the burning.   It is claimed that this method is quicker and more effective than any other, though in cases of very severe burning which might prove fatal the treatment might have to be kept up continuously, day and night, for some time.

247

lemon juice. An enema of normal salt solution and of blood temperature should be administered as soon as possible. Wet packs applied to the neck, trunk or extremities will also draw the blood into the surface and thus relieve inner congestion and promote elimination of toxic substances. A full hot bath of body temperature of from ten to fifteen minutes' duration may give quick results in serious attacks. This should be followed by a brisk cold salt water rub. In convulsions of infants the body first becomes cold and rigid, then the skin breaks into a clammy perspiration, and pulse is weak and rapid. This is followed by convulsive movements and later by a semi-comatose condition which usually passes into natural sleep.

After the first aid measures herein described have given temporary relief, the underlying causes must be overcome by natural methods of treatment.

(b) Uraemic convulsions frequently occur in the course of Bright's disease and of diseases which cause prolonged retention of the urine in the bladder. In such cases it is imperative to increase the activity of the skin in order to compensate for lessened elimination through kidneys and bladder. The best way to do this is to apply the bed sweat bath described under Sec. XIV, No. 5. Sufficient hot water bags, bottles or heated bricks must be placed outside of the whole body pack and under the outer blanket covering so as to produce free perspiration. The patient remains in the pack from fifteen to thirty minutes, as long as he can endure it. After the removal of the pack he is quickly rubbed down with cold water, either in a bathtub, spray room or in bed. He is then covered well with blankets in order to induce free "after perspiration". This procedure is repeated as often as the patient can endure it and react to it properly. After the pack has been applied, the patient should drink freely of hot lemonade made with brown sugar or honey. This will promote free perspiration. Expert massage and neurotherapy treatment should be given to stimulate the circulation. Juniper berry tea (Sec. XIX, No. 5) will stimulate the activity of the kidneys. Fasting is imperative. It must be extended for days or weeks, according to the nature of the disease back of the convulsions. In cases of serious ailments such as Bright's disease, inflammation of the bladder, subacute and chronic prostatitis, the fasting must be followed by raw food diet for weeks or months at a time. Hot, normal salt enemas should be given to cleanse the lower intestines and to stimulate vital activities.

For treatment of epileptic convulsions see No. 14, below.

11. **Cuts and Wounds.** Small cuts or wounds should be thoroughly cleansed with warm or cold water and then treated with dilute lemon juice. Air and light are the best of all healers. It is injurious to close cuts with

adhesive plaster, because it prevents elimination and shuts off air and light. However, in case of large wounds, the edges may be held together with narrow strips of adhesive tape just sufficient to keep the lips together but to allow drainage. When the bleeding has stopped, the wound should be left uncovered if this can be done without exposing it to the pollution of impurities; or, the covering should consist of just enough porous gauze to protect it. If the wound should prove painful or become inflamed, frequent bathing in cold water, or allowing a stream of cold water to run over it, is the best remedy. If the wound is large enough to cause serious or dangerous haemorrhage, appropriate treatment must be applied. For this see "Haemorrhages", No. 18 (c).

12. **Disease, Sudden Onset of.** The simplicity of the natural treatment enables us to apply the most efficient treatment at the sudden onset of any disease whatever. While the medical man has to wait for days and sometimes for weeks before he can find out what the exact nature of the trouble is and apply his specific remedy, the natural therapist gives the most effective treatment from the first manifestation of symptoms. In that way he may be able to abort or even to avert many serious diseases which might end fatally if neglected for a few days.

At the first appearance of great weakness, of aches and pains in any part of the body, of increased temperature and quickening pulse rate, a normal salt enema (Sec. XVIII, No. 4) of body temperature should be administered in order thoroughly to cleanse the lower intestine. This should be followed by a full sheet pack (Sec. XV, No. 7) or by a trunk pack or, if reaction is unsatisfactory, by a full sheet bed sweat bath (Sec. XIV, No. 5). Fasting must be enforced from the appearance of the first symptoms of malaise or acute inflammatory activity. If there are signs of poisoning or of severe inflammation of the stomach and intestines, vomiting should be induced immediately by means of drinking copious quantities of lukewarm water, either pure or mixed with salt or mustard. If vomiting cannot be induced in this way, tickle the throat with a feather or piece of cloth drawn over a sliver of wood. After thus thoroughly cleansing the stomach, allow the patient to drink freely of water mixed with the juice of acid fruits. Neurotherapy treatment should be given at once to promote heat radiation, elimination of morbid matter, and to correct mechanical lesions. A few days of such natural treatment will suffice in most cases to restore the system to normal condition. If an acute disease should develop, it will run a much milder and safer course after prompt natural treatment, and the results obtained will be infinitely better than under the old time drug treatment.

Carefully observe the following warnings, though you may find contradictory advice in books on naturopathic and physical culture treatment: In acute conditions never apply hot water applications nor the ice pack; neither give cold water enemas. They are very dangerous, as they may suppress the inflammatory process and bring about fatal collapse. In cases of serious shock or collapse where the vitality is too low to react to cold applications, alternating hot and cold fomentations are in order, and the wet packs may be wrung out of hot water instead of cold water. If the hands and feet remain cold and bloodless, the best remedy for drawing the blood into the extremities is good magnetic massage. After the manipulative treatment, firmly hold the hands of the patient or grasp the feet around the ankles and will the blood to flow into the extremities. The magnetic treatment must be continued until the hands or feet warm up. The hot bath or hot water bag treatment produces warmth temporarily but is followed, in accordance with the law of action and reaction, by cold reaction; therefore the anaemic condition of the extremities is only made worse by such hot applications.

13. **Ears, Foreign Bodies in.** Locate the foreign body by using an ear speculum and head mirror. Turn the patient to the affected side and use a syringe from below; to straighten the canal, pull the outer ear up and back. In some cases forceps made of fine wire may be necessary. Living insects in the outer canal may be killed by the injection of alcohol or oil and then removed by syringeing or by the wire loop. In cases of peas or beans, do not use water; it will make them swell. Use a wire loop or attach a strip of adhesive plaster to the foreign body and pull it out that way.

Foreign bodies in the nose may be removed in similar manner.

14. **Epileptic Convulsions.** Nothing must be done to check or suppress the convulsions; this would be very injurious. All that can be done during an attack is to place the patient in a comfortable position and to elevate the head slightly. A neurotherapist should give firm inhibitory treatment over the upper cervical vertebrae and at the base of the skull. Immediately apply rectal dilatation. If the fit occurs in the house, the patient should be exposed to a draught of fresh air. Push the lower jaw forward so that the lower row of teeth projects over the upper. This will keep the windpipe open and prevent choking and suffocation. Push a piece of wood padded with a cloth, a cork or a rolled handkerchief between the teeth in order to prevent biting of the tongue. The opening of the clenched hands is useless. After the attack the patient should rest until its effects have worn off. The treatment for the cure of the disease must be administered between the attacks. Two-thirds of such cases that have come under our treatment made permanent recoveries.

15. **Eye Injuries.** (a) *Black Eye.* Caused by external injury, blows, etc. Treatment: Cold application applied immediately will prevent discolouration and will alleviate inflammation.

(b) Foreign bodies in the eyes, such as cinders, bits of sand, etc. These are usually found embedded in the cornea or in the lid. Pull the lid outward and bend it backward over a toothpick, match or other bit of wood, thus exposing the inner surface. Then remove the obstacle with a bit of cottonwool if it is embedded in the lid; or if necessary with a toothpick or sharp instrument if it is located in the cornea. Treat inflammation with cold compresses and cold eye baths.

(c) Perforating wounds of the eyes should be treated with cold compresses and cold eye baths. The patient must remain absolutely quiet and not expose the eyes to any strain whatever. If the sight is lost and symptoms of sympathetic inflammation appear in either eye, removal of the affected eye may become necessary, but this will seldom be the case if the cold compresses and the potato compress and cold ablutions are applied faithfully from the start (Sec. XV, Nos. 1, 4). In any case of injury do not use Vaseline, atropine or antiseptics.

For burns see No. 8, above.

16. **Fainting — Insensibility.** Find out first whether the unconscious one is alive and breathing. Hold a mirror, piece of glass, bright piece of metal or a feather before the mouth and nose. If the patient is still breathing, the bright surface will be dimmed by the breath, or the feather will move. Another test is to raise the eyelid and touch the white of the eye. If life is not extinct, the eyelid will twitch.

(a) Observe the odour of the breath. It will indicate such poisons as alcohol, chloroform, ether, etc. If the tongue has been bitten it indicates epilepsy. If the eyes are sensitive to touch and light, there is no brain injury. Unequal contraction of the pupils indicates brain trouble. Pupils contracted to pin points indicate opium poisoning. Slow, weak breathing indicates collapse or shock. Snoring or stertorous breathing and slow, weak pulse indicate brain trouble. Rapid pulse points to sunstroke. A hot skin and rapid pulse indicate sunstroke or high fever. Cold skin and weak pulse may be the result of fainting, freezing, or of acute alcoholism. High fever should be treated as described under treatment of acute diseases (Sec. VIII).

(b) If the patient is still breathing, place him in a comfortable position, the head somewhat lower than the rest of the body. Open or cut the clothing wherever it constricts the body and expose the patient to a draught of fresh air; if in the open, fan the air over his face.

(c) In order to stimulate heart action, apply alternate hot and cold compresses to the chest; sprinkle or dash cold water over the face and neck; also apply alternate hot and cold fomentations to the spine. Massage and apply passive movements to the extremities. If the breathing is very slow and faint, apply artificial respiration (No. 3). Dash cold water on the neck and on the soles of the feet. Give cold salt water rubs all over the body. Administer a warm normal salt enema. Do not try to administer water or stimulants while the patient is unconscious; it would only choke him.

(d) When he revives, do not give alcoholic liquors or other poisonous stimulants. The reaction might prove fatal. Give sips of fresh water mixed with acid fruit juices, or black coffee or tea in small quantities; repeat until full consciousness has been restored.

(e) Try to find out what caused the unconscious condition. It may be the result of any one of the following causes: fainting, collapse, shock, asphyxiation by gas, drowning or other means, acute alcoholism, opium, chloroform, ether or other drugs, sunstroke, apoplexy, epilepsy, convulsions, injury to the brain by concussion or fractured skull, or it may be caused by certain diseases of the heart, stomach or kidneys. Treat accordingly.

17. **Fractures.** In case of fracture, a physician or surgeon must be secured without delay. In the meantime excessive bleeding may be stopped as described under "Haemorrhages". Swelling may be reduced by wet packs and cold ablutions.

18. **Freezing.** Frozen limbs, ears, nose or other fleshy parts of the body should be rubbed vigorously with ice water or snow. Great care, however, must be taken not to break the frozen parts; they are brittle and may break easily. If a person has become unconscious through freezing, he must be taken into a cold room and treated with cold rubs by means of ice water or snow, until the circulation in the various parts is restored. As before stated, great care must be taken not to break the frozen parts. If breathing and heart action are very low, artificial breathing, with due precautions, must be at once resorted to. The individual condition must determine the best method to be employed. When normal breathing commences, place the patient in a cold bed and heat the room very gradually. When the body becomes warm, rub with warm flannels, but the frozen parts must still be treated with cold applications and snow rubs. Warm the body from within by giving hot lemonade with brown, unrefined sugar or honey. Black coffee with lemon juice will stimulate heart action and circulation.

To drink alcoholic liquors in order to keep warm is extremely dangerous. The benumbing after-effects of this and other strong stimulants will induce numbness and sleep when wakefulness is necessary to resist the freezing.

19. **Heat Exhaustion.** This is usually the result of injudicious diet in summer, excessive clothing, and of working in close, hot, ill ventilated rooms. The principal symptoms are faintness of syncope, a cold and

252

damp skin and a rapid and feeble pulse. When death results it is due to heart failure, but most cases recover. It is not as often fatal as sunstroke.

(a) The patient should be removed to a cool place. Hot lemonade will stimulate heart action; a brisk, cold rub and wet packs, if necessary reinforced by hot water bottles (see "Bed Sweat Bath", Sec. XIV, No. 5), will restore the activity of the skin.

(b) Both in sunstroke and heat prostration the head should frequently be laved with cold water. If the body temperature is subnormal and death seems imminent, the legs should be wrapped in woollen blankets saturated with hot water. Care must be taken not to scald the flesh; around the wet blanket wrap several layers of dry sheeting or dry blanket in order to retain the heat. The patient should take at intervals small quantities of hot lemonade.

20. **Haemorrhages.** (a) *Haemorrhages from the Mouth.* When the blood is of dark colour and looks as if it were mixed with coffee grounds or food materials it comes from the stomach and the haemorrhage is caused by cancer. If the blood is mixed with food materials but looks bright red, the haemorrhage is caused by ulcers of the stomach. If the haemorrhage is from the stomach, the patient should be placed in a recumbent position. A trunk pack will draw the blood away from the stomach and relieve congestion. The patient should sip at frequent intervals small quantities of cold water mixed with lemon juice, and should be allowed to rest.

(b) *Haemorrhage from the Lungs.* When the blood is bright red and foamy and free from food materials, it comes from the lungs and is caused by breakdown of the lung tissues. It is not necessarily directly fatal. Under natural treatment of lung diseases, haemorrhages frequently occurs during the crisis periods and is then a form of elimination. In many cases, recovery from tuberculosis has been preceded by copious haemorrhages. The patient should be kept in bed in order to give the disrupted tissues a chance to heal. The treatment must be directed to the underlying disease.

(c) *Haemorrhages from Cuts and Wounds.* If the blood is bright red and comes in spurts, it is an indication that some important artery has been severed and a ligature should be applied without delay above the wound, between it and the heart. Any solid object, a piece of rock, wood or anything convenient, held in position firmly by a bandage or belt will serve the purpose (Figs. 35, 36).

(d) If the blood is dark in colour and flows smoothly, then some vein has been opened and the ligature should be applied just below the wound (Fig. 37). Any strap, rope or handkershief may be used for this purpose, but a rubber hose, if it can be procured, is best suited on account of its

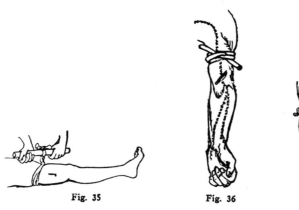

Fig. 35   Fig. 36   Fig. 37

elasticity.   The ligature may be applied more tightly by inserting a stick, pipe or similar object below the knot and twisting it (Fig. 35).

Do not try to remove any clots of blood; they are nature's provision for stopping the haemorrhage.   Haemorrhages from large arteries may be stopped temporarily by compressing the blood vessel with the fingers.   In order to do this, one must know where to find the arteries.

(e) For an injury on the side of the upper part of the head, the temporal artery must be compressed with the thumb.   This artery is located about three-quarters of an inch in front of the opening of the ear underneath the temporal bone (Fig. 38).   If the injury is in the back of the head, the occipital artery must be compressed with the thumb.   It is located about an inch from the centre of the back of the ear (Fig. 39).   The facial arteries can be compressed by exerting strong pressure at a point one inch in front of the angle of the lower jaw (Fig. 40).   The arteries pass over the jaw at these points.   They should be pressed at the same time on both sides.

The common carotid artery can be reached at a point one and a half

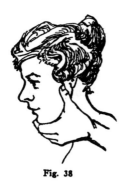

Fig. 38

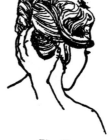

Fig. 39

254

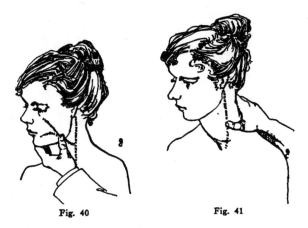

Fig. 40   Fig. 41

inches above the joint between the breast bone and the collar bone. Pressure may be exerted inward and backward (Fig. 41).   The subclavian artery can be reached at a point behind the middle of the clavicle or collar bone where the hump of this bone is felt.   First lower and draw the shoulder forward, then press downward and backward with the thumbs or with the finger tips of both hands.   The pressure must be firm and persistent (Fig. 42).

The axillary artery can be compressed by first raising the arm, pressing it outward and backward, and then compressing the artery on the inner surface of the upper arm (Fig. 43).   The brachial artery passes along the inner border of the biceps muscle.   First extend or raise the arm, then

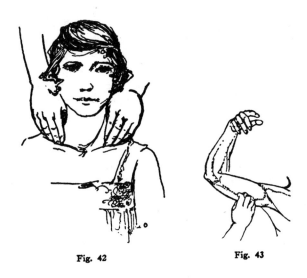

Fig. 42   Fig. 43

255

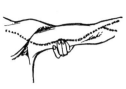

Fig. 44

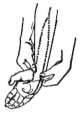
Fig. 45

press outward and backward (Fig. 44). The radial and ulnar arteries in the wrist may be compressed readily with the finger tips (Fig. 45).

The popliteal artery can be reached by strong pressure in the central part of the ham, applied while the patient is lying on his stomach, directly downward.

The wounded part should always be raised as high as possible. Cold water is very effective for stopping haemorrhages. If possible it should be allowed to run over the wound in a constant stream. This inhibits the circulation and favours the clotting of the blood. However, care must be taken not to run the water directly on the wound as this might prevent the forming of clots. In order to accomplish this it may be well to place a cup or saucer or some other protecting object directly over the wound. Only boiled or aseptic bandages should be applied to the wound. Clay or mud must never be applied to open cuts or wounds. Water mixed with lemon juice applied directly to the wound acts as a natural antiseptic and astringent, thus favouring clotting.

21. **Hiccough or Hiccup.** This is a spasm of the diaphragm, caused by nervous irritation of some kind. It may be due to digestive disturbances or to irritation caused by systemic or drug poisons. In chronic form we find it frequently associated with mercurial, phosphorus and other drug poisoning. Ordinary hiccough requires little or no special attention; one of the best remedies is continuously to sip and swallow water until one or two of the spasms have been missed; anything that will break the regularity of the spasm will stop it. Out of this fact grew the old custom of "frightening the hiccough" by a sudden motion or exclamation. It its most serious form, in cases of drug poisoning, we have always succeeded in alleviating and in most instances overcoming the spasms by the natural treatment. Certain neuropathic moves give good results, particularly inhibitory pressure exercised on the phrenic nerve.

22. **Lightning Stroke.** If a stroke of lightning results in shock or collapse, treat as described under "Shock". If it results in burns, treat as described under "Burns and Scalds".

256

23. **Mania.** A sudden maniacal outbreak, whether the result of an attack of insanity, of acute alcoholism or of great emotional excitation, is best treated by cold applications such as cold sprays, cold sitz bath, hip bath, quick submersion under cold water, or by cold wet packs. Soothing manipulative and magnetic treatment is very effective. It is wrong to submerge such patients for hours or days in warm or hot water. Such sedative treatment is as weakening as opiates and hypnotics and will only aggravate the underlying conditions which are always negative in character. Such patients should have nothing but vitalizing, up-building treatment. Sedative drugs and long continued submersion in hot water will only aggravate the negative conditions and make the underlying ailments more chronic and incurable.

24. **Mental Disorders.** At the first appearance of symptoms of mental disorder, the patient should be placed in an institution for natural healing, where surroundings and treatment are favourable for early recovery.

25. **Nose.** (a) For treatment of foreign bodies in the nose see "Ears", above.

(b) *Nose Bleed.* Sniff cool water mixed with lemon juice. This has an astringent effect upon the capillaries. Compress the nostrils temporarily, throw the head backward, and avoid vigorous blowing of the nose. Apply cold compresses to the neck at the base of the brain. Repose on a chair or couch, perfectly relaxed, in a sitting position and remain that way until the bleeding ceases. Refrain from any movement of the body. Cause someone else to catch the running blood in a basin or cloth. This is the best way to facilitate clotting of the blood. If this is not sufficient to stop the bleeding or if it should grow worse have small plugs of cotton-wool or muslin inserted tightly into the nostrils. However, it must be remembered that the bleeding may be a form of elimination. It often occurs as a form of healing crisis and should, therefore, not be interfered with unless necessary to avoid excessive weakening and collapse.([1])

26. **Poisoning.** (a) The first thing to be done in any case of poisoning, whether or not the exact nature of it be known, is to empty the stomach. This may be accomplished by the swallowing of large quantities of warm water containing the appropriate antidote, and by tickling the palate with the finger or a feather, thus causing copious vomiting. The washing of the stomach must be repeated several times. If mouth and throat are not burned, a rubber tube may be pushed down the throat into the stomach. By means of a funnel, warm water is poured through the hose until it

([1])
It is a remarkable fact that there is a very definite connection between nose bleeds and lesions of the left sacro-iliac joint. This is a thing which was discovered by Daniel Mackinnon, the disciple of Lindlahr. In very many cases it has been found possible to stop nose bleed by nothing more than making the necessary pelvic adjustments.

overflows. The end of the hose outside is then suddenly lowered below the level of the stomach and water syphoned out of it. This may be facilitated by making the patient assume a position prone upon the face during the draining of the stomach.

(b) In emergency cases, mustard, common salt or powdered alum may be given as emetics in proportion of one teaspoonful to a glass of water. A lukewarm solution of soap in water is a simple and efficacious emetic. If no emetics are available, cold water should be taken freely and vomiting induced by tickling the throat.

After washing of the stomach, white of egg, milk or sugared water should be given freely. They are soothing to the inflamed membranes and give the poisons something to work on. Blood warm enemas of normal salt solution (Sec. XVIII, No. 4) should be given repeatedly in order to eliminate the poison from the intestines. When the patient is strong enough, bed sweat baths followed by cold ablutions will stimulate elimination through the skin.

(c) In corrosive sublimate or other forms of mercurial poisoning, retained rectal enemas of milk or white of egg beaten up in warm water will help to neutralize the destructive action of the metallic poison.

(d) In all cases, fasting, with dilute fruit juices, should be enforced until the system has eliminated the poison and the injured membranes have been repaired. Where the latter have been severely burned, fruit juices may cause burning pain unless very much diluted with water. In the mild dilute form they will antidote the destructive effects of the poisons.

(e) So-called antidotes are effective only when administered immediately. The general rule is, against acid poisons administer water mixed with baking soda or fresh lime; other good antidotes are white of egg, rich milk or oil. These substances neutralize the acids.

(f) Alkaline poisons must be antidoted with dilute vinegar, milk, white of egg and other albuminous substances which neutralize alkaline poisons as well as acid poisons by diluting them and giving them something to work on besides the tissues of the body.

(g) Narcotic poisons like opium, morphine, belladonna, digitalis, poisonous mushrooms, ptomaines, alcohol, strychnine, etc., cause loss of consciousness, stertorous breathing, redness of the face, cramps and delirrium. If the victim of poisoning is unconscious, artificial breathing must be resorted to (No. 3), and the neck, chest and other parts of the body should be sprinkled with cold water. A brisk, cold salt water rub is very efficacious in reviving the vital activities. As a stimulant administer small doses of strong black coffee.

(h) Arsenic, phosphorus, Paris green, vitriol, carbolic acid, hydrochloric acid and lye do not as a rule cause unconsciousness, but give rise to violent pains in the oesophagus, stomach and abdomen, followed by choking and vomiting. Some of these poisons burn the lips, oesophagus and stomach; such burns may be treated with a solution of baking soda or powdered chalk. The treatment otherwise is the same as given for alkaline and acid poisoning.

In cases of poisoning a physician should be called in as soon as possible.

(i) Ptomaine poisoning results from eating putrefying or decayed meats, fish, cheese, ice cream or other animal food products. The usual symptoms are collapse, subnormal temperature and pain in the digestive tract. Nature generally tries to remedy the trouble by vomiting and diarrhoea. Both these forms of natural elimination must be encouraged by the swallowing of warm water in large quantities and by warm salt enemas (Sec. XVIII, No. 4). The treatment of ptomaine poisoning is very much the same as that of other forms of poisoning. The stomach and intestines must be emptied and cleansed as thoroughly as possible by induced vomiting and by salt water enemas, as described above. After that the patient should drink copious quantities of fresh water mixed with acid fruit juices. This is much better than the taking of poisonous antiseptics. While the temperature is subnormal, the bed sweat bath by means of the trunk pack or full sheet pack will promote elimination through the skin. When the subnormal condition is followed by inflammation and fever, cold packs and ablutions are in order and the treatment in general is the same as that for acute inflammatory conditions described under Sec. VIII.

(j) *External Poisons.* Poisons which affect the human body from outside include poison ivy, poison oak and poison sumac. Poisoning by insects, snakes and rabid animals has been considered above. Poison ivy and the other poisonous plants owe their toxic qualities to the odourless, transparent oil found on the leaves, bark and twigs, which is insoluble in water. These poisons are powerful irritants. Contact of the skin with these plants causes insufferable itching, swelling and vesicular eruptions. In severe cases there may be vomiting, colicky pains, fever and delirium. Parts of the body or the entire cutaneous surface may be covered with eruptions.

The U.S. Department of Agriculture recommends the application of a solution of acetate of lead to be applied to the itching skin. This, however, is a powerful suppressant. While the eruption disappears rapidly under this treatment, it drives the plant poison plus the drug poison into the system, and wherever these concentrate the morbid soil is prepared for chronic disease. The poison in its outward symptoms, as well as its internal chronic after-effects, resembles very closely the psora or itch taint. Its suppression in the acute stages broadens the scurf rim and frequently produces itch spots in the iris. The best homoeopathic antidotes in acute and chronic cases are rhus tox, psorinum or sulphur. The homoeopathic rhustoxicana is a trituration of the ivy poison.

The Natural Treatment. First, it must be remembered that the itchy, burning eruptions represent nature's effort to eliminate the poisons from the system and that therefore it should not be checked or suppressed by any means whatever. The natural treatment includes everything which will promote elimination of the poison through the skin and other organs of depuration. If water is immediately accessible a good, thorough scrubbing of the skin with soap and water, or, if in the open, with sand, tufts of grass or any other scrubbing material, may be sufficient to remove the poison before it will do any harm; at any rate it will greatly reduce the bad effects. The preliminary cleansing should be followed as soon as possible by a whole sheet pack or a bed sweat bath, and cold ablutions. This may be repeated several times, if necessary, or followed by partial packs. Otherwise, the treatment is the same as for acute diseases (Sec. VIII). Fasting and raw food diet are especially beneficial. The cold packs, compresses and ablutions are the best means for allaying the intolerable itching and burning.

(k) *Antidotes for Acute Poisoning.* By lead: magnesia; soda; or chalk water.

By phosphorus: thick liquid gum; white of egg; flour; bread; magnesia and cold water, for the purpose of enveloping and isolating the poisoning. Do not give milk or liquids containing alcohol or oily matter.

By caustic acids, such as sulphuric, muriatic, carbolic or nitric acid: large quantities of soap, salt, chalk, lime water or milk.

By copper and verdigris, frequently contracted by foods or drinks prepared in copper vessels or by drinks from soda fountains when the copper has become exposed through the wearing away of the zinc lining: dilute white of egg; milk; water mixed with honey or sugar.

By iodine: starch or flour paste.

By nitrate of silver: strong salt water solution; white of egg.

By oxalic acid: chalk or lime water.

By strychnine: meat burned to a cinder; decoction of acorn coffee; tan or gall apple.

By arsenic: warm milk; sweetened water.

27. **Seasickness.** The unpleasant sensations accompanying this disorder are undoubtedly caused by a disturbance of the centre of equilibrium in close proximity to the left ear, which in turn affects the entire nervous organism and especially the nerves supplying the digestive organs, causing intense nausea and vomiting. So far no effective remedy has been discovered for this peculiar disorder. The following directions have in many

instances either prevented or greatly alleviated its symptoms. Those who intend to travel on the sea should prepare themselves by a brief fast and light raw food diet. This should be continued on board ship. The heavy, rich, greasy foods served in overabundance on board seagoing vessels undoubtedly have much to do with bringing on the gastric disturbance. The invigorating effects of a sea voyage might be greatly enhanced by a prolonged fast beginning a day or two before taking passage and extending for a week or more, according to the vitality and recuperative powers of the individual. The best remedy, aside from these dietetic measures, and according to my experience the most efficient, is getting into harmony with the motion of the vessel or car. Many times outside patients have come to me saying they could not continue coming for treatment because the benefits were offset by nausea and vomiting caused by the shaking of the cars. I have instructed the sufferers from car sickness as follows: Instead of tensing yourself physically and mentally against the violent vibrations caused by the rolling of the vessel or car, relax completely. Do not oppose and fight the motions but let yourself go with them. A good way to do this is to hum a tune in harmony with the oscillating motion of the ship or car. In many instances the very first trial of my remedy has given relief and after a few attempts no discomfort whatever was experienced. Those who are naturally immune to car or seasickness probably practise this form of relaxation and rhythmic adjustment unconsciously. It is another proof of the truth and practicability of the maxim of the Master, "Resist not evil." Those who most fear this form of evil and tense themselves against it are most affected by it, while the person who thoroughly enjoys sea travel and to whom the rolling of the vessel is a pleasure naturally relaxes to it, enjoys the sensation, and therefore feels no discomfort.([1])

28. **Shock.** Shock is characterized by collapse and frequently by loss of consciousness. It may result from excessive loss of blood or physical injury, or it may be caused by emotional depression resulting from mental and nervous excitation such as sudden fright, grief, anxiety or anger. In many instances it is the shock rather than the actual physical injury which causes death. If the collapse is due to haemorrhage, this must be stopped as quickly as possible. Cool behaviour and reassuring suggestions are necessary to dispel fear and anxiety. The same tonic treatment must be administered as described under "Fainting — Insensibility", etc.

([1])
Seasickness is another condition in which good results can often be obtained by making sure that the pelvic bones are in proper alignment. Lesions of the sacro-iliac joints (in this case particularly of the right sacro-iliac) can produce an irritation which affects the sympathetic nervous system in such a way as to cause nausea and vomiting under the stress of the unusual motion to which the nervous system cannot accommodate as well as it should.

29. Sprains, Strains and Dislocations. Sprains and dislocations must be attended to as quickly as possible by a competent physician, preferably a neurotherapist, osteopath or chiropractor. If, however, a physician is not immediately available and the injury results in swelling, then cold packs must be applied to reduce inflammation and to facilitate the adjustment. If swelling or pain make it impossible to remove parts of the clothing or the shoes and stockings, these should be cut away with a sharp knife. The affected part must have absolute rest before and after the adjustment. Do not apply hot applications of any kind.

30. Sunburns. Sunburns are frequently the result of imprudent exposure in the sun baths and are best treated by cold compresses and cold ablutions or by olive oil and soda mixture.

31. Sunstroke. Sunstroke is caused by exposure to the direct rays of the sun in a heated atmosphere. Loss of consciousness is caused by the direct action of the rays upon the brain and the cardiac and respiratory centres in the medulla.

(a) The onset is sudden. The most prominent symptoms are unconsciousness, pallor, feeble pulse and rapid failure of the heart and respiration. Death is common, recovery often only partial, leaving the brain permanently injured.

(b) Under natural treatment few cases end fatally. The patient should be quickly undressed and cold water poured all over his body, also over the head. This should be followed by brisk salt water rubs; or the body should be wrapped in a wet sheet which must be kept wet by pouring cold water over it from time to time. If collapse has taken place and vitality is greatly depressed, the patient must be put to bed and well covered with blankets so as to produce a warm reaction.

32. Thermic Fever. This may arise by night or by day through exposure to artificial or solar heat. Premonitory symptoms are malaise, nausea, diarrhoea, giddiness, sleeplessness, after which the temperature rises quickly to 108° to 110°F. or even higher. Prominent symptoms are lividity of the face, dyspnoea and delirium. These are often followed by coma and death within a few hours. If recovery takes place it is slow and incomplete. Cold, wet packs, followed by cold ablutions, must be applied. The drinking water should be cool and mixed with acid fruit juices (see the usual treatment for acute diseases, Sec. VIII). Under natural treatment few cases end fatally.

33. Transporting an Injured Person. To lift or carry an injured person in the wrong way may cause permanent injury or even death; therefore, carefully examine the victim of an accident in order to ascertain whether he has sustained a fracture or serious internal injury. First aid should be administered at once and on the spot; but if removal is necessary, a

262

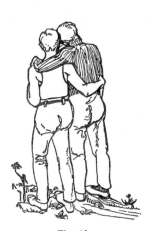
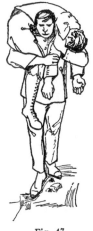
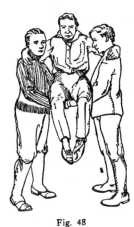

Fig. 46   Fig. 47   Fig. 48

stretcher may be improvised out of a board, a door, bed spring, or anything else convenient for the purpose (Fig. 49).   Care must be exercised
not to drop the injured one.   If a patient must be transported by carrying,
the following methods will be found practical:

(a) If the injured one can walk, let him put his sound arm around your
neck and with one hand grasp his hand hanging down from your shoulder
and with your other arm firmly support his body (Fig. 46).

If the patient is unconscious, the following methods will be found most
convenient:

(b) You may carry the patient in an upright position, placing your right
shoulder under his armpit and your right arm around his waist, his left
arm back of your own neck and over your shoulder, taking hold of his left
wrist with your left hand.   In this way you can either help him to walk, as
previously described, or carry him entirely (Fig. 46).

(c) If an adult person is unconscious and requires immediate removal,
it would be impossible for one person to carry him in his arms.   In such
an emergency, the pick-a-back method is the most practical.   Stoop down
and place the patient well up on your back; then pass your right arm
around his right knee and with the other hand grasp firmly the wrist of his
right hand drawn over your left shoulder.   In this way he is in a safe
position to be carried for a considerable distance and weight is fairly
distributed and balanced over your back and shoulders.

(d) The third method of carrying an unconscious person is similar to
(c), the only difference being that your right hand, after passing around
the upper part of the right leg of the patient, grasps his right wrist,
drawing his right arm over your left shoulder and firmly across your chest

263

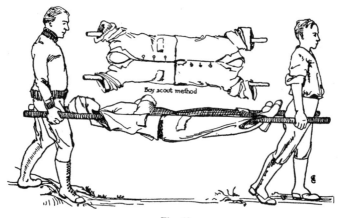

Fig. 49

as illustrated in Fig. 47. This position leaves your left arm free for other employment, if desired.

(e) If two persons are available for transportation they may support the injured one on their locked hands while he places his arms about the necks of his carriers (Fig. 48).

(f) Fig. 49 illustrates an improvised stretcher. Two poles have been slipped through the sleeves and body of two buttoned coats. Other improvisations may be made by means of a board, door, shutter, mattress, etc.

SECTION XLIII

CARE OF THE TEETH

1. Disease of the teeth, generally speaking, is the result of two causes: first, malnutrition, which causes deterioration and destruction of the teeth from within; second, corrosion caused by systemic acids and other corroding substances which attack, from without, the enamel of the crown and the hard covering of the neck and roots.

Dentists and books on hygiene deal almost esclusively with the last named factor. They have a great deal to say about the regular and thorough cleansing of the teeth, of dental treatment, but seldom mention the influence of food materials, nutrition and constitutional disease on the

264

condition of the teeth. That this is not as it should be is proved by the fact that animals living on natural food, as well as savage races, and people who live in primitive surroundings and subsist largely on products of the soil not demineralized and devitalized by modern manufacturing processes, have splendid teeth and retain them to the end of life without tooth brush, dentifrice or attention of a dentist. The teeth of animals and humans who live on natural food well adapted to their needs gradually wear off to the gums with advancing age but do not decay or fall out; neither are they troubled with abscesses, pyorrhoea or other diseases produced by unnatural and artificial ways of living.

Regular examinations of children in our schools disclose the fact that in spite of tooth hygiene taught in the schools and enforced in the homes, 85 percent or more are suffering from defective teeth. Of 1,694 children examined in six clinics during the year 1913 by Dr. A. F. Foot, only eleven were found to possess normal teeth. His report to a Dental Society in New York is as follows: "The six-year molars of nearly every child were broken down wholly or in part. In many instances the molars were decayed to the gums. So extensive and far advanced were the defects that corrective treatment, even if applied, would have been of little value."

2. This almost universal decay of the teeth is caused:

(1) by wrong food combinations;
(2) by devitalized and demineralized food;
(3) by the action of corrosive substances from within and without;
(4) by the softness of the food materials and by their excessive heat and coldness.
(5) by hereditary and congenital influences.

Examining these pathogenic factors separately we find that the ordinary diet customary in the home, hotel, restaurant and boarding house, consisting almost entirely of cooked foods, is excessively rich in starches, sugars, fats and proteins, but very deficient in the mineral salts. This is true of these foods even in their natural condition, as they come from the soil; but the discrepancy between negative food elements and positive mineral elements is much greater after the cereals, rice, sugar-cane sap and beet sap have passed through the modern milling and refining processes. These leave the white flour, polished rice, decorticated corn products, pearled barley, corn starch, white sugar and corn syrup in a devitalized and demineralized condition. Together with the all-important mineral food elements, the foods have been robbed also of their vitamins or life elements. What little is left of the vitamins is destroyed and dissipated by boiling, roasting, frying or fermenting.

Unnatural food combinations, which predominate in acid and pathogen forming negative food substances and are very deficient in the acid neutralizing and eliminating mineral elements or alkaline bases, produce excessive amounts of acids, ptomaines, leukomaines, xanthines and other pathogenic substances which corrode and tear down the outer enamel covering and internal dentine structure of the teeth. The destructive effect of acids upon bone tissue can readily be demonstrated by submerging a piece of bone in hydrochloric acid. Within a few days the lime salts constituting the solid framework will be dissolved and abstracted, nothing being left but a soft cartilaginous and gelatinous mass. Submerge an egg shell in strong vinegar; within a few days it will be completely dissolved. In similar manner, acids in the blood and mouth fluids, and acids which form in decaying matter clinging to the teeth and in the hollow spaces between them, will gradually destroy the enamel and dentine. Refined sugars act very much the same as do acids. Having been robbed in the refinery of their positive mineral elements, the remaining negative elements, hydrogen, carbon and oxygen, by chemical affinity leech the minerals from the bones and tissues, thus causing gradual decay.

The sturdy Scots owe their tall and large boned bodies to the highly mineralized cereal, fruit and vegetable products of their mountain valleys, the soil of which is enriched every season by the mineral wash from the rocky hillsides. As long as they lived on wholemeal barley bread and oatmeal porridge made from home-grown and home-milled cereals, they had splendid teeth. During the last few generations, however, since they began to abandon their primitive foods for white bread, white sugar and devitalized breakfast foods, dentists have become more numerous among them.

3. **Gingivitis and Pyorrhoea.** These ailments are so injurious, not only to the teeth, but also to the general health of the body, and they are increasing in frequency with such alarming rapidity that they deserve special attention. Allopathic medical science declares that gingivitis and pyorrhoea, like all other inflammatory diseases, are caused by germs, and has vainly tried to cure these common ailments by the application of antiseptics and germ killers. We find that as usual the germs are secondary effects, that we must look for the true causes in other directions. These are:

(1) lack of exercise for the teeth and the connective tissues which hold them in place;
(2) inflammation of the gums, caused by hyperacidity of the system and other pathogenic conditions;
(3) the corroding action of mineral deposits on the teeth.

Dr. Robert Aiston, a prominent Chicago dentist, who for twenty years has made pyorrhoea a special study, says he is positive that lack of exercise for the teeth and the connective tissues which hold them in place is the principal cause of pyorrhoea. In an interview which I had with him he said: "No man living has made a more exhaustive study of pyorrhoea than I have, and I am convinced that the principal cause is the predominance of soft, mushy, cooked food in the customary diet of our American people." The reasons with which he backs his opinions are very convincing. I shall condense them as follows: The roots of the teeth are held in place by ligamentous tissues and these remain strong and sound as long as they are subjected to normal strain from the push and pull exerted by vigorous mastication. When this ceases as a result of the continuous consumption of soft, cooked foods, then the dental ligaments and other connective tissues begin to weaken and decay. Stagnation and putrefaction set up inflammation; this produces inflammatory exudates rich in calcareous salts and these in turn form seruminal calculi on the roots of the teeth, so called because these mineral incrustations are precipitated from the blood serum. The doctor showed me a number of teeth which were thickly covered with these rough, earthy deposits. I fully agree with Dr. Aiston that local stagnation, due to lack of exercise, is one of the primary causes of inflammation and destruction of dental ligaments, but I believe this is greatly facilitated and aggravated by pathogenic materials and disease taints in the circulation, and in the very beginning by mineral incrustations on the surface of the teeth. Elsewhere I have mentioned that in several cases pyorrhoea entirely disappeared after the patients had been cured, by natural methods, of smallpox, gonorrhoea, syphilis and other acute, eliminative diseases. Healing crises eliminated the disease taints, raw food diet reduced the "calcareous exudates" and scoured the teeth of slimy and earthy deposits. In this connection I would mention that after the adoption of a raw food diet mineral deposits on the teeth at first increase. This is caused by the neutralization of large amounts of acids. But as the acidity, under the influence of alkaline diet, diminishes, mineral precipitation ceases, inflammation subsides, the incrustations on the teeth are gradually absorbed and the gums have a chance to heal. Pyorrhoea, as well as other chronic ailments, can be cured only by restoring the entire organism to a clean, normal condition.

Gingivitis. The mineral deposits on the crowns of the teeth, usually light grey in colour, are commonly called tartar. Dentists speak of them as salivary calculi, because they are formed by earthy precipitates from the saliva. These tartar deposits may encroach under the borders of the gums, and this, together with slimy, mucoid accumulations, gives rise to inflammatory, destructive processes in gum tissues. This is commonly called gingivitis. It is the forerunner of pyorrhoea. The only difference between the two ailments is that in pyorrhoea the mineral deposits form on the necks and roots of the teeth, and that these seruminal calculi are blacker, harder and more destructive than the tartar on the crowns. The sharp earthy crystals help to corrode the dental ligaments, aggravate the inflammatory processes, and thus in turn increase the inflammatory exudate of calcareous matter. Filthy, putrefying matter could not accumulate around the teeth and under the gums if the food contained sufficient coarse, scouring material. Thus it will be seen that the two causes, stagnation due to lack of exercise, and mineral precipitation due to hyperacidity of the system, seesaw in the causation of gingivitis and pyorrhoea.

The Rational Treatment of Gingivitis and Pyorrhoea. It is well enough to scrape from the teeth the earthy incrustations which cause the gums to recede and to putrefy, but what good does this do when the hyperacid condition of the system makes new deposits? Many people have the idea that they can safely eat meat, eggs and large amounts of starchy foods as long as they consume with them plenty of the mineral salt foods, such as fruits and vegetables. As explained in Vol. 1 of this series, in Chap. XXXIX, this is a mistake. The intake of too much starchy and protein food leads to the excessive production of acids and other pathogenic substances. Though these are neutralized by alkaline mineral elements, more earthy salts are thus formed than can be properly eliminated through the skin and kidneys. These salts collect on the teeth as tartar, or they may form deposits in the joints resulting in rheumatism.

4. In order to prevent these and a host of other acid diseases, it is not enough to adopt a vegetarian diet, but the intake of vegetables, starches and proteids must be kept within normal limits. How to accomplish this I have explained under the heading of food combinations in Sec. I, No. 10.

Normal consistency of the food also has much to do with the preservation of the teeth. The perfect condition of the teeth of wild animals and of primitive man is partly due to the fact that they consume their foods in the natural raw condition, thus giving the teeth plenty of wholesome exercise by the gnawing, grinding and crunching of bones, grasses, raw cereals, fruits and nuts. While savage or primitive people cook some of their food, they use much more raw food than do their civilized cousins. Cooked food, in which most of the vitamins have been destroyed, is much more prone to acid formation than live, raw food. Physicians and dentists frequently warn against acid and subacid fruits "because they destroy the enamel of the teeth". This is a mistake. The live organic acids of fruits and vegetables, charged with vitamins, have not a destructive effect upon the bony structures as do the disease-producing acids formed by abnormal food combinations and putrefactive processes. The malic and citric acids of the fruits are highly organized and help to dissolve the earthy deposits in the joints, and the tartar on the teeth.([1])

Unless the diet contains liberal proportions of raw vegetables, fruits, roots and nuts, which are splendid scourers and cleansers, the teeth are bound to deteriorate and decay. Even the teeth of cows become loose and fall out when the animals are fed continually on the soft, sloppy, devitalized and demineralized cereal offal of breweries and distilleries. To begin the day and to end it with the munching of an apple or some other raw fruit or vegetable relish is the best way to keep the teeth in a perfectly clean and sound condition.

Another reason why dentistry in civilized countries is one of the best paying professions is the habit of swallowing food and drink, either very hot or extremely cold. Not infrequently the piping hot soups and other viands are washed down with iced water or immediately followed by ice cream, sherbet or other chilled desserts. The sudden expansion and contraction due to contact with excessive heat or cold causes the enamel to crack and thus exposes the dentine of the teeth to the destructive activity of acids and other corroding substances.

When prospective parents have destroyed their teeth by unnatural practices, how can they expect to produce offspring with sound bones and teeth? When the blood of the mother is utterly deficient in the bone-building mineral elements, is it any wonder that the newborn comes into the world handicapped for life with a dwarfed, defective bony framework? The formation of tooth substance begins in the embryo after the sixth week and continues all through gestation. This further reveals how important is is that the food of the mother contains sufficient amounts of the bone and teeth making elements. This is possible only when her diet includes an abundant supply of fruits and vegetables, hulls of grains and other mineral salt foods, classified under Group V of the Food Table. I have observed in many instances that when the prenatal structure and chemical composition of the teeth are abnormal, natural feeding after birth cannot always make good for the defective foundation. An imperfect, cankered seed will not produce a perfect tree, even though the soil in which it grows contains abundant nourishment.

5. **Cleaning the Teeth.** By the foregoing I do not wish to depreciate the importance of keeping the teeth in a clean and sweet condition by careful scrubbing several times a day, particularly in the morning and before retiring. If convenient it should be done after every meal. However, we

([1])
It should be noted that acids act differently on dead and living tissues. The hydrochloric acid secreted by the stomach in normal solution does not affect this organ injuriously, while it readily decomposes the stomach of a dead animal. The same principle holds true in relation to the action of fruit acids on dead and live teeth. [Author's note.]

do not favour for this purpose the use of preparations containing poisonous antiseptics. These are readily absorbed by the tender tissues of the mouth and in time will cause trouble in the body. Practically all tooth powders, pastes and lotions sold in the drug stores contain such deleterious substances. These are not only decidedly harmful, but entirely superfluous because the best tooth wash is fresh, cool water made slightly acid with lemon juice. Brisk scrubbings of the teeth with this natural dentifrice will keep the gums and teeth in clean and sweet condition. This should be followed by rinsing the mouth with fresh water. The scrubbing should be done from above downward and from below upward. This will tend to pull the gums over the teeth and to cleanse the crevices between the teeth from food particles and slimy accumulations. Another good treatment is to dip the forefinger into cold water and give the gums, inside and outside, a good rubbing and kneading. Always finish by rinsing the mouth thoroughly with water as cool as the gums will endure.

If there is a tendency to the formation of tartar, the teeth may be thoroughly scoured a few times a week with ground pumice stone, whiting or oyster shell, but this must not be repeated too often because it might injure the enamel. It goes without saying that the teeth should be looked after by a competent dentist at least every six months, and that defects of any kind should be attended to promptly. Many a tooth can be saved by a timely filling, a well fitted crown or good bridge work. These matters must be left to the skill of the dentist. The better he understands his art, the more economical will be his services in the long run.

6. **Foci of Infection and their Suppression.** The latest theory of medical science is that rheumatism and a number of other acute and chronic diseases are caused by gum infection from suppurating tonsils and adenoids, from abscesses in the teeth, and ulceration and pyorrhoea in the gums. These short-sighted deductions are the natural outgrowth of the germ theory and of the local and symptomatic conception of disease. We find in our institutional work that the aches and pains of rheumatism, headaches and asthmatic spasms, etc., come and go, rise and fall in exact proportion to the increase and decrease of acids and other pathogenic materials in the circulation. I do not deny for a moment that the pathogenic materials in these foci of infection may start or aggravate acute conditions in other parts of the body, but is it sufficient to suppress the foci of infection with antiseptics and surgical treatment? The question is, what causes the foci of infection, the suppurating tonsils and adenoids, the abscesses in the teeth, the ulcerating gums and jawbones? Does medical science imagine that the suppression of these foci of infection with poisonous antiseptics and surgical operations solves the problem? Why cannot they see that this also is rank suppression and not cure? Can a healthy

270

body, endowed with pure blood, normal tissues and perfect mechanical structural alignment, develop such foci of infection? What is the use of suppressing these symptoms of constitutional disease in one place and having them bob up at another place in more destructive form? Of such nature are the great achievements of modern medical science.

7. **This latest craze** has led in innumerable instances to the pulling out of whole sets of teeth because one or more were abscessed or because of the presence of so-called pyorrhoea, which frequently is nothing but a raw condition of the gums induced by incrustations of tartar on the roots of the teeth. I meet almost daily with people who have been robbed of sound teeth, sometimes of entire sets, on the assumption that it would cure their rheumatism or other constitutional disease. To their sorrow they find that the cruel sacrifice has brought no relief so far as their chronic ailments are concerned. Such criminal experimentation is on a level with tearing out sound ovaries with the idea of curing epilepsy or other chronic diseases. I have known of a number of such uncalled for mutilations. In no instance has the unnatural treatment benefited the patient; it has only served to aggravate the chronic ailment and to hasten physical, nervous and mental breakdown. The constant suppression of symptoms of disease by drug poisoning and surgical mutilations creates chronic invalidism, hereditary disease, and defectives. Is it not more rational to put the system, through natural living and treatment, in such a pure and wholesome condition that it cannot develop inflammation and suppuration of the tonsils, teeth, gums and jawbones? Such is the practice of the new school of healing.

8. **Toothache.** One of the most excruciating tortures that man inflicts upon himself by wrong living is the toothache. All the causes I have enumerated and described help to create it, and avoidance of the causes is the best prevention. There are two general types of toothache, the acute inflammatory, accompanied by heat and swelling, and the cold neuritic or neuralgic.

(a) The acute inflammatory may be due to congestion and irritation of the blood vessels and nerves of a tooth or row of teeth by systemic poisons, in the same manner that inflammations arise in other parts of the system as the result of pathogenic obstruction and irritation. Acute inflammation may arise when the nerve of a tooth becomes exposed through decay of the bony structure. In that the case the attention of a dentist may be necessary, but care must always be taken not to cover decaying particles with a filling or crown. The parts to be covered must be carefully cleansed of all materials that might cause further putrefaction.

(b) Treatment. The acute inflammatory toothache is best treated by retaining cool or cold water in the mouth until it warms up, when it should be spat out and replaced. At the same time cooling compresses or packs should be applied to the cheek on the affected side. The pack as usual consists of a piece of muslin, folded from three to six times, and wrung out in cold water; the cold compress by one or several folds of dry flannel or woollen cloth. The compress or pack may be kept in place by one of the bandages described above. An acute congestive toothache may be greatly relieved by gentle downward massage movements along the veins and lymphatics of the neck. Thorough drainage of these vessels will do much to relieve the congestion in the affected parts. While giving the massage movements also use your mental power to combine with the mechanical treatment the magnetic effects. Osteophatic, chiropractic and naprapathic treatments prove very effective in many cases. In serious cases the local water treatment may be reinforced by a whole sheet pack, bed sweat bath, or body or leg packs followed by cold ablutions (Sec. XV). During the night the sufferer may at intervals take a cold rub and go under the bed covering without drying. All these water applications draw the blood away from the congested area into the surface and thus relieve the local congestion and excruciating pain. They also promote the elimination of the pathogenic materials which are the primary cause of the trouble.

If acute inflammation within and around the teeth were always treated in this way it would seldom come to the formation of acute or chronic abscesses. The pathogenic materials would be absorbed and eliminated immediately. Of equal importance with the water treatment is fasting. From the first appearance of a toothache, absolutely no food should be taken until it has ceased entirely, and even then the fasting should be continued for a day or two in order to clear up the constitutional condition which caused the local inflammation. Fasting alone in many instances has cured the severest toothache. I would warn strongly against the use of poisonous pain killers. They only serve to paralyse the nerves and do not in any way remove the underlying causes of the trouble. They add drug poisons to disease poisons and thereby accelerate the destruction of the teeth and gums.

(c) Neuritic Toothache. This type of toothache is not accompanied by great heat and swelling as is the inflammatory kind. It is usually caused by the exposure of a nerve, or by the irritating effect of some systemic or drug poison. If caused by defects of the teeth and by exposure of a nerve, proper dental attention is of course indicated. This type of toothache is much more stubborn and does not yield to treatment as easily as does the acute inflammatory kind. Cold water, magnetic and manipulative treatment give but momentary relief. The reason is that the pain will continue or will return at intervals until the poisonous irritant is removed or until

272

the nerve is killed or protected. Sometimes the jawbones and cheek bones are more affected by these neuritic toothaches than are the teeth themselves. This is usually due to the action of some irritating poison.

(d) Treatment. In these cold, persistent forms of toothache, hot applications sometimes give better relief than the cold applications, though the relief is temporary. A remedy worth trying when cold treatment fails consists in the application of a muslin bag partly filled with hot salt and held in place by a bandage. The salt should be as hot as it can be endured. The only way in which these neuritic toothaches can be permanently cured is by eliminating the poisons which are at the root of the trouble. In many cases we have found mercury, iodine, arsenic, quinine or other drugs to be the real cause of the disturbance. Elimination of these hidden enemies can be accomplished only by a thorough systemic treatment and natural methods of living. Many dentists are in the habit of using large doses of iodine, arsenic or other powerful poisons for killing the nerves. They should be warned not to use any more of these destructive poisons than is absolutely necessary. If the work can be accomplished without using them at all, so much the better. I would also warn strongly against amalgam fillings. The amalgam or silver filling, so called, contains about 50 percent of mercury. Acids in the blood and in the fluids of the buccal cavity have a tendency to dissolve the mercury and to create bichloride of mercury and other mercurial salts which will accumulate in certain parts of the body for which they have a special affinity, particularly in the brain and spinal cord. I am aware that such warnings are pooh-poohed and ridiculed by many dentists, but practical experience tells a different story. The blackening of the teeth indicates the formation of mercurial salts. In numerous cases, we have observed pronounced symptoms of mercurial salivation, such as metallic taste in the mouth, ulceration about the necks of the teeth, foetid breath and abnormally increased flow of salvia, which did not disappear until the amalgam fillings were removed from the teeth and replaced by gold or porcelain. Gold filling, whenever it is practicable, is undoubtedly the best of all. I know skilled dentists who have discovered these facts for themselves in the course of practice and who have discontinued the use of amalgam fillings on this account. Of late I have met with several cases of paresis which showed distinctly the sign of mercurialism in the iris. Enquiry revealed that these patients were dentists who for many years had been in the habit of mixing the amalgam and alloy in their bare palms. Mercury had thus been absorbed and was responsible for the destruction of brain substance.

SECTION XLIV

WHY GROW OLD?

"What a question," you exclaim. "We grow old because we cannot prevent it; because nature has decreed it so." Of course we shall grow old in years, but if we live in harmony with nature's laws we need not grow old in mind or heart nor lose our physical energy and our alertness and suppleness of body and mind long before the expiration of our allotted time. While growing older in years we should grow younger and more robust as far as our intellectual, emotional, moral and spiritual qualities are concerned.

As regards longevity and the possibility of retaining our youthful qualities to very old age, we meet with two extremes of opinion. Many mental scientists and new thought people tell us in their lectures and writings that it is not impossible to achieve immortality and perpetual youth in the physical body on this earth plane; that we die long before our time because we imagine we must; that a short-lived existence was necessary for animals and human beings in the early stages of evolutionary development, but that now since the physical body has become more perfect the necessity for dying has passed away and that as soon as we can exterminate the old age and death thought which has become race habit, the "last enemy" will be vanquished and immortality and perpetual youth in the flesh will become the common heritage of humankind. However, the majority of mankind entertains an entirely opposite and somewhat pessimistic opinion as regards longevity and the preservation of youth. They are convinced that growing old and decrepit, that losing the enthusiasm, beauty and efficiency of youth is inevitable. They argue that growing old or dying young, health or disease, depend upon heredity, environment, colds, draughts, germs and other accidental circumstances over which we have little or no control. One prominent physician recommended the chloroforming of people over sixty years of age.

These two opposing views were brought home to me quite vividly some time ago, while attending a lecture by a well known mental scientist. His subject on this occasion was "Perpetual Youth". In alluring language, scintillating with plausible argument and beautiful metaphor, he proved to his own satisfaction the possibility of perpetual youth and life everlasting in the physical body. After the audience had given fevent expression to its approval of his lofty idealism, an elderly gentleman in the audience arose and delivered his views on youth and longevity in a pessimistic wail which was taken in shorthand by a stenographer present in the audience. He said: "This subject of perpetual youth as put forward by our speaker is a beautiful theory. It is a wonderful theory, but I am very clear that it does not work out in life. I do not believe that there is such a thing as perpetual youth. It is an ideal belief. You cannot by any process known to human science or human ingenuity turn back the wheels of time or stay them in their revolutions. This fountain of perpetual youth old men have sighed for, old women have prayed for, and in search for it from time immemorial young women have appropriated their husband's wages and poured their money into the cash box at the drug store; but they have never yet found it. It is true that by right thought and right action you can probably postpone old age, but you can postpone it only to a very limited degree. The speaker stated that seventeen hundred people in the United States had reached the age of one hundred years, but he did not tell you how many of them are paralysed, how many of them are palsied, how many are more dead than alive. He tells you that with advancing age the arm of the blacksmith grows stronger. This is true for a certain time, but its strength reaches its zenith, then it grows weaker and weaker until it hammers no more. Young man, you cannot turn back the wheels of time and you cannot stay their revolutions. The time that is past is laid to rest in eternal sleep; it is buried in the mysterious realm of oblivion. Time robs the bridal wreath of its beauty. Time writes wrinkles upon the brow of the aged. You may wreathe garlands and place them around the brow of youth, but the onward march of time sees them wilt and mingle with the dust. The birds that sing so sweetly will return in the spring. The flowers will return and bloom again, but, ah, my friends, youth is gone. It is past, forever. It never returns, but age is real and forever — perpetual youth is no more than a beautiful dream."

As regards the possibility of life everlasting on this earth plane, I for my part would gently but firmly decline it. The idea of living in the same old place forever and forever is not attractive to my mind. I imagine in time it would become monotonous. To me, life is a great school; a school of personal effort for the development of our latent god-like faculties, capacities and powers. This school takes in all there is in the sidereal universe. Its course in length of time is eternity; its class rooms and laboratories are the solar systems and their planets. Whenever we have learned all there is to learn, all there is to be acquired of knowledge, wisdom and experience in this great school of life, then it will be time for us to die. The only death I know of is stagnation and retrogression. Life is growth; growth is change, continual perpetual change — senescence and rejuvenescence, as science calls it. Death is only a phase in this continuous process of change. The majority of mankind look upon death as the greatest evil in life. They think of it with despair and terror. Some commit suicide because they are afraid to die — a strange paradox, inspired by fear, fear of something which is in reality the greatest of all blessings, the birth into a new and brighter world with new life, new youth, new and broader possibilities, after we have acquired all there is to be learned in one brief earthly pilgrimage. Why grieve for the loss of loved ones who have made the great transit before us? Shall we not be glad to meet them when we arrive on the other shore? If we had to travel on a long journey to a foreign country, wouldn't we be pleased to meet with friends among strangers in a strange land? Life on earth is only the kindergarten in the great school of the universe. Even the greatest and wisest of men who live on this earth are only in the lower grades of the great Cosmic University. Why should we fear to pass on? Nobody would like to remain in the primary grades all his life when there are so many more interesting, useful and beautiful things to be learnt in the higher grades.

One New Thought philosopher argues that immortality in the flesh, or at least a prolonged term of life on this earth, is necessary in order to acquire all there is to be learned and experienced in this beautiful world of ours and in order to permit the law of compensation to work out the great chain of cause and effect. How much more reasonable and beautiful than this idea of continuous existence on earth is the philosophy of Karma and reincarnation of the ancient wisdom religion. Is it not better to have the arduous training of earth life alternate with vacations in the spirit land, and to return oblivious of previous existences with their depressing burdens of errors, sins and sorrows? Thus death on one plane of life becomes birth into another, and vice versa. In this continuous change from the old age of one life to youth in another life, lies for me the true solution of rejuvenescence, of immortality and of perpetual youth.

If we look upon life from this higher and brighter viewpoint, how can we grieve at growing old? How can we fear death? Those who are in conscious touch with life on the spiritual planes tell us that beings of high spiritual development appear in a condition of youthful maturity, combining the wisdom of millenniums of spiritual and celestial existence with the beauty of perpetual youth. It is not knowledge, wisdom and experience that causes premature senility and death, but wrong thinking, feeling and doing. Aside from unnatural physical habits of living, nothing promotes senile decrepitude like fear of disease and death, bred through ignorance of life's great laws. He who looks at life from the higher and brigher viewpoint enjoys advancing life in ever greater serenity of soul and happiness of spirit. He rejoices in ever greater expansion of mind and deeper understanding of life's mysteries. He is justly proud of every year added to a life of usefulness to himself and to his fellow beings. Such a one has only pity for the pessimist's wail previously recited. Such gruesome thinking and feeling is the very essence of black magic that ages and stiffens the body and pencils wrinkles on the brow. To grow younger as we grow older, we must practise white magic. The body is an electrotype of our mental images. Physical matter convolutes to the mental and psychical or soul pattern. "As a man thinketh in his heart, so is he," or as Gautama Buddha expressed it, "I am today what my past thoughts and feelings have made me." See yourself in your mind's eye as always beautiful, vigorous and active, as in the prime of youth, for, "A man is never older than he feels, and a woman never older than she looks." "But," you ask, "how shall we keep our looks young?" That is simple. Bathe daily in the sparkling waters of serenity of mind and of cheerfulness and in the milk of human kindness. Learn to relax completely in body, mind and soul and never entertain discordant and destructive thoughts and emotions.

Physical Causes of Senescence

Mental magic alone, powerful as it may be, is not sufficient to prevent the ageing of body and mind. We must live in harmony with the laws of the physical. No matter how good a watch you have, if you allow it to fill up with dust, dirt and corroding acids, it will lose time and finally stop entirely. This is exactly what happens to the human clock when it "grows old". As philosophy has two divergent opinions concerning the prolongation of life, so has physical science two theories concerning the causes of senescence or senile deterioration. According to one of these theories, the animal and human being is endowed at birth with a certain amount of vitality, or with a certain momentum of vital force. When this is gradually spent in course of time our powers begin to wane; as a result of lowered vitality the vibratory power to expel waste declines; blood and lymph vessels become obstructed, joints stiffen, brain and nerve matter hardens and we grow old and decrepit. Certain facts in nature favour this viewpoint. Even under the most favourable conditions in the freedom of nature animals live only to a certain age limit. Each species and family of creatures seems to have its own allotted lifetime or age limit. When this limit is reached they suddenly decline and die. I say "suddenly" advisedly. They do not spend a third or a half of their lifetime in getting old and in dying like the average human being. They retain their full vigour and beauty of form almost to the end of life. It is of rare occurrence that a hunter kills an animal that is found to be diseased or deformed. Among antelope, deer and elk the oldest bucks are usually the leaders of the herd. In order to maintain their supremacy they must fight and vanquish their younger rivals. So human beings when living the natural life, physically, intellectually, morally and socially, will reach the

277

age limit fixed by nature for the human species in full possession of their faculties, capacities and powers, and will depart from life peacefully. Death will be as painless and sweet as sleep. I believe that in higher reaches of evolutionary development yet to be attained by mankind, the transition from earth life into spiritual life will not mean the passing "through the valley of the shadow" but that human beings will make the transition in full possession of their waking consciousness.

The opposite theory advanced by physical scientists as regards the causes of senescence, postulates that vital energy is generated by the cells, tissues and organs of the body, and that as these with advancing age deteriorate and disintegrate, vital energy ceases to be generated and the constituent elements of the body become unfit to carry on the vital activities.

Natural Therapeutic philosophy teaches that the physical body is an instrument for the manifestation of the great life force which is divine life, intelligence and creative power. God or Nature evidently does not intend us to live on this earth forever in one continuous stretch of life and therefore has wisely limited the supply of vital force as well as the durability of the physical body in accordance with the laws governing incarnation and reincarnation on the physical and spiritual planes of life. As before stated, even the healthiest animals living in the most congenial surroundings in the freedom of nature do not much exceed their allotted span of life, nor do they fall much below it. As a rule, the longer the period between birth and maturity, the longer the life of the animal. All the different families of mammalia, when living in freedom, live closely up to the life period allotted to them by nature. Man is the only exception. It is claimed that according to the law of longevity his average length of life should be considerably over one hundred years, while according to life insurance statistics the average is at present about forty years. This shows an immense discrepancy between the possible and the actual longevity of man. Even this brief average span of life means for the majority of mankind little else than weakness, physical and mental suffering, premature senility and death. Visiting physicians of the public schools in our large cities report that 75 percent of all school children show defective health in some way. Diagnosis from the eye proves that the remaining 25 percent are also more or less affected by hereditary and acquired disease conditions. Christian Science says: "There is no disease." Nature's records in the iris of the eye prove there is no perfect health.

These established facts of greatly impaired longevity and universal abnormality of the human race would of themselves indicate that there is something radically wrong somewhere in the life habits of man, and that there is ample reason for the great health reform movement which was started about the middle of the last century by the pioneers of Nature

278

Cure in Europe and which has since swept, under many forms and guises, all portions of the civilized world. When people in general grow better acquainted with the laws underlying prenatal and postnatal child culture, natural living, and the natural treatment of disease, human beings will approach more closely the normal in health, strength, beauty and longevity. However, to reach this ideal of perfect physical, mental and moral health, succeeding generations will have to adhere to the natural ways of living and treating their ailments. It cannot be attained by the present generation. Those enthusiasts who claim that they can, by their particular methods, achieve perfect health and live the full term of human life are destined to disappointment. We are so handicapped by the mistakes of the past that the best which most of us adults can do is to "patch up", to attain a reasonable measure of health and to approach somewhat nearer nature's full allotment of life. Growing old consists in the accumulation of waste and morbid matter, earthy deposits, destructive acids and alkaloids, causing the stiffening and hardening of joints, bones, veins and arteries and the gradual loss of physical and mental energy.

Do you ever stop to think how this clogging and corroding of the wheels of life is promoted and accelerated by wrong habits of eating and drinking? Food chemistry as taught by the school of Natural Therapeutics clearly shows that excessive use of starchy and proteid foods is the most prolific cause of disease and of premature old age. These classes of food create in the body a large variety of destructive acids, ptomaines and alkaloids, such as uric acids, sulphuric acid, oxalic acid, indican, xanthine, creatine, etc. Flesh foods especially favour these morbid accumulations because they are already saturated with all the waste products of the animal carcass. The poisonous xanthines of coffee and tea are almost identical with uric acid. While at first they overstimulate the organism, the second and lasting effect is to benumb and paralyse heart and nerves and to retard elimination, thus causing directly and indirectly retention and accumulation of waste matter in the body. For these reasons, we of the Natural Therapeutic school realize that the only way to keep the system pure and sweet and its vibratory activities vigorous and harmonious is to reduce in the daily dietary the allowance of starchy and proteid food and to use a larger proportion of fruits and vegetables whose alkaline elements tend to dissolve and eliminate the acid crystallizations and deposits in the tissues. When we pass the meridian of life, growth ceases; there is much less physical activity and therefore much less need of starchy, fatty and albuminous elements. Therefore, as we advance in years these foods should be reduced in amount and replaced by the dissolving and eliminating fruits and vegetables, though conventional habits and the doctor's advice usually favour the opposite course.

"You are growing older," says the doctor; "you must have plenty of strengthening foods — meats, eggs, fish, fowl — and you need some stimulants. Coffee or tea is all right and an occasional glass of beer or of 'Duffy's Old Malt' won't hurt you either." Frequently a patient tells us: "All the young people in our house are now living on the natural diet, but you know father and mother are growing old and they must have their soup and meat, their coffee and beer, in order to keep up their strength." Reverse the prevalent ideas on hygiene and you are just about right; so in this regard the very opposite policy should be adopted. The older we grow, the less we need of the heavy clogging foods and the more of the light and purifying. The majority of people eat too much anyway. Habitual stuffing practised through many generations has made it second nature. Many consume the best part of their available vital force in endeavouring to digest and eliminate superfluous quantities of food and drink. Every ounce of food in excess of actual need wastes vital force. A Roman proverb said: "Plenus venter non studet libenter" — a full stomach does not like to study. Vital energy required to remove useless ballast cannot be transformed into physical or mental energy. Vital force is a primary force. It cannot be eaten. It comes from the source of all life and is independent of the physical body just as electricity is independent of the bulb which it fills with light. Food can only furnish fuel material for the flame of life and keep the human organism in such condition that vital force can manifest itself in it and through it. If food and drink could give life they should prolong it indefinitely; in that case the glutton and drunkard would live the longest, but common experience teaches us that the man temperate in all things best preserves his physical and mental vigour and lives the longest.

The beauty about all this is that Nature Cure philosophy does not confine itself to visionary theorizing, but that it "delivers the goods". If we can take all sorts of chronic incurable disease and within four or five months or a year's time work a wonderful transformation and actually cure the majority of such patients and give them a new lease of life, why should it be impossible to prolong life to its natural limit and to retain to the last, unimpaired, our faculties, capacities and powers of body, mind and soul?

How much greater would be the possibilities for health and longevity if human beings were brought into life and treated in the natural way from the beginning; that is from the time of mating and conception through the prenatal and postnatal periods and on through youth to maturity. Within a few generations the offspring of such natural heredity would live the full allotted time of a hundred and fifty years in perfect health, strength and beauty, thoroughly efficient in the business of life, a true aristocracy.([1]) Many of our young people are now beginning to carry out this great plan for the creation of a better, healthier and more beautiful humanity. They are seeking partners among those who have been educated and trained in the ways of natural living. If the offspring of such naturally mated couples do likewise and select their partners in turn from among those who are the product of natural heredity, what a different humanity will inhabit this earth within a few generations. This is not vain dreaming. It is marvellous how the youth of this country have taken hold of these new ideas; how many are adopting the new life in harmony with Natural Therapeutic philosophy, physical culture teachings and other systems of natural living and healing. Quite frequently young couples come to me, saying: "Doctor, we want to get married; but before we do give us a thorough examination and, if necessary, we intend to take a course of treatment in order to put our bodies in right condition for the great responsibilities of matrimony and procreation." What wisdom — what a glorious promise of a better, healthier and happier humanity.

How to Grow Younger

Keep in the light — cultivate the air and light bath — nothing sweet or beautiful grows or ripens in the darkness. Avoid fear in all its forms of expression; it is responsible for the greater part of human suffering. The only thing to fear is fear. Don't live to eat, but eat to live. The cook is the chief executioner of King Death. In the morning do not say: "I am another day older and so much nearer the end" — say "I feel one day younger." How can we grow old with all eternity before us? The wise man tells us that in the higher life the good ones always appear in the vigour and beauty of mature manhood and womanhood. What difference makes it if this old suit of ours grows a little shabbier? We shall soon wear a new and better one. Be as a child, live simply and naturally, steer clear of too much money and too much worry. Cultivate the spirit of content; nothing ages the face and furrows the brow so quickly as nagging discontent, suspicion and jealousy. Before going to sleep, throw off all the cares and anxieties of the day and attune your physical, mental and psychical vibrations to harmonies of rest and peace and love.

([1])
A good deal of evidence seems to be accumulating that the natural span of human life is much more than the three score years and ten spoken of by the psalmist. We learn from travellers and researchers that there are remote places where the inhabitants live in splendid health and activity for more than a hundred years. These are places where there is a good climate, a good alluvial soil and a good traditional system of agriculture and diet. Examples are to be found in the Himalayas, the Caucasus, the Andes and elsewhere. As a rule these peoples are wholly or mainly vegetarian. Books by Dr. G. T. Wrench and "The Recovery of Culture" by Henry Bailey Stevens (C. W. Daniel) point to the conclusion that these peoples are the remnants of very ancient cultures which were happier and more healthy than our own, though no doubt less sophisticated and less "advanced" in certain ways.

APPENDIX I

THE MENSTRUAL CYCLE

While it would be rash to contend that there is not still much to be learnt with regard to the physiology of ovulation and conception, it would appear that research and observation, much of it since Lindlahr's time, do enable us to be reasonably certain about the normal reproductive cycle, although undoubtedly many abnormalities and irregularities do occur.

(1) It seems to be established that there is normally a twenty-eight day cycle which commences with an ovulation (and not, as is frequently thought, with menstruation). If this ovulation is not followed by fertilization and conception, then menstruation will take place between twelve and sixteen days after ovulation. The object of this menstruation is to prepare the uterus and fallopian tubes to be in a fit state for conception and implantation when the next ovulation occurs.

(2) It is also established that normally ovulation takes place alternately in the two ovaries so that in one month it will be in the right ovary and in the next month in the left.

(3) It is generally believed on very good evidence that the actual time of fertility during the monthly period is extremely short, neither the ovum nor the spermatozoon normally living for more than three days in the female tract. (There is evidence that spermatozoa may sometimes remain alive for rather longer periods up to as much as ten days, especially in cold areas, but actually this is rare and it is doubtful whether they ever remain fertile for this length of time.)

It is obvious that if this knowledge is to be used for the encouragement or discouragement of conception it is important first to establish the menstrual pattern of the woman because there are many cases in which menstruation is irregular and/or in which it is habitually at periods either shorter or longer than the normal twenty-eight days. Not until the pattern has been ascertained by keeping records for a period of some months is it possible to arrive at a reliable estimate of the days during which ovulation is to be expected. When this estimate has been obtained it is then possible to make use of it either to secure conception or to avoid it. It is possible also to be more certain of the time of ovulation by making use of the slight change in temperature which takes place at the actual time of ovulation. Some women, too, appear to have sensations of various kinds at the time of ovulation and such sensations may also give a guide as to which ovary is ovulating, the sensation being referable to one side or the other. Iridiagnosis is another method by which it is possible to pinpoint the exact time of ovulation though this does require a high degree of skill in the diagnostician. It may be noted that many of the abnormalities of menstruation, including great shortness and irregularity of periods, are due to bad health or to pathological or psychological conditions, and when these are corrected, normal, regular periods of twenty-eight days or near that will be established. It should also be mentioned that there appears to be some evidence that the time of ovulation may sometimes be advanced by a few hours by the excitation and stimulation of sexual intercourse taking place shortly before the expected time.

It is on the basis of this information that Ogino-Smulders and, following them, Mr. Murray Davey and others have based the system for the control of contraception which they advocate and which would appear to be reliable and sound.

APPENDIX II

BIRTH CONTROL

Lindlahr's attitude towards contraception, which would now be considered very out of date, does not allow of any interference whatever with the reproductive process by artificial means, either mechanical or chemical. In this he would appear to join hands with the official attitude of the Roman Catholic Church, if, perhaps, for somewhat different reasons. He does recognize that this is a hard doctrine, and while he maintains that "from the highest and best viewpoint" sexual intercourse should be considered as a sacred function to be exercised only for the propagation of offspring, he does allow that "temperate indulgence" may not be wholly condemned in "our present stage of ethical and moral development". On the other hand, he also considers that limitation of families in accordance with individual and social circumstances and responsibilities is right, proper and desirable even though the only legitimate methods of birth control are "abstinence or common cleanliness", by which he presumably means the use of the douche. In a general way his attitude is that we should go in for quality rather than quantity in our reproductive efforts. This is certainly an attitude which should commend itself to us in our times when overpopulation has become a real problem in many parts of the world and when there is so much sub-standard health which bodes ill for the future of the race, in spite of the fact that for the time being there is greater longevity among the so-called "advanced" peoples, and less in the way of infant mortality and destructive epidemics than there used to be. It now seems to be generally accepted that there should be limitation of offspring and that procreation of children should be deliberate and voluntary and not a matter of chance or a sort of by-product of sexual intercourse indulged in for other reasons.

Although much may have changed since Lindlahr's time it is, I believe, right to take a good square look at his view of proper conduct in sexual relations although it may seem antiquated and puritanical, because it does have much to be said for it on a good many grounds. Lindlahr maintains that we are in need of getting back to the idea that the natural purpose of sexual intercourse is the production of offspring and that the desires and pleasures and satisfactions connected with it are nature's provision for the continuance of the race. When something which exists for one purpose is pursued and indulged in for other purposes one begins to get on dangerous ground. There may be an analogy here with another of men's appetites, that of eating. The object of our feelings of hunger and our pleasures in eating is to ensure that we seek and enjoy the food which we require. When we acquire unnatural tastes in food and drink and go in for overeating we begin to get into trouble; and civilized man has in fact got into serious and disease-producing trouble in this way. The same may perhaps apply if we start to use or indulge sexuality for purposes other than reproduction, although civilized man has been doing this, or trying to do it, for centuries. At the very least to do so will tend to produce a sort of dichotomy in which we are doing something which derives its glory and joy from being a great creative act concerned with the creation of new life, and, at the same time, taking steps to avoid its being creative.

It may well be that a time may be approaching when we shall begin to look on sexual activity in a very different light from what we do at present. Lindlahr and Mackinnon have pointed out that sexuality is conditioned very much by all sorts of factors such as diet, season, periodicity, the marital behaviour of parents, the emotional states and upbringing both of parents and children, and that an obsessive occupation with sex and a tendency to constant sexual activity and desire are not really natural. Moreover, it is clear that, while sexual repression is capable of being very harmful in various ways, moderation and the disciplining or sublimation of the sexual urge is desirable and necessary both for individuals and for the race and makes for good health and the conservation of energy, as well as being of significance in the development of the intellectual and spiritual faculties. All societies and races have in fact developed laws and customs of marriage and sexual behaviour designed, if for no other reasons, to secure the orderly procreation and upbringing of children. The health of societies, as well as of the individuals which compose them, is very much bound up with the goodness or badness of such laws and customs and their fundamental soundness and suitability.

However, though there is much to be said for Lindlahr's views on contraception and on the desirability of a high degree of sexual abstinence, we must face the fact that there are many who conscientiously and with reason take a different view, and also we must recognize that we live in a time when birth control is being practised almost universally and is being encouraged and even legally enforced in some countries. So, if it is felt that there are desirable reasons for sexual love and intercourse other than the production of children and that, in any case, greater evils can result from suppression and denial of sexuality than from its reasonable indulgence, it is desirable that those who are concerned with health and therapeutics should take a critical look at the various methods of birth control which are used and advocated and seek to make up their minds which are best to be used or are least to be avoided.

There is not very much doubt that Lindlahr is right in contending that all artificial methods of birth control are to some degree objectionable on physiological grounds and are likely to be harmful and disease-producing in the long or short term. However, it would appear that mechanical methods must be regarded as preferable to chemical methods and that there are very great dangers in the use of oral contraceptives which operate by their effects on the endocrine system. The most desirable method of birth control would certainly seem to be that which is based on the discovery and use of the so-called "safe" periods. Though progress has been made in this direction it is to be hoped that further research may make it possible to fix with greater ease and certainty the exact time of ovulation.

APPENDIX III

SEX DETERMINATION

Lindlahr was a believer in the possibility of the predetermination of sex, and he based his ideas on the theory which appears to have originated with Rumley Dawson according to which it is believed that one ovary (usually the right) produces male offspring, and the other female. This theory, coupled with the fact that the two ovaries normally work alternately, should make it possible to choose the sex of offspring once the first pregnancy has established which ovary is functioning in a particular month. (Thus after the birth of a male child the first ovary to ovulate will be the "female" ovary. The first menstruation will therefore be a sign that the "female" ovary has ovulated. If a female child is desired intercourse should therefore take place in the month after the second menstruation.)

It appears that this method has been used with some success both with animals (notably cattle) and with man, but it does seem to be totally contrary to accepted scientific opinion at the present time. It is now generally held that the sex of offspring is entirely determined by the male, some spermatozoa being male-producing and some female-producing, and that the ova are neutral and all the same. This view is supported by the fact that some spermatozoa have an X chromosome and some do not in about equal proportions, and this is regarded as the sole determining factor. However, it is not impossible that these apparently contradictory theories may be capable of being reconciled. It may be that a male-producing sperm may not normally be capable of being attracted to and of fertilizing any but a "male" ovum. It may also be possible that the male sperms are produced by one of the testes and female by the other. (If this view is correct it would then be expected that if a woman has lost her right ovary or if her husband has no functioning right testis, they would be incapable of producing male offspring, and vice versa. Certain cases of absolute sterility could also be explainable on the basis that one partner is incapable of producing males and the other incapable of producing females.) Mackinnon also suggests that where there is an abnormal reproduction of an hermaphroditic nature, mosaic or otherwise, this can

287

be explained by a fertilization of a "female" ovum by a "male" type of sperm (producing a masculine type of female) or of a "male" ovum by a "female" type of sperm (producing a feminine type of man). This may also have a bearing on the problem of homosexuality or the tendency towards it.

The desire of mothers to be able to predetermine the sex of their children is a very understandable one and has a very long history. Generally the desire has been to produce sons, especially in societies where it is customary for kingships, titles and property to pass in the male line, but sometimes a girl is very much wanted in a family of several boys. Also it has been observed that while in a general way families will produce children of both sexes in fairly equal proportions, there are some women who produce only boys or girls and this would seem to imply that in such cases there must be a reason why this is so. Over the years various theories have been put forward as to how the sex of a child might be predicted or predetermined, some of which would seem to be bizarre or superstitious, but others of which can claim to be supported by research and evidence of a scientific kind. It is difficult to read Rumley Dawson's book "The Causation of Sex in Man" (published about 1920) without feeling that this writer has arrived at least at a part of the truth. Unfortunately his ideas were never very generally studied and now they have been entirely discredited because he said that the male played no part in the causation of sex and that this was determined entirely by the female, one of whose ovaries produced "male" ova and the other "female". Now, it having been discovered that the spermatozoa of the male are of two kinds differing in their chromosomes, and that all ova appear to be the same under the microscope, it is held that the determination of sex is entirely a matter of chance and operates through the male only. It should also be noted that Rumley Dawson, like Lindlahr his contemporary, seems to have thought that ovulation takes place at the time of menstruation or a little before or a little after. It now seems to be established without doubt that the cycle starts with an ovulation which takes place some sixteen to twelve days before menstruation. This knowledge, however, would not seem to invalidate Rumley Dawson's basic idea that the sex of a child will depend on the ovary from which it comes. In fact, a more exact knowledge of the time of ovulation and consequently of conception should make it easier to calculate the exact time when a child of the desired sex can be conceived.

It would appear very desirable that Rumley Dawson's ideas should be seriously studied by persons desiring to produce a child of a particular sex and by doctors who advise such persons. It must be admitted that it is not always easy to apply his method in individual cases. Abnormalities and irregularities of menstruation and ovulation do occur and consequently mistakes can be made in calculating the time at which a child of the desired sex can be conceived. Also, when twins of different sexes have been born it can be regarded as implying that both ovaries have functioned in the same month and this may make it difficult to say which of the two ovaries should be the next to ovulate. Also, critics of Rumley Dawson's theory have pointed out that some women have produced children of both sexes (or of the sex not to be expected) in cases where surgery has been performed on one ovary. All these and other points are very fully discussed by Rumley Dawson in his book where he gives numerous case reports. (For instance, he firmly maintains that if a really complete ovariotomy is performed it will afterwards be impossible for children of both sexes to be conceived by that woman, but he also maintains that in many cases the ovariotomy, either by accident or by design, is not complete and that some ovarian tissue remains.)[1]

Other theories about sex determination have been advanced and are still being so. A very old belief exists that sex can be determined by what is known as "lateral decubitus". This means that if a woman desires a male child she turns on her right side directly after coition but that if she desires a female she should lie on her left. According to Rumley Dawson there is a modicum of truth in this idea because lying on one side will encourage a guiding of the seminal fluid and the spermatozoa towards the right or left fallopian tube as the case may be and so encourage fertilization if there is an ovum in that tube. Another theory is that males tend to be conceived in the earlier part of the month soon after menstruation and females later shortly before menstruation. Rumley Dawson did not believe that there was any validity in such ideas, but it may be possible that there is a tendency in certain individuals for one ovary to ovulate earlier than the other. There has been a considerable amount of publicity recently in the newspapers and on radio about methods of sex determination by which, it is claimed, sex can be predetermined by diet or by directly changing the chemistry of the vagina or uterus in an acid or alkaline direction.

Finally, in connection with the two subjects of the menstrual cycle and sex determination, I feel that attention should be drawn to two books written some fifty years ago by Lady Monteith Erskine entitled "Sex at Choice" and "Nature's Law of Birth Control". To me these books constitute something of a mystery because the physiological theories put forward in them would seem to be utterly untenable and yet the practical application of those theories appears to have led to success in a very large

[1]
A book entitled "Son or Daughter?" by D. Murray Davey (published by The Wales publishing Co., 26 Charing Cross Road, London W.C.1) gives directions on the practical application of Rumley Dawson's theory. It is uncertain whether this book is now obtainable.

number of cases, as is evidenced by numerous case reports and letters from grateful patients. Lady Monteith Erskine had a very large following and was encouraged and approved of by eminent gynaecologists of the time, and she shows evidence of having, in a very honest and thorough way, given much thought, study and observation to her subject before writing her books and putting forward her theories. Put briefly, her contention is that one ovary (the male) ovulates after menstruation and the other (the female) before menstruation. There is therefore one totally infertile month in which conception cannot normally take place at all and one fertile month in which a male child can be conceived in the second week and a female child in the fourth week.

APPENDIX IV

DIAGNOSIS AND TREATMENT

Lindlahr states in more than one place in his writings that treatment is more imporant than diagnosis. In both acute and chronic conditions it is possible and desirable to apply treatment, in the one case to help the body through a crisis and in the other to arouse it to the point when it can begin to get rid of its troubles and encumbrances. Such treatment may in many cases be good and successful without a differential diagnosis of the orthodox medical type being made at all. However, there are a number of diseases, conditions and symptom complexes which are grave, complicated and sometimes mysterious and difficult either to understand or to treat. Lindlahr recognizes that this is so and that some cases will require to be treated in an institution or sanitorium in which the patient can be watched and given the right kind of attention and care from day to day. Also it is clear that Lindlahr's works are not complete and that he did intend to produce two further volumes, one of which would have given more information on a number of obscure and difficult conditions and the special way in which they should be approached.

There are, for instance, a number of diseases of the central nervous and circulatory systems many of which are regarded as incurable. Lindlahr took the view that we should never regard a particular disease as incurable, though he admits that there may be incurable cases in which the degeneration of cells and tissues has gone too far to be stopped or reversed. In dealing with such conditions it is very desirable to know what the principal factor has been in bringing them about. Is the basic problem simply one of a kind of poisoning due to wrong feeding or poor elimination; is it due to drug poisoning from the suppressive treatment of earlier diseases or other causes; is it due to a specific lack of some essential vitamin or mineral element in the body chemistry; is it due to some endocrine deficiency or imbalance and, if so, what is the cause of that? Obviously if an answer can be found to these questions it is going to be a useful guide in the application of the natural treatments most appropriate to the case. It must also be recognized that inherited and congenital diseases and abnormalities present a special problem. How can these be

291

avoided or prevented from occurring and, if they have occurred, how far can they be treated or cured? Lindlahr quotes some cases in which he obtained very remarkable results in this field which at least give a hint of how such conditions may be caused and how they may be dealt with satisfactorily.

Parasitism is another phenomenon which raises problems. Lindlahr, as we have seen, denies that the ordinary run of acute infectious diseases are parasitic in character, but there are some troubles which seem obviously to be due to parasites, especially in tropical countries. However, even in these cases it is becoming clear that true parasitism may be much rarer than at first appears and is generally believed to be. Lindlahr maintains that people who are thoroughly clean and healthy within and without will not be apt to harbour parasites to any serious extent, and he goes further by contending that in many instances parasites are fulfilling a useful function in the body of the host by assisting a process of elimination or cleaning up. For instance, he quotes cases in which head lice and pubic lice have appeared as part of a healing crisis and have disappeared spontaneously when the crisis was over. There is evidence, too, that intestinal worms live only in an unhealthy intestine and can be made to disappear by dietary, homoeopathic and other measures which do not attack or kill the parasite directly so much as cause it to starve or go away; whereas the giving of powerful vermifuges may be suppressive and very harmful. In the case of malaria too, which is regarded as a purely parasitic disease, Lindlahr maintains that while it may be a good thing to destroy offending mosquitoes as far as possible, the real secret of avoiding and treating malaria is not to be found in the use of drugs for prophylaxis or treatment but in following a largely fruitarian diet and keeping covered at night sufficiently to produce a certain degree of perspiration (see "Iridi-agnosis", Chap. XIII). To what extent this kind of approach is applicable to all forms of parasitism is no doubt a matter which should be the subject of research and enquiry, but it is clear that in dealing with parasites care should be taken not to use means which are damaging to the tissues or body functioning of the host.

Finally, it is certain that much research, study and observation are needed to discover more about the causes of many diseases and chronic conditions, but it is doubtful whether the kind of research which is now being conducted into this disease or that by orthodox medical scientists will generally produce very fruitful results. This research is for the most part too much concerned with pathology rather than health, and with seeking to discover more germs and viruses and more and more drugs. The germs and viruses may indeed be existent and associated with certain diseases, but the much more important question of how and why they have arisen and what causes the body to harbour them is very much neglected. Lindlahr and others have, however, pointed out a number of methods and lines of enquiry which should be kept alive, developed and followed up. For instance, Lindlahr maintained that poliomyelitis was a disease of fairly recent origin and that it was not unconnected with the almost universal introduction of vaccination during the nineteenth century. He also maintained that many of the serious organic diseases of the central nervous system and of other parts and organs of the body were the result of poisoning by drugs used in medication or of contamination of persons engaged in certain trades and occupations. The effects or metals such as mercury, lead and zinc, and probably also aluminium, can be especially bad, but other substances such as iodine, arsenic, quinine, bromides, coal-tar products and sulphur in various inorganic combinations can be responsible for serious chronic conditions. Lindlahr was able to discover the effects of this kind of poisoning in many of his cases by means of iridiagnosis as well as by careful case taking. It is important that the art of iridiagnosis should be kept alive and developed and it also seems that we may be coming to a time when radionic and other new forms of diagnosis will be capable of giving the same kind of information. It is obviously desirable that much more serious attention should be paid by official research bodies and by medical scientists in schools and universities to the clinical results obtained and the theories and methods of treatment advocated and used by individual practitioners both outside and inside the medical profession. These people are in fact carrying out very valuable clinical research and this should be recognized and sympathetically studied and investigated and, if necessary, either confirmed or shown to be valueless or unsound by further research of a more organized kind. Also, when we look at the general picture of medicine as it is practised today we see that many changes and developments have taken place since Lindlahr's time. These should be critically examined and evaluated by those who are interested in Natural Therapeutics to see whether they are good or bad. An enormous number of these changes and developments are undoubtedly impossible to reconcile with the principles laid down by Lindlahr and his school of thought, and can be condemned on the ground that they are suppressive or damaging in one way or another. On the other hand, there are some which may be good and of permanent value and there are others which, although they would appear to be doubtful or wrong in principle, seem to produce results which are apparently very successful and which one must therefore condone or accept at least until such time as a better way can be found. To take some examples: (1) Leprosy is a disease in connection with which the picture seems very much to have changed in recent years. There are some

293

interesting passages in Lindlahr's works in which he affirms, quoting from the writings of Hahnemann, the founder of Homoeopathy, that leprosy is a condition arising basically from the suppression, for many generations, of psora. He no doubt would have treated leprosy in the same way as any other chronic condition, but it must be acknowledged that the present form of treatment by sulphur drugs appears to have produced a striking measure of success. Such treatment must undoubtedly be suppressive and we do not know what the long-term effects of it may be, but, in the meanwhile, it is perhaps hard to say that it should not be used until something better can be found, tested and put into general use. (2) In the realm of so-called immunology an enormous number of vaccines and serums have been elaborated in the last fifty years and are very widely used. Here again there can be very little doubt that practically all of them are to be deplored from the point of view of Natural Therapeutics and there is even much room for uncertainty as to their effectiveness for the purpose for which they are intended. Lindlahr affirms that orthodox vaccine and serum treatments constitute an aberration, distortion or mis-application of homoeopathic principles and methods and it is along genuine homoeopathic lines that we may hope to bring about a greater degree of immunity of a specific kind to a number of diseases. It may be noted that there does seem to be a slight sign that some immunologists are beginning to move in the homoeopathic direction by such things as greater attenuation and administration per mouth (see notes and appendix in Vol. 1). (3) The very wide use of blood transfusions in all sorts of circumstances is something which has become a very important part of treatment in all modern hospitals. While it would seem that there are occasions on which it saves life there are obvious objections to it and there is a strong probability that it is being overused. There are practitioners who maintain that, if transfusion does seem desirable, the use of normal saline is as good or better in most cases, if not in all.

In conclusion, it may be affirmed that a very much wider understanding and use of homoeopathy and of herbal medication could lead to a realization that symptoms can be controlled in a manner which does not suppress, involve bad side effects or long-term effects, or add to the toxicity with which the body has to contend.

REFERENCE INDEX

APPENDICITIS—fasting imperative in appendicitis, 24.
APPETITE—loss of appetite indicates need for fasting, 68.
ARMY—use of serums, a case, 4–6.
ARSENIC—produces congenital defects in offspring, 168; poisoning, treatment, (h) 258; poisoning, antidotes, 260; injurious effect of arsenic on teeth, 273.
ARTERIES—where to apply ligature in case of severed artery, 253; where to apply pressure in cases of injury to artery in various parts of the body, 254–256.
ARTIFICIAL RESPIRATION—description and illustration of various methods, 240–242.
ASPARAGUS TEA—directions for making, 104.
ASPHYXIATION—suffocation, treatment, 242–243.
ASTIGMATISM—natural method of curing astigmatism, 134.
AUTHOR—history of author's son, 37–41.
AUTOINTOXICATION—caused by meat, white bread, coffee and white sugar, 55; caused by inactivity of eliminating organs, 136; cause of insanity, 171–172.
AUTOPSIES—failure of medical diagnoses in Mass. General Hospital as shown by autopsies, 20.

BABY—umbilical cord, 214; care of the newborn, 215; bathing, cold baths, 216; injurious effect of powders, oil, creams, 216; air baths, 216; constipation and diarrhoea, 217; bandages, clothing, 217; diapers, 217–218; wet nurse, 218; care of eyes, mouth, ears, nose, 218; care of genital organs, 219; how to lift the baby, 219; prenatal feeding of baby, 219–223; normal weight of newborn, 222; feeding has improved in last ten years, 223; bottle-fed babies, 223; why rachitis is common among babies, 223; the right way to feed babies, 225–227; when and how to feed, 227; grain extracts for baby, constipation and diarrhoea, 228; baby's natural medicines, 228; weaning, 228–229; feeding after first year, 229–231; exercises for baby, 231; high chair and toys, 232.
BABY'S AILMENTS—hernias, umbilical, ventral, congenital, 233–234; colic, 234; convulsions, 235; ailments of teething, 235; acute catarrhal diseases, 235–236; convulsions, 247–248.
BACTERIA—develop from microzymes, 2.
BANDAGES—wet bandages, how made and applied, 87; vinegar and Epsom salt, 88; head, throat, chest, trunk, 90–91; for baby's navel, 217; triangular bandage, figure of eight bandage, roller bandage, double roll bandage, T bandage, 243–245.
BAREFOOT WALKING—outdoor, 81; indoor, 81; magnetic effects of barefoot walking, 108.
BATHS—morning air and cold water, 10; cold water bath in acute disease, 26–28; foot bath, leg bath, 81; limb bath, 82; upper and lower body bath, 82; hip bath, cold morning bath, sitz bath, head bath, 82–83; tepid bath, tepid sitz bath, warm and hot bath, Turkish, Russian and electric light bath, 84–85; bed sweat bath, 85–86; mud or clay bath, 94–95; Epsom salt bath and sitz bath, 96–97; how to take an air bath, 106–107; sun bath, 107–108.
BATHING—outdoor bathing and swimming, 81; injurious effects of warm bathing, 104; baby, cold baths, 216; air bath, 216–217.
BECHAMP—discoverer of microzymes and their relation to disease, 2.
BED—breathing exercises, 113–114.
BEDTIME—value of pre-midnight sleep, 17.
BELLADONNA—poisoning, treatment, (g) 258.
BILIOUS—vomiting in fasting, 74–75; headaches, cause and treatment, 142–143.
BIRTH AGE—definition, effect on offspring, 194–195.
BIRTH CONTROL—as affected by economic independence of mothers, 195–196; many methods injurious, natural means the only safe and legitimate way, 200–201 and Appendix II.
BIRTHMARKS—denied by medical men, 205–206; how to guard against, 205–206.
BIRTH RANK—determined by birth age of offspring, 194.
BITES—of animals, treatment, 245–246.

BLEEDING—internal bleeding, 253; from cuts and wounds, how to stop, 253–256; from nose, 257.

BLINDNESS—often caused by poisons absorbed from dandruff cures and hair tonics, 83.

BLOOD—chronic patients improving under natural treatment show decrease in white and increase of red corpuscles, 3; richness of blood depends on positive mineral elements, 55; circulation stimulated by cold water, 79–80; table of comparative blood analyses, animal and human, 221.

BODY—whole body pack, 89–90.

BOTTLE-FED BABIES—223.

BOWELS—normal frequency of movements, 136; injurious effects of laxatives and carthartics, 136–137; causes of constipation, 137; see also Intestines.

BRAIN—effect of pathogenic materials on brain, 207; insensibility from concussion of brain, treatment, 251–252; moulding likened to the making of phonographic records, 206.

BREAKFAST—fruit and vegetable breakfast, 58; when luncheon foods should be taken for breakfast, 58; raw food breakfast, 59; milk breakfast, 66.

BREAKING—of water bag, 214.

BREATHING—laboured breathing (dyspnoea) danger symptom in fever, 27–28; bad effects of shallow breathing, 109–110; general directions for corrective breathing exercises, 110–111; proper standing position, 111; breathing exercises, 111–113; diaphragmatic breathing, 113; internal massage, 113; exercises in bed, 113–114; rhythmical breathing, 114; alternate breathing, 115; warning in connection with Yoga breathing, 115–116; methods of restoring breathing, 240–242.

BRIGHT'S DISEASE—treatment of convulsions in, 248.

BRONCHITIS—treatment of acute breathing in baby, 234–236.

BRUISES—treatment, 246.

BRUSH—dry brush rub, 108.

BUMPS—treatment, 246.

BURNS—treatment, 246–247.

CABBAGE—how to cook, 56.

CABOT, Dr.—on inaccuracy of diagnoses in Mass. Gen. Hosp., 20.

CALOMEL—effects of on intestinal tract, 137.

CANCER—case cured by natural treatment, 19; how to treat haemorrhage caused by cancer of stomach, 253.

CARBOLIC ACID—poisoning, treatment, (h) 258–259; poisoning, antidotes, 260.

CARRYING—an unconscious person, 262–264.

CAR SICKNESS—remedy for, 260–261.

CAT-BITES, treatment, 245–246.

CATARACT—due to pathogenic obstruction, 132–133.

CATHARTICS—effects of cathartics and laxatives, 136–137.

CAULIFLOWER—how to cook, 57.

CAUSTIC ACIDS—poisoning, antidotes, 260.

CEREALS—whole grain cereal necessary to health, 55.

CEREBRO-SPINAL—relation of cerebro-spinal nervous system to the pelvic outlets of body, 145.

CHEMICAL—causes of nervous diseases, 156–158.

CHEST—bandage and pack, 91.

CHILD-BEARING—not dangerous under natural methods of living and treatment, 201.

CHILDBIRTH—coccygeal lesions sustained at childbirth, 153–154; three stages of labour, 212–213; safety and ease of childbirth under natural living, 213–214; preparation for delivery, 214; no anaesthetics, 214; breaking of water bag, 214; umbilical cord, 214; afterbirth, 215; lying-in period, 215; care of newborn, 214–216; suffering in childbirth not God-ordained, 219–220; childbirth among primitive peoples, 219–220.

CHILDREN—examination in schools show 85 per cent with defective teeth, 264–265.

297

CHILLS—cold water treatment, 44.

CHLOROFORM—treatment for insensibility from, 251–252.

CHOKING—methods for removing objects in throat, 247.

CHRONIC DISEASES—treated by uniform methods, 51; treatments to be applied by patient and by Natural Therapist, 51–52; list of chronic diseases, 52–53.

CLAY—packs, 93–94; baths, 94–95.

CIRCULATION—stimulated by cold water, 79–80.

CIRCUMCISION—barbarous and unnecessary practice, 146–147.

CLITORIS—hooded clitoris, natural treatment, 147–148.

CLOTHING—injurious effects of tight clothing, 109; during pregnancy, 210; for baby, 217.

COCCYGEAL—relaxation, 154–155.

COCCYGEAL LESIONS—anatomy, occurrence of, 153; causes of, 153–154; effects of, 154.

COFFEE—injurious influence on system, 55, 279.

COLD FEET—cure for, 81.

COLDS—flaxseed tea and rutabagas as remedies for, 26; bed sweat bath for, 29; practical application of natural treatment for colds, 42–47; treatment of babies' colds, 235–236.

COLD WATER—why we favour, 79; see also Hydrotherapy.

COLIC—cause and treatment, 234.

COLLAPSE—causes, treatment, 251–252.

COLON—flushing, directions, 101; flushing in constipation, 141.

COMPRESS—extra compress in local inflammation under pack, 30; hot compress or fomentation, when indicated, 86–87; vinegar and Epsom salt, 88; potato, 88; eye, 92; Epsom salt, 96.

CONCEPTION—prevention of disease must begin with conception and mating, 192; how it occurs, 208.

CONCUSSION—of brain, treatment of insensibility from, 251–252.

CONDIMENTS—injurious, 55–56.

CONGENITAL—mental and emotional disorders, 168; deficiency of ductless glands, 170.

CONGESTION—how cold packs relieve inner congestion, 31–32.

CONSTIPATION—caused by white bread, coffee, meat and white sugar, 55; why milk causes constipation, 61; use of enemas in, 98; importance of manipulative treatment in, how administered, 98–99; general prevalence of chronic constipation, often result of medical treatment, 136; effects of laxatives and purgatives, 136–137; causes of, 137–139; remarkable case, 139; effects of constipation, appendicitis, autointoxication, etc., 139–140; treatment, diet, 140–141; a natural laxative, 140–141; colon flushing only a beginning of treatment, 141; hydrotherapy for, 141; exercises for, 141; massage, neurotherapy, 141; cure of constipation aided by rectal dilatation, 142; treatment of constipation in babies, 217.

CONTROL OF HEREDITY—Redfield quotation, 196.

CONTUSIONS—treatment, 246.

CONVULSIONS—of baby, cause and treatment, 235; cause, general treatment, 247–248; of infants, 248; uraemic convulsions, 248; epileptic convulsions, 250.

COOKING—vegetables, 56–57.

COPPER—poisoning, antidotes, 260.

CORD—umbilical, 214.

CORNARO—experience of with limited food allowance, 68–69.

CORROSIVE SUBLIMATE—treatment for poisoning by, 258.

CORSETS—how injurious, 109–110.

COTTON MOUTH—in fasting, 74.

COUGH—flaxseed tea and rutabagas as remedies for, 26; treatment for baby's cough, 235–236.

CRETINISM—(Idiocy) caused by mercury, salvarsan, arsenic, iodine, potassium, etc., 168.

CROUP—flaxseed tea, etc., as remedies, 26; form of elimination, treatment, 235–236.

CUTS—treatment, 248–249; haemorrhages from, 253; how to stop bleeding from, 253–256.

DANDRUFF—form of elimination, danger of "cures", 83–84.
DANGER—point in fever, 44–45; signals in fasting, 70–71.
DEAD—tests to determine whether dead, 251.
DEAFNESS—often caused by dandruff cures and hair tonics, 83–84.
DELIRIUM TREMENS—description and treatment, 238–239.
DELIVERY—ease of under natural living, cases cited, 213; preparation for, 214; no anaesthetics, 214; breaking of water bag, 214; umbilical cord, 214; after delivery, 214–215.
DENTIST—mainly considers attacks on teeth from without, 264–265; teeth should be examined every six months, 270; dentist contracts paresis from mixing amalgam in bare hands, 273.
DETERMINATION—of sex, 201 and Appendix III.
DEW—walking, 81.
DIAGNOSIS—statistics of medical diagnosis, 20 and Appendix IV.
DIAPERS—care of, 217–218.
DIAPHRAGMATIC—breathing, exercises, 113.
DIARRHOEA—treatment of in babies, 217.
DIET—correct diet for wholesome living, 11–13; proper proportions of various kinds of food, 12–13; effects of wrong diet, 53–54; wholesome diet of European peasants, 54; proper proportions of foods, 54; number of eggs per week, 55; proteins, 55; general vegetarian diet, sample menus, 57–59; raw food diet, menus, 59; dry diet, 60; milk diet, 60–63; straight milk diet, 64; milk diet for fleshy people, 64; buttermilk diet, 64–65; sour milk, clabber or sumik diet, 65; natural milk diet, 65; milk and acid fruit diet, 65; milk and fruit diet, 65–66; exclusive meat diet, 66; Salisbury meat diet, 66–67; combination meat and vegetable diet, 67; modified meat and vegetable diet, 67; hot water drinking in meat diet, 67; for constipation, 140–141; effect of diet during pregnancy, 219–222; table of percentages of minerals in cow's milk and other materials, 221; influence of diet on the teeth, 265.
DIGESTION—and assimilation at standstill during fasting, 24.
DIGITALIS—poisoning, treatment, (g) 258.
DILATATION—beneficial effects of dilatation of sphincter muscles, 145–146; of the lower orifices of the body, 148–149; technique of rectal dilatation, 150; mechanical dilatation, 150–151; dilatation of sphincters and tubes of genital organs, 151–152; dilatation of sphincters of female organs, 152–153; dilatation by neurotherapy, 153; of nasal orifices, 155.
DILATORS—how to use rectal dilators, 151.
DINNER—vegetarian dinner combinations, 59.
DIPHTHERIA—quickly relieved by wet packs, 31–32.
DISEASE—regimen for prevention of, 9–18; uniformity of acute disease makes possible uniform treatment, 20–21; natural treatment may be applied from beginning, 20–21; fresh air of special importance in acute disease, 22–23; effect of mental and emotional attitude on acute disease, 34–36; effect of mental and emotional attitude of friends and relatives, 36; how to treat sudden onset of disease, 249–250.
DISEASES—list of acute diseases, 49; list of chronic diseases, 52–53; baby's diseases, 233–236; see also Nervous Diseases.
DISLOCATIONS—first aid, 262.
DISTILLED—water, injurious, 76.
DIZZINESS—often caused by poisons absorbed from dandruff cures and hair tonics, 83–84.
Dr. X—history of esperience with serums in army, 4–6.
DOG—bites, treatment, 245–246.
DRINK—morning, 10.
DRINKING—general principles of right eating and drinking, 11–13; flushing fad a mistake, 14; cause of abnormal thirst, 14–15; amount of water necessary, 15; at meals, 15; excessive drinking in febrile diseases weakening, dilute fruit juices used, 25–26; water should be natural temperature, never very cold or hot, 57; hot water drinking in fasting, 73–74.

DROPSICAL SWELLING—during pregnancy, 211.
DROWNING—resuscitation, 240–242.
DRUGS—as cause of insanity, 175–176; insensibility from drugs, treatment, 251–252.
DRUG POISONS—cause of chronic headaches, treatment, 145; produce congenital defects in offspring, 168–169.
DRY—diet, 60; brush rub, 108.
DUCTLESS GLANDS—congenital deficiency of ductless glands in relation to insanity, 170.
DYES—hair dyes poisonous, often affects brain, 83–84.
DYSENTERY—fasting imperative in dysentery, 24.
DYSPEPSIA—little known among peasants in Europe, 54.
DYSPNOEA—(laboured breathing) danger sign in fever, 27–28.

EARS—care of baby's ears, 218; foreign bodies in, 250.
EARTH—magnetism, with air bath, 108.
EATING—general principles of right eating, 11–13; suppresses healing crises, 72–73.
EGGS—how many, 55; when and how to be given to children, 229.
ELECTRIC LIGHT BATHS—85.
ELECTROMAGNETIC—effect of cold water, 32–33; forces in body increased by positive attitude of mind and will, 34–35; effects of cold water, 78–80; effect of salts in sea water, 81.
ELIMINATION—of waste and morbid matter during fast, 24; promoted by cold packs, 32; active elimination of vital importance in fasting, 75–76; of impurities by cold water, 79; importance of skin for elimination shown in iris, 105–106.
EMETICS—in case of poisoning, (b) 258.
EMOTIONAL—effect of mental and emotional attitude of friends of patient, 34–36; causes of nervous diseases, 159–167; disorders, see Insanity.
EMOTIONS—effect of emotions upon disease, 34; destructive emotions poison body secretions, 34–35.
ENEMAS—in acute disease, 30–31, 43; cold water enemas dangerous, 32; habitually taken have weakening effect on intestines, 98; should only be used when specially indicated, 98; danger from cold enemas, 99; temperature of, 99–100; positions for application of enemas, 100–101; knee-chest position, 100–101; directions for giving enemas, and for colon flushing 100–101; use in acute diseases, 101–102; while fasting, 102; use of enemas in constipation, 140–141; in cases of poisoning, (b, c) 258.
ENVY—Injurious effects of, 165.
EPIDEMICS—explained, 3–4.
EPILEPSY—treatment of insensibility and convulsions from, 250, 251–252.
EPSOM SALT (MgSO₄)—treatment, 30, 95–97; bandages and compresses, 88; has tendency to form deposits, a case, 95; how to eliminate accumulations caused by use of sodium, magnesium, etc., 96; use of Epsom salts sometimes temporarily advantageous, 96; baths, packs and compresses, 96–97; whole body rub, 97.
ETHER—treatment for insensibility from, 251–252.
EXERCISES—daily, 10; while fasting, 74; sweating by exercises, 86; breathing exercises, 111–112; diaphragmatic breathing, 113; internal massage, 113; breathing exercises in bed, 113–114; rhythmical breathing exercises, 114–115; alternate breathing exercises, 115; philosophy of exercises, 116–117; general rules for physical exercises, 119–120; corrective exercises, 120–122; for muscles of abdomen and ribs, 120; for chest stretching, 121; for scrawny necks and hollow chests, 121; for muscles of chest and upper arm, 121; for sluggish liver, 121; for strengthening abdominal muscles and pelvic organs, 122; supplementary exercises, 122–123; for reducing flesh, 123–124; for invalids, 124; beneficial effects of exercises increased by use of intelligence and will power, 125–126; effects of psychological exercises on mental and psychical ailments, 126–127; natural exercises, 127–128; eye exercises, 135–136; for constipation, 141; during pregnancy, 209–210; in infancy, 231–232.
EYE—bath, 10; potato compress, 92; constitutional causes of diseases of eye, 132–133;

cataract due to pathogenic deposits, 133; aims of natural eye treatment, 133; water treatment, 133–134; massage and vibratory treatment, 134; massage, 134–135; eye gymnastics, 135–136; trouble caused by uric acid, 142; danger of resorting to glasses, 142; care of baby's eyes, 218.

EYE INJURIES—burns, 246–247; black eye from external injury, treatment, 250; removal of foreign bodies, 251; inflammation, 250; perforating wounds, 251.

FAINTING—how to determine whether life extinct and cause of fainting, treatment, 251–252; alcoholic liquors dangerous, 252.

FAST—breaking the fast, 25; of six weeks in typhoid-malaria, 24.

FASTING—of primary importance in acute febrile conditions, 23; why fasting is necessary, 24; used to cure colds, headaches, etc., 68; experience of Cornaro, 68; physiology of, 69–70; examples of long fasting, 70; danger signals in fasting, 70–71; how long, 71; danger of too long fasting, 71; preparation for, 72; fruit juices in fasting, 73; hot water drinking in, 73–74; exercises while fasting, 74; gas formation, temperature, cotton mouth, 74; bilious vomiting, 74–75; offensive perspiration, 75; fear of fasting unfounded, 75–76; regimen, 75–77; importance of keeping elimination active, 75–76; necessary to economize vitality in fasting, 76; distilled water injurious, 76; the regular fast, 76; dry fast, 76–77; seven day fast, 77; long fast, 77; breaking the fast, 77–78; use of enemas in fasting, 102; in cases of acute poisoning, (d) 258; for tooth-ache, 272.

FAT—excessive fat formation in pregnancy, 222; fat babies not normal, 222.

FATHER—age at conception of offspring is called birth age, 194; chances of offspring better as age of father advances, 195.

FATS—proper proportion to be used in diet, 55.

FEAR—effect upon heart action and respiration, 34; fear of fasting unfounded, 75; a cause of nervous diseases, 160–162; is faith in evil, 161–162.

FEEDING—artificial feeding of infants, orthodox methods, 223–225; the right way, 225–227; when to feed, 227; how to feed, 227; night feeding, 228; amount of food, 228; grain extracts for baby, 228; feeding after first year, 229–231.

FEMALE ORGANS—dilatation of sphincters, 152–153.

FEVER—cold water treatment, 26–33; must not be checked or suppressed, 27; danger symptoms, 27–28; subnormal temperature, 28; management of packs in high fever, 88.

FIRST AID—alcoholism, 237–239; apoplexy, 239–240; artificial respiration, 240–242; asphyxiation, 242–243; bandages, 243–245; bites, 245–246; bruises, bumps, contusions, 246; burns and scalds, 246–247; choking, 247; convulsions, 247–248; cuts and wounds, 248–249; sudden onset of disease, 249–250; foreign bodies in ears and nose, 250; epileptic convulsions, 250; signs of life, 251; exhaustion, 252–253; haemorrhages, 253–256; hiccough, 256; lightning stroke, 256; mania, 257; mental disorders, 257; nose bleed, 257; poisoning, 257–260; shock, 261; sprains, strains, dislocations, 262; sunburns, 262; sunstroke, 262; thermic fever, 262; transporting injured, 262–264; unconsciousness, 251–252.

FIXED IDEA—see Monomania.

FLAXSEED TEA—valuable in colds, croup and catarrhal diseases, 26.

FLOUR—white, deficient in minerals, vitamins, ferments, 55; whole grain flour necessary to health, 55.

FLUSHING—directions for colon flushing, 101.

FOCI—of infection and their suppression, 270–271.

FOMENTATIONS—hot fomentations or compresses, when indicated, how applied, 86–87.

FOOD—see Fasting; fallacy of strengthening patient by nourishing food or stimulants during acute fevers, 23; vital force not derived from, 23; should not be taken when over-tired or excited, 57; raw food diet, 59; dry food diet, 60; destructive effect of food on teeth, 265–266, 268–269.

FOODS—proper proportions of various kinds of food, 11–13.

301

FOOT—cold foot bath, 81; spray, 81; sweat must not be suppressed, 81.
FOOT, Dr. A. F.—report on children's teeth, 265.
FRACTURES—procedure, 252; fractures of the skull, 252.
FREEZING—treatment of person unconscious through freezing, 252.
FRUITS—raw fruits after fast, 25; juices of acid fruits in water natural tonic in acute diseases; 25–26; proper proportion to be used in diet, 55; juicy fruits and leafy vegetables not improved by cooking, 56; juices of fruits in fasting, 73; acid and subacid fruits not destructive of teeth, 268.
FUNCTIONAL—disorders cause of insanity, 171.

GAS—formation in fasting, 74; asphyxiation by gas, treatment, 251–252.
GASTRITIS—fasting imperative, 24.
GENERAL—regimen for wholesome living, 9–18.
GENITAL ORGANS—dilatation of tubes of, 151–152; care of baby's genital organs, 219.
GERM—allopathic germ theory of disease, 1; new theory of germ activity, 2–3.
GINGIVITIS—an ailment of the teeth, allopathic explanation, 266; description, 267–8; rational treatment, 268; prevention, 268–269.
GYMNASTICS—eye gymnastics, 135–136.

HAIR—cause of loss or discolouration, 83; tonics, dandruff or eczema cures, or hair dyes dangerous, 83–84; hair should be cut in first quarter of moon, 84 note.
HEAD—treatment for excessive pain in head, 45; bath, 83; bandages for headaches and earaches, 90; bandage described, 245.
HEADACHE—often caused by dandruff cures and hair tonics, 83–84; body and other packs better than head bandages, 90; a symptom of disease, 142; wearing of glasses often prevents removal of underlying causes, 142; uric acid common cause of headache and eye trouble, 142; migraine, 142; bilious or sick headache, 142–144; anaemic headache, cause and treatment, 144; nervous, 144; caused by mechanical lesions and drug poisons, 144–145.
HEALING—mental and spiritual, 188–191.
HEALING CRISES—suppressed by eating, 72–73.
HEART—how to stimulate heart action, 251–252.
HEAT—radiation promoted by cold packs, 31.
HEAT EXHAUSTION—causes, symptoms, treatment, 252–253.
HAEMORRHAGE—how to determine where haemorrhage is located, 253; from the mouth, 253; from the lungs, 253; from cuts and wounds, treatments described and illustrated, 253–256.
HAEMORRHOIDS—benefitted by rectal dilatation, 151.
HEREDITARY—mental and emotional disorders, 168.
HEREDITY—use heredity, 194–197; pernicious heredity, 197.
HERNIA—umbilical, 233; ventral, 233–234; congenital, 234.
HICCOUGH—cause and treatment, 256.
HIGH CHAIR—when and how to be used for baby, 232.
HINDUS—racial purity in higher castes, 194.
HOODED CLITORIS—description, natural treatment, 147–148.
HOT—food and drink, 13–14; hot baths weakening and enervating, 85; hot water applications injurious in inflammation, 28–29; compresses or fomentations, when indicated, how applied, 86–87.
HOT WATER—drinking, 67; drinking and fasting, 73–74; applications not to be used in acute conditions, 249–250.
HYDROCHLORIC ACID—poisoning, treatment, (h) 258–259.
HYDROTHERAPY—in acute disease accomplishes beneficial effects ascribed to drugs, 26–27; objects to be obtained by hydrotherapy, 26–27; baths and ablutions, 27–29; enemas, 30–31; danger of suppression of inflammation and fever by cold water, 44;

good effects of cold water, 79; stimulation of circulation, 79; why we favour cold water, 79–80; danger of prolonged or excessively cold applications, 80; outdoor bathing and swimming, 81; foot and leg bath, barefoot walking, 81; indoor water treading, 81; foot spray, 81; partial ablutions, 81; limb bath, 82; upper and lower body baths, 82; hip bath, 82; morning cold rub, 82–83; evening sitz bath, 83; head bath, 83–84; water treatment for eyes, 133–134; for constipation, 141; in orificial treatment, 155; value in pregnancy, 213–214; cold water treatment for toothache, 271–272.

LEG BATH—instructions for, 81.
LEMON—juice should be used for salads, promotes digestion, 55; valuable as a dentifrice, 269–270.
LESIONS—158–159; see also Coccygeal Lesions.
LETTER—from Dr. X in army hospital, 4–6.
LEUCOCYTES—true nature and function, 3.
LIFE—tests to determine whether life is extinct, 251.
LIFE FORCE—independent of physical body, 69; source of life force, 69; how acquired, 110.
LIGATURES—how to apply in cases of wounds, venous and arterial, 253–254.
LIGHTNING STROKE—burns from lightning stroke, 246, 256; shock on collapse, 256, 261.
LIMITATION OF OFFSPRING—injurious effects of many methods, 200–201; poisonous antiseptics dangerous, only natural methods safe, 201.
LONGEVITY—various opinions regarding longevity, 274–277.
LOVE—creative alchemy of love, 197; importance of love in production of perfect offspring, 198–199.
LUNCHEON—foods, 58; limited variety best, 58; combinations, 58; raw food luncheon, 59; milk luncheon, 65–66.
LUNGS—effect of corsets and tight skirt bands on lungs, 109; relation of lungs to the body, 108; process of breathing, 109; how to distinguish haemorrhage from lung, treatment, 253.
LYE—poisoning, treatment, (h) 258–259.
LYING-IN—period, 215.

MAD DOG—bite, treatment, 245–246.
MAGNETISM—of earth, good effects in connection with air bath, 108.
MALNUTRITION—long standing malnutrition and indigestion need sanatorium treatment, 57.
MANIA—causes, treatment, 257.
MANIPULATIVE—treatment in acute disease, 46–47; treatment for constipation, how applied, 98–99; treatment for retention of urine, 102; treatment for constipation, 141–142; treatment for bilious or sick headache, illustrated, 142–144; for anaemic headache, illustrated, 144.
MARRIAGE—early marriage detrimental to offspring, 194; advantages of later marriage, 194–196; importance of love as a basis, 198–199; comparison of peoples marrying early and late in life, 196.
MASSAGE—internal massage, exercise, illustrated, 113; massage and vibratory treatment for eyes, 134; massage movements for eyes, 134–135; for constipation, 141–142; movements for toothache, 272.
MASTICATION—thorough mastication important, 57.
MATING—prevention of disease must begin with conception and mating, 191; importance of correct mating, 193; should take place only between descendants of same sub-race, 193–194.
MEALS—frequency of, 13; heavy meal not best between working hours, 57.
MEAT—exclusive meat diet, 66; Salisbury meat diet, 66–67; hot water drinking with meat diet, 67; danger from meat diet, 67; combination meat and vegetable diets, 67; detrimental to children, 230; influence on age, 279.
MECHANICAL—causes of nervous diseases, 158–159.
MECHANICAL LESIONS—cause of headaches, treatment, 144–145.
MEDICAL—practice in army, effects of serums, treatment in hospital, 4–7.
MENSTRUATION—cold water treatment during menstruation, 46 and Appendix I.
MENTAL—adjustment, 9; attitude, 16; power increased by concentration of will, 35; effect of attitude of friends of patients, 36; ailments benefited by psychological exercises, 126–127; mental and emotional causes of nervous diseases, 159–160; mental and

emotional disorders due to organic degeneration of brain and nerve matter, 176–177; mental healing, 188; prenatal influence, 203–205; mental disorders, 257; see also Insanity.

MENUS—sample vegetarian menus, 57–59; raw food menus, 59–60.

MERCURY—produces congenital defects in offspring, 168; injurious effect of mercury on teeth, 273; amalgam filling contains 50% of mercury, 273; serious results produced on system by amalgam fillings, 273; absorbed by dentists from mixing amalgam in bare palm, paresis resulting, 273.

MEXICO—mongrelized population of Mexico example of miscegenation, 194.

MICROZYMES—relation to disease germs, 2; relation to germ activity, 2–3; in serums, antitoxins and vaccines develop into bacteria, 6; of procreative elements as a factor in use heredity, 194.

MIGRAINE—uric acid headache, 142.

MILK—diet, 60; analysis of cow's milk and human milk, 60; effect of food on milk, 60; effect of long continued forced milk feeding, 61; why milk causes constipation, 61; acid fruit juices and milk, 62; injurious effects of Weir-Mitchell treatment, 62–63; importance of purifying blood and tissues before prescribing milk diet, 63; straight milk diet, 64; milk diet for fleshy people, 64; buttermilk diet, 64–65; sour milk diet, 65; natural milk diet, 65; milk and fruit diets, 65–66; table of comparative percentages of mineral in cow's milk and other food materials, 221; more sodium, calcium and iron in cow's than in human milk, 223; milk from healthy cow better for infants than impoverished milk of scrofulous mothers, 224; cow's milk should not have additions of water, salt, soda and inorganic lime, 224; why the "top milk" mixture not good for babies, 224–225.

MIND—influence of mind in acute disease, 34; effect of positive attitude on electromagnetic forces, 35.

MISCEGENATION—evil results of, 193–194.

MONGREL—disapproved by nature, 193–194; Mexican population, 194.

MONOMANIA—causes, effects, 178–180; treatment, a case, 181.

MORAL—power increased by concentration of will, 35.

MORBID—accumulations develop bacteria and parasites, 2–3; matter eliminated during fast, 24; materials eliminated through skin by packs, 32.

MORNING—drink, 10; cold rub and air bath, walk, 10.

MORNING SICKNESS—during pregnancy, 211–212.

MORPHINE—poisoning, treatment, (g) 258.

MORTALITY—in 1918 epidemic greater in soldiers than civilian population, 6–7; comparison of mortality from disease and wounds in late war, 7.

MOTHER—influences offspring through use heredity, prenatal influence and postnatal training, 194–195; reproductive function best below thirty-five years, 195; why statistics seem to prove birth age of mother less important than that of father, 195–196; benefits to offspring of increased professional and commercial activity of mother, 195; economic independence will help solve birth control problem, 196; sexual intercourse during pregnancy crime against mother and child, 199–200; prenatal influence of mother, how effected, 202–205; pathological condition of mother's blood has injurious effect on infant in womb, 207–208.

MOUTH—cotton mouth in fasting, 74; care of baby's mouth, 218; haemorrhages from, 253.

MUCOID MATTER—all acute diseases start with obstruction by mucoid matter, 3.

MUD—and clay treatment, 93–94; baths, 94–95.

MURIATIC ACID—poisoning, antidotes, 260.

MUSHROOMS—poisoning, treatment, (g) 258.

NAP—noon-day, 17–18.

NAPOLEON BONAPARTE—example of prenatal influence, 205.

NARCOTIC—poisoning, treatment, (g) 258.

NASAL—dilatation of nasal orifices, cold water sniffing, 155.

NATURAL REGIMEN—9-18; advantages in pregnancy, 222-223.

NATURAL THERAPEUTICS—What it is, 1; explanation of germ activity, 1-2; shows marvellous results in acute diseases, 19-20; teaches prevention as well as treatment of disease, 191-192.

NATURAL TREATMENT—in acute diseases, 19-21; of acute diseases insures largest percentage of recoveries, 21; leaves no chronic after-effects, 21; Otto Lindlahr's case, 37-41; practical application of natural treatment in acute diseases, 42-47; treatment for pain in head, 45; in mild fever and low temperature, 45-46; for constipation, 140-142.

NERVE—various causes of nerve waste, 148-149; how to stop the leaks, 149-150.

NERVOUS—disorders traced to use of foot powders and antiseptic washes, 81; headaches, 144.

NERVOUS DISEASES—chemical causes of, 156-158; mechanical causes of, 158-159; mental and emotional causes of, 159-160.

NERVOUSNESS—what is it, 156.

NEURALGIA—often caused by poisons absorbed from dandruff cures and hair tonics, 83-84.

NEURASTHENIA—Chicago nerve specialist's definition of, 156.

NEURITIC TOOTHACHE—cause, treatment, 272-273.

NEUROTHERAPY—what it includes, 47.

NEW—interpretation of acute disease, 3-4.

NEWBORN—care of, 215-219.

NIPPLES—care of, 218.

NITRATE OF SILVER—poisoning, antidotes, 260.

NITRIC ACID—poisoning, antidotes, 260.

NOSE—care of baby's nose, 218; foreign bodies in, see Ears, 250; nose bleed, treatment, 257.

OLD—no need to grow old if living in harmony with Nature's laws, 274; differing opinions as to growing old, 274-277.

PACKS—whole body or sheet packs in fever, 29; alternating packs, 29; bed-sweat bath, 29-30; purpose of wet packs, 30; number of wrappings at varying temperatures, 30; protection of bedding, 30; oilcloth or rubber coverings not to be used, 30; local compresses with packs, 30; how cold packs promote heat radiation, 31; how cold packs relieve inner congestion, 31-32; how cold packs promote elimination, 32; effects of whole body packs in a case of pneumonia, 41-42; how used in influenza, cold, pneumonia, etc., 43-44; alternating packs, renewal, 44; in case of chills, 44; ablutions after packs, 44; procedure in great weakness, 44; danger in reducing temperature too rapidly, 44; use of packs as temperature declines, 45; in case of pain in the head, 45; in mild fever and low temperature, 45-46; use during menstruation, 46; number of wet wrappings, 46; cleansing the packs, 46; wet packs, how made and applied, 87; number of wet and dry wrappings, 88; how often renewed, 88; whole body pack illustrated, 89; throat, chest, trunk packs illustrated, 91-92; ankle, knee, hand, leg and T packs illustrated, 91-92; shoulder or Scotch pack illustrated, 93; clay pack, 93-94; Epsom salt packs, 97; wet packs for toothache, 271-272.

PAINKILLERS—danger of use for toothache, 272.

PARANOIA—causes and treatment, 178-180.

PARAPHYMOSIS—description, natural treatment, 147.

PARIS GREEN—poisoning, treatment, (h) 258-259.

PATHOGEN—see Morbid.

PEASANT—diet of European peasant, obviates need for dentists, 54.

PEPPER—injurious, 55.

PERITONITIS—fasting imperative in, 24.

PERNICIOUS—heredity, 197.

PERSPIRATION—offensive perspiration in fasting, 75.

PHILOSOPHY—of exercise, 116–117.

PHIMOSIS—natural treatment, 146–147.

PHOTOGRAPHIC RECORDS—making of photographic records likened to brain moulding, 206–207.

PHOSPHORUS—poisoning, treatment, (h) 258–259; poisoning, antidotes, (k) 260.

PHYSICAL—power increased by concentration of will, 35.

PHYSICAL INFLUENCE—prenatal, 206–207; a case, 208.

PHYSIOLOGY—of exercise, 118–120; of fasting 69–70.

PLACENTA—does not filter poisons from blood of mother, 207–208.

PNEUMONIA—natural treatment, my first case, 41–42; practical application of natural treatment, 42–47.

POISONING—emptying stomach, (a) 257–258; emetics and enemas, (b) 258; corrosive sublimate, (c) 258; fasting, (d) 258; antidotes, (e, f, g, h) 258–259; ptomaine poisoning, (i) 259; external poisoning from poison ivy, oak and sumac, (j) 259; antidotes for acute poisoning by lead, phosphorus, caustic acids, copper, etc., (k) 260.

POPCORN—used in breaking fast, 25, 77.

POSITIVE—effects of positive attitude of mind and will, 35–36.

POTATO—compress, 88, 92.

POWDERS—foot powder injurious, 81; injurious to baby, 216.

PREGNANCY—sexual intercourse during pregnancy a crime against mother and child, 199–200; exercise during pregnancy, 209–210; clothing, 210; dropsical swelling, 211; uraemia, 211; morning sickness, 211–212; duration of, 212; effects of diet during pregnancy, 219–220; results of faulty diet in pregnancy, 220–222; excessive fat formation, 222; advantages of natural regimen, 222–223; formation of tooth substance in foetus begins after sixth week, 269.

PREGNANT—congenital disorders of offspring due to injuries of abdomen of pregnant woman, a case, 169–170.

PREMATURE OLD AGE—causes, 279.

PRENATAL FEEDING—219–223.

PRENATAL INFLUENCE—medical science denies prenatal influence, 202; how prenatal influence is transmitted to infant in womb, 203–204; mental and psychical prenatal influence, 203–205; an example from history, 205; birthmarks, 205–206; physical, 206; likened to the making of phonographic records, 206–207; a case, 208.

PREPARATION—for fasting, 72; for delivery, 214.

PREVENTION—better than cure, 1–3; of disease, regimen, 9–18; of disease taught by natural therapeutics, 191–192; must begin with mating and conception, 191–192.

PROCREATION—without love produces degrading tendencies in offspring, 197–199.

PROCREATIVE—function confers highest possible benefits only when sex attraction operates on higher planes of being, 199.

PROSTRATION—from heat, treatment, 252–253.

PROTEINS—meat, eggs, 55.

PSYCHIC—insanity or abnormal psychism, 182–187.

PSYCHICAL—ailments benefitted by psychological exercises, 126–127; prenatal influence, 203–205; disorders, see Insanity.

PSYCHOLOGICAL—exercises, described and illustrated, 128–132.

PTOMAINE—poisoning, treatment, (i) 259.

PURGATIVES—effects of purgatives and laxatives, 136–137.

PYORRHOEA—causes of, 266; opinion of Dr. Aiston, 266–267; disappears under successful natural treatment of acute diseases, 267; can be cured only by restoring entire organism to normal condition, 267.

QUININE—paralysing effect on digestive tract, 137; injurious effect on teeth, 273.

RABIES—treatment for bite of dog affected with, 245–246.
RACIAL PURITY—constructive results of, examples, 193–194.
RADIATION—how cold packs promote heat radiation, 31.
RAW FOOD—diet, 59–60.
RECTAL—technique of rectal dilatation, 150; mechanical dilatation, 150–151; how to use rectal dilators, 151.
RECTUM—contraction of sphincters of the rectum, injurious results, 150; causes of tight sphincters, 150.
RED BLOOD CORPUSCLES—see Blood.
REDFIELD, CASPER LAVATER—quotation from Control of Heredity, 196.
REDUCING—exercises for reducing flesh, 123–124.
REGIMEN—for wholesome living, 9–18; general vegetarian regimen, sample menus, 57–59; fasting regimen, 75–76.
RELAXATION—importance of daily relaxation, 16; coccygeal relaxation, 154–155; orificial relaxation by cold water treatment, 155.
RESPIRATION—artificial methods for restoring, 240–242.
RESUSCITATION—in cases of drowning, asphyxiation, etc., 242–243.
RHEUMATISM—of the mind, 207; fallacy of removing teeth to cure rheumatism, 270–271.
ROLLER BANDAGE—described, illustrated, 244–245.
RUB—see Bath.
RUSSIAN—baths, 85.
RUTABAGAS—remedy for colds, croups, catarrh, how prepared, 26; how to cook, 57.

SALADS—should be dressed with lemon and olive or other vegetable oil, 55–56.
SALIVA—must be thoroughly mixed with starchy foods, 57.
SALT—should not be used at table, 55–56; sanatorium treatment needed to overcome long standing indigestion and malnutrition, 57.
SCALDS—treatment, 246–247.
SCHROTH CURE—modification of, 60.
SCURF RIM—its relation to skin and other systemic conditions, 105–106.
SEA SALT—electromagnetic effect upon the body, 81.
SEA SICKNESS—remedy, 260–261.
SELF PITY—psychological phthisis, cause of nervous diseases, 163–165.
SENESCENCE—physical causes of, 277.
SERUMS—use in army, effects, a case, 4–6; relation of serums treatment in army to influenza outbreak of 1918, 6–7.
SEX—perversion often the result of sexual treatment of the mother during pregnancy, 200; sex determination, 201–202 and Appendix III.
SEX FLUID—carrier of the life force, 199.
SEXUAL INTERCOURSE—effects of forced sexual intercourse on the woman, 199; during pregnancy, crime against mother and child, 199–200; benefits from continence, 199; frequency of, 199; harmful effects of frequent indulgence, 199; not a necessity to manly vigour, 200.
SEXUAL ORGANS—mutilation of inexcusable, 147; natural methods attain desired results, 147; dilatation of sphincters of, 151–153.
SHOCK—treatment, 261; see also Haemorrhage, 253, and Fainting, 251.
SHOULDER OR SCOTCH PACK—described, illustrated, 93.
SICK HEADACHE—cause and treatment, 142–144.
SIGNS OF LIFE—see Fainting, 251.
SITZ BATH—evening sitz bath in daily regimen, 11; tepid, 85; when tepid sitz bath indicated, 85; Epsom salt sitz bath, 97; for retention of urine, 102.
SKIN—cause of poor skin action, 104–105; an organ of absorption and excretion, 105; condition shown by scurf ring in iris, 105; importance of skin as organ of elimination, 105; examination of skin favourite method of diagnosis by Father Kneipp, 106.

SKULL—treatment of insensibility from fractured skull, 251–252.

SLEEP—necessary for storage of vital energy, 16; rules for inducing sound sleep, 17; bedtime, 17; duration of sleep, 17; noonday nap, 17–18.

SMALLPOX—truth about smallpox in late war, 7.

SNAKE—bites, treatment, 245–246.

SOLDIER—experience of soldier with serums, 4–6.

SPHINCTER—treatment in spasm of sphincter muscle and rectum, 99; effect of over-tension of sphincter muscles, 145–146; effects of dilatation, 146.

SPHINCTERS—contraction of sphincters of rectum and causes, 150; dilatation of sphincters and tubes of genital organs, 151–153.

SPICES—irritating to mucous linings of intestinal tract, 55–56.

SPINAL LESIONS—see Lesions.

SPIRITUAL—the secret of spiritual healing, 190–191.

SPRAINS—and strains, first aid; 262.

STANDING—proper standing position, 111.

STARCHES—proper proportion to be used in diet, 55.

STIMULATION—of circulation by cold water, 79–80.

STOMACH—how to distinguish haemorrhages in stomach, treatment, 253; emptying and washing stomach in cases of poisoning, (a) 257–258; emetics, (b) 258.

STRANGULATION—methods of resuscitation, 240–243.

STRYCHNINE POISONING—antidotes, 260; treatment, (g) 258.

SUBLUXATION—of hip bones, see Innominate.

SUBNORMAL—temperature, treatment, applying packs, 44–45.

SUDDEN ILLNESS—how to treat, 249–250.

SUFFOCATION—treatment, 242–243.

SUGARS—proper proportion to be used in diet, 55.

SULPHURIC ACID—poisoning, antidotes, 260.

SUMAC—poison, symptoms and treatment, (j) 259–260.

SUMMARY—of natural methods for treating acute disease, 48–49.

SUN—baths in daily regimen, 11; importance of sun and air to the body, 104–105; bathing, beneficial effects, necessary precautions, 107–108.

SUNBURNS—treatment, 262.

SUNSTROKE—insensibility from sunstroke, 251–252; treatment, 253, 262.

SUPPRESSION—danger of suppression of inflammation and fever by cold water, 44; of healing crises by eating, 72–73.

SURGICAL—effects of surgical orificial treatment, 155.

SWEATING—in bed, 85–86; by exercise, 86.

SWIMMING—beneficial if reaction is good, 81.

SYMPATHETIC NERVOUS SYSTEM—controls involuntary functions of the body, 145–146.

SYMPTOMS—caused by fasting, 74–75.

SYPHILIS—drugs, not syphilis produce congenital defects in offspring, 168–169.

TABLES—Dietetics in a nutshell, 312; of mental and psychic diseases, varieties and causes, 169; of comparative percentages in cow's milk and other food materials, 221.

TARTAR—on teeth, how formed, 267; prevention of tartar formation, 268–269; removal with pumice stone, 270.

TEA—injurious effect on system, 55, 279.

TEAS—flaxseed, rutabaga, etc., 26; to promote flow of scanty urine, 26, 104; directions for making juniper berry and asparagus teas, 104.

TEETH—cause of decay, 54, 265–266, 268–269; ruined by icy or over-hot food and drink, 57, 269; causes of diseases of teeth, 264–265; teeth of animals and humans living on natural food do not become diseased, 265; defective in 85 per cent of children in public schools, 265; report of Dr. Foot on children's teeth, 265; not injured by acid fruits, 268; raw vegetables, fruits, roots and nuts necessary to prevent decay,

269; formation of teeth substance begins in foetus after sixth week, 269; cleaning of teeth, 269–270; powders and pastes injurious to teeth, lemon juice best natural dentifrice, 270; use of ground pumice stone to remove tartar, 270; as foci of infection, 270–271; theory of medical science that rheumatism results from abscessed teeth, 270; fallacy of removing teeth to cure rheumatism, 271.

VEGETARIAN—general vegetarian regimen, sample menus, 57–60.
VEINS—how to apply pressure in case of severence of veins, illustrated, 253–254.
VENTILATION—why good ventilation necessary in sick-room, 22; methods of ventilation of sick-room, 22–23.
VENTRAL HERNIA—see Hernia.
VERDIGRIS—poisoning, antidotes, 260.
VIBRATORY—and massage treatment for eyes, 134.
VINEGAR—and condiments injurious, 55–56; bandages and compresses, 88.
VITALITY—important to economize vitality in fasting, 76.
VITRIOL—poisoning, treatment, 258–259.
VITAL FORCE—not derived from food, drink, medicines, etc., 23–24.
"VITAMINE"—how prepared, 59–60.
VOMITING—bilious vomiting in fasting, 74–75.

WALK—morning, 10.
WALKING—proper walking position, 111.
WATER BAG—breaking of, 214.
WATER SNIFFING—effects, etc., 9–10, 155.
WATER—hot water drinking, 67; hot water in fasting, 73–74; distilled water injurious, 76; hot water applications injurious in inflammation, 28–29; electromagnetic effect of cold water, 32–33; increase of oxygen and ozone by cold water, 33; drinking water should not be icy or very hot, 57; see also Hydrotherapy.
WEIGHT—losing weight, 15–16; normal weight of newborn baby, 222.
WET—bandages and packs, how made and applied, 87–88; see also Bandages and Packs.
WET NURSE—preferred to artificial feeding, 218.
WHITE BLOOD CORPUSCLES—see Leukocytes, and Blood.
WHITE FLOUR—see Flour.
WHOLE BODY PACK—described, illustrated, 89–90.
WHOOPING COUGH—treatment, 235–236.
WHY EPIDEMICS—3–7.
WILL—effect of positive attitude of will on electromagnetic forces, 34–35; concentration of will increases physical, moral and mental powers, 35–36.
WOUNDS—treatment, 248–249; perforating wounds of eye, 251; haemorrhages from wounds, 253; how to stop bleeding from wounds, illustrated, 253–256.

YOUNGER—how to grow younger, 281.

22. Dietetics in a Nutshell

	Food Classes	Predominant Chemical Elements	Functions in Vital Processes	Foods in which the Elements of the Respective Groups Predominate
GROUP I Carbohydrates	Starches and Dextrines	Carbon Oxygen Hydrogen	Producers of Heat and Energy	**Cereals:** The inner, white parts of wheat, corn, rye, oats, barley, buckwheat and rice **Vegetables:** Potatoes, roots, sweet potatoes, pumpkins, squashes **Fruits:** Bananas **Nuts:** Chestnuts
GROUP II Carbohydrates	Sugars	Carbon Oxygen Hydrogen	Producers of Heat and Energy	**Vegetables:** Melons, beets, sorghum **Fruits:** Bananas, dates, figs, grapes, raisins **Dairy Products:** Milk **Natural Sugars:** Honey, maple sugar **Commercial Sugars:** White sugar, syrup, glucose, candy **Nuts:** Cocoanuts
GROUP III Hydrocarbons	Fats and Oils	Carbon Oxygen Hydrogen	Producers of Heat and Energy	**Fruits:** Olives **Dairy Products:** Cream, butter, cheese **Nuts:** Peanuts, almonds, walnuts, cocoanuts, Brazil nuts, pecans, pignolias, etc. **Commercial Fats:** Olive oil, peanut oil, peanut butter, vegetable-cooking oils The yolks of eggs
GROUP IV Proteids	Albumen (white of egg) Gluten (grains) Myosin (lean meat)	Carbon Oxygen Hydrogen Nitrogen Phosphorus Sulphur	Producers of Heat and Energy Building and Repair Materials for Cells and Tissues	**Cereals:** The outer, dark parts of wheat, corn, rye, oats, barley, buckwheat and rice **Vegetables:** The legumes (peas, beans, lentils), mushrooms **Nuts:** Cocoanuts, chestnuts, peanuts, pignolias (pine nuts), hickorynuts, hazelnuts, walnuts, pecans, etc. **Dairy Products:** Milk, cheese, eggs **Meats:** Muscular parts of animals, fish and fowls
GROUP V Organic Minerals	Organic Mineral Elements	Sodium Na Ferrum (Iron) Fe Calcium (Lime) Ca Potassium K Magnesium Mg Manganese Mn Silicon Si Chlorine Cl Fluorine F	Eliminators; Blood, Bone and Nerve Builders; Antiseptics; Blood Purifiers; Laxatives; Cholagogues; Producers of Electro-magnetic Energies	The red blood of animals **Cereals:** The hulls and outer, dark layers of grains and rice **Vegetables:** Lettuce, spinach, cabbage, green peppers, watercress, celery, onions, asparagus, cauliflower, tomatoes, string-beans, fresh peas, parsley, cucumbers, radishes, savoy, horseradish, dandelion, beets, carrots, turnips, eggplant, kohlrabi, oysterplant, artichokes, leek, rosekale (Brussels-sprouts), parsnips, pumpkins, squashes, sorghum **Fruits:** Apples, pears, peaches, oranges, lemons, grapefruit, plums, prunes, apricots, cherries, olives **Berries:** Strawberries, huckleberries, cranberries, blackberries, blueberries, raspberries, gooseberries, currants **Dairy Products:** Milk, buttermilk, skimmed milk **Nuts:** Cocoanuts

312

Quantitative and Qualitative Analysis of Milk

	I	II	III	IV		V				VI					VII	VIII
		Water parts per 100	Negative, gaseous and earthy elements acid forming. Parts per 100. Nitrogenous food elements C O H N P S	Negative, gaseous and earthy elements acid forming. Parts per 100. Carbohydrates C O H		Negative, gaseous and earthy elements acid forming. Parts per 1000. Negative, earthy or mineral elements				Positive mineral elements acid binding and eliminating. Parts per 1000					Totals per 100 of the negative elements in the proteid and carbohydrate foods in columns III & IV	Totals of the positive elements K, Na, Ca, Mg, Fe as given in columns under VI
Standard Foods				Fats Oils	Sugars Starches Dextrin	P	S	Si	Cl	K	Na	Ca	Mg	Fe		
Human Milk..........		87.02	2.36	3.94	6.26	7.84	0.33	0.07	6.38	11.73	3.66	6.80	0.75	0.75	12.56	23.69
Cow's Milk..........		87.42	3.55	3.70	4.88	15.79	0.17	0.02	8.04	13.70	5.34	12.24	1.69	0.30	12.13	33.27